Praise for
Evolutionary Herbalism

"Sajah Popham powerfully presents a holistic model of plant medicine that weaves traditional knowledge, science, and an integration of the heart and mind to guide you toward transformational health."

—ROSALEE DE LA FORÊT, author of
Alchemy of Herbs: Transform Everyday Ingredients into Foods and Remedies That Heal

"Popham crystallizes complex healing traditions and modalities, simplifying and making them palatable. Practical tips abound on merging observations of the human and differentiating to match the plant to that human, whether in relation to astrology, elements, principles, holism, or whichever concept is being shared. Chapters are infused with Popham's own delightful herb profiles. His humor grounds the education shared, creating a sense of ordinary, necessary knowledge. Essential for serious practitioners."

—MARGI FLINT, RH, author of
The Practicing Herbalist

"Popham's evolutionary approach to herbalism provides a detailed blueprint to guide aspiring herbalists as well as those already walking the Green Path in the bringing together of plants and humans to inspire wholeness and affect healing. Firmly grounded in ancient wisdom and expertly distilled by the author before being recombined with his own clinical experiences, *Evolutionary Herbalism* offers medicine for transforming the root of our individual and cultural dis-ease."

—SCOTT KLOOS, author of *Pacific North-west Medicinal Plants: Identify, Harvest, and Use 120 Wild Herbs for Health and Wellness*

"An incredibly beautiful weaving of herbal and esoteric traditions creating a rich tapestry of what author Sajah Popham calls Universal Herbalism. This is a comprehensive study of not only the principles of various modalities but also the patterns inherent within them and how they intersect with each other. This is a must-read for anyone looking to have a comprehensive understanding of the expansive nature of healing and how to move into a new herbalism."

—PAM MONTGOMERY, author of *Plant Spirit Healing* and founder of Organization of Nature's Evolutionaries (ONE)

"A tireless confederacy of dedicated souls strive to preserve and pass forward our collective herbal, alchemical, and astrological knowledge. Within each generation a few pioneers arise to forge new schools or mediate divergent approaches. Sajah Popham has achieved a remarkably synthetic paradigm, integrating previous historic stages of herbal practice with his profound understanding of energetic systems, Eastern and Western."

—JUDITH HILL, producer of the Renaissance Medicine Conference and author of *Medical Astrology: A Guide to Planetary Pathology*

EVOLUTIONARY
HERBALISM

EVOLUTIONARY
HERBALISM

*Science, Medicine, and Spirituality
from the Heart of Nature*

SAJAH POPHAM

FOREWORD BY MATTHEW WOOD

North Atlantic Books
Berkeley, California

Published by
North Atlantic Books
Huichin, unceded Ohlone land
Berkeley, California

Cover photo © Tyler Penor
Cover art directed by Sajah Popham
Book design by Happenstance Type-O-Rama

Printed in Canada

Evolutionary Herbalism: Science, Medicine, and Spirituality from the Heart of Nature is sponsored and published by North Atlantic Books, an educational nonprofit based in the unceded Ohlone land Huichin (Berkeley, CA) that collaborates with partners to develop cross-cultural perspectives; nurture holistic views of art, science, the humanities, and healing; and seed personal and global transformation by publishing work on the relationship of body, spirit, and nature.

MEDICAL DISCLAIMER: The following information is intended for general information purposes only. Individuals should always see their health care provider before administering any suggestions made in this book. Any application of the material set forth in the following pages is at the reader's discretion and is their sole responsibility.

North Atlantic Books's publications are distributed to the US trade and internationally by Penguin Random House Publisher Services. For further information, visit our website at www.northatlanticbooks.com.

Library of Congress Cataloging-in-Publication Data

Names: Popham, Sajah, 1986- author.
Title: Evolutionary herbalism : science, spirituality, and medicine from the
heart of nature / Sajah Popham.
Description: Berkeley, California : North Atlantic Books, [2019] | Includes
index.
Identifiers: LCCN 2018042878 (print) | LCCN 2018044579 (ebook) | ISBN
9781623173142 (e-book) | ISBN 9781623173135 (paperback)
Subjects: LCSH: Herbs—Therapeutic use. | Traditional medicine. | Mind and
body. | BISAC: HEALTH & FITNESS / Herbal Medications. | NATURE / Plants /
Flowers. | BODY, MIND & SPIRIT / Healing / Prayer & Spiritual.
Classification: LCC RM666.H33 (ebook) | LCC RM666.H33 P65 2019 (print) | DDC
615.3/21—dc23
LC record available at https://lccn.loc.gov/2018042878

6 7 8 9 MQ 26 25 24

This book includes recycled material and material from well-managed forests. North Atlantic Books is committed to the protection of our environment. We print on recycled paper whenever possible and partner with printers who strive to use environmentally responsible practices.

For Whitney,
my root and flower,
whose never-ending love like
an infinitely unfolding Rose
has made me into a better man.

READ THIS FIRST!

First off, thank you so much for purchasing my book!
To show you my gratitude, I'd love to give you a free integration guide.
To download it in PDF format, visit:

www.evolutionaryherbalism.com/book-bonuses

This guide will help you take what you learn throughout my book and integrate and implement it in your work with plants and your unique plant path.

CONTENTS

FOREWORD

Despite beliefs to the contrary, animism—the experience of Nature as a living being—is not long dead and finished in the Western world. While it has been declared extinct by the high priests of the universal Muggle church (called "science"), it has enjoyed a persistent existence, literature, and educational system of its own. Recently, conventional science has come to similar conclusions about the natural world: it is infused with intelligence and communication binding it into whole communities that operate as if self-aware.

Idea: what if this newly discovered world of science is the Living Nature of the animists? This is where our journey begins, under the able guidance of Sajah Popham, who, despite his youth, carries the experience necessary to travel this path. He is one of the only people I know who has been trained in herbalism, alchemy, astrology, and conventional science, and he has integrated them together, discovering the common and foundational roots uniting them. But all of that would amount to nothing if he were not also a citizen of the Living World. For animism is not a belief but an *experience.*

The traditional name for the Living Nature of Western animism is *anima mundi,* translated as the "Soul of the World" or the "Living Nature." The animists found the world to be alive and aware, like a person. When we experience our own soul, that of another, and then of many others, we gradually move to an experience of the Soul of the World. And she is a person.

This experience comes to us through our heart. We feel the Living Nature when we experience a soul connection with someone we love, belongingness to a community, or love for our Mother Earth. This, as Sajah explains, conforms to the findings of modern science. The physical heart, it turns out, can perceive the surrounding environment with precision in ways that the brain cannot. This awareness is not as complicated as one would think, for it is based on a simple principle. The heart is an electromagnetic oscillator and is able to synchronize with other biological oscillators, such as another person or even a plant. This synchronization gives us the experience of feelings that are based on similarity, harmony, and empathy, and it can also give us the opposite experience: aversion and antipathy. Our deepest choices are based on the feeling perceptions of the heart.

The perception of the heart also gives rise to what we call intuition, that is, our ability to see patterns, for both love and intuition are based on similarity and difference. From patterns we build the experience of the whole, so the heart is the seat of holistic awareness as well as love, aversion, and choice. In the "aha moment" of an intuitive perception, we also feel that we are experiencing truth. So the heart is the source of our experience of love, holism, and truth. This method of perception was known as the "Light of Nature" by the animist philosophers. The accumulation of knowledge based on this emotionally secure, holistically complete truth-seeing was known as the Wisdom of Nature, or *natura sophia*.

Now we begin to see that there is an animistic educational system, which is traditionally called the School of Nature. This is the platform upon which Sajah constructs the rest of this wonderful book. He draws on the innate intelligence of the natural world, both Earth and Sky.

The subjects in this schoolhouse include alchemy, astrology, and herbal medicine. If Nature is not a dead thing but alive, then our science must be based upon the incarnation of the spirit and soul into the body. The study and application of these transformations is what we call alchemy. If there are patterns within the Living Nature, then we must have a vocabulary, and this is where astrology comes in, not just as a predictive art but also as a language of energy patterns. And finally, our co-walkers in the Living Nature—minerals, plants, and animals—want to interact with us as peers, teachers, and healing agents. So Sajah shares his herbal experience with us, based on more than a decade of direct herbal, clinical, and alchemical laboratory experience. All these teachings come together, for herbs are prepared alchemically, described elementally and astrologically, and administered holistically to heal the whole person. Sajah slowly develops this remarkable vision of natural wholeness from a pearl to a living globe of energetic architecture.

But there is an additional implication. The Living Nature is loving, holistic, and comprehensive, so it is always expanding and attempting to enlarge the experience and spirituality of her established citizens, and to solicit new associates. This means she is *evolutionary,* or even *coevolutionary,* for she is always working through her citizens—mineral, plant, animal, and human. The whole is always influencing the parts, and each part influences the whole.

As Sajah once said to me, "As we heal, our soul evolves, and as our soul evolves we must heal; these are two sides of the same leaf." This synergy of plant medicine, alchemy, astrology, and the Living Nature ultimately culminates as a model of *evolutionary herbalism.* This is the holistic healing so many people seek and need in our modern world, which is so far removed from the Living Nature, yet so close to it. But *Evolutionary Herbalism* is not limited to herbalism; this book carries other implications, like a little ship loaded with spices and gems, sailing from magical, faraway lands to enrich the planet, in many disciplines and directions.

Matthew Wood
Sunnyfield Herb Farm
Wherever-that-may-be

ACKNOWLEDGMENTS

I first must acknowledge my most important teachers: the plants themselves, whose living intelligence and healing power have turned me into who I am.

Second, I must acknowledge my family: my mothers, Elizabeth and Kathy, who always encouraged me to follow my own path and showed me what unshakable faith looks like; and my fathers, Arthur and Tracy, who always told me to keep my eye on the ball and showed me the importance of strength, discipline, and determination.

Third, I must acknowledge my teachers. Most important is Matthew Wood, who patiently held my hand as I wrote this book and whose insights and perspectives were crucial in making it what it is today. Judith Hill helped me refine the astrological portions, and Robert Bartlett as my guide in humbly preserving the alchemical tradition. Alex Turtle and Chenoa Egawa for their precious teachings, powerful prayers, and good medicine. Jason Scott and Tyler Penor for their philosophical, alchemical, and astrological inspirations and insights. Steven Harrod Buhner and Pam Montgomery for revealing the Light of Nature within plants to my heart. Other highly influential people whose work made this possible include Paul Bergner, Michael Tierra, Rosemary Gladstar, Margi Flint, David Hoffman, David Winston, Todd Caldecott, Vasant Lad, David Frawley, Ted Kaptchuk, Mark Stavish, Manfred Junius, and Jane Ridder-Patrick, among many others.

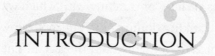

INTRODUCTION

Ancient Teachings for a
New Paradigm of Plant Medicine

A plant has stood up in the forest
and called your name

Now more than ever, humanity needs the healing power of medicinal plants. And not just as alternatives to over-the-counter or prescription drugs that put Band-Aids on symptoms. We need *true healing* that changes the way we live on this Mother Earth, healing that touches our hearts and minds, that helps our consciousness return to the natural order of life. For there is a spiritual sickness pervading humanity, lying at the roots of the problems we face individually and collectively, casting the illusion that we are separate from Nature. This spiritual sickness spreading through our true hearts, infecting our natural minds, and contaminating the purity of our bodies is ultimately destroying the planet itself. In this way, we need transformational healing not only for ourselves but for the Earth itself, for we are a part of the Earth.

Yet wherever there is sickness, there is a medicine. And the medicine needed for these times of crises will not take the form of a pill or some other invention of the human mind. As Albert Einstein is reported to have said, "The significant problems we have cannot be solved at the same level of thinking with which we created them." It is the kind of thinking dominant in our modern world that has created this sickness in humanity and the Earth. The medicine to heal it can only come from something greater than our own inventions, something vastly more intelligent than isolated molecules produced in a laboratory. That something is medicinal plants, the living, healing intelligence of the Earth.

And they have called you. You didn't hear the call with your ears but instead felt it in your heart, something unexplainable yet irrefutable. This calling, this pulse from the heart of Nature that touches the souls of certain people, has been heard since time immemorial. It is a calling from the natural world for the people to heal. It is a calling from the plants in an ancient language for their people to reenter the wild territories of the Earth so their medicine can be carried into the world and take root in the heart of humanity.

All across the world there have long been herbalists, plant people, those who have heeded this calling from the depths of Nature, been instructed in its wisdom, and shared the healing potency of the botanical kingdom. The medicinal power of the plants is not simply a removal of bodily symptoms, not just a replacement for a pill; it is a deeper level of doctoring within the territory of the human spirit and soul. For when we perform our medicinal art well, the plants move through us and transform someone's life.

When we attend to this calling of the plants, we open ourselves to the wisdom of the Earth and reweave the pattern of Nature into the fabric of the human organism, which has over time become replaced by technology and human ingenuity. The plants are calling us to heal ourselves so we can heal others. They are calling us to reenvision how we live on this Mother Earth so we can exist in harmony with the tapestry of Nature, of which we are a mere thread. The plants beckon us to become instruments for their medicinal power to reach out and heal the world.

This calling of the plants is deeper than a profession or a hobby. The true herbalist is not designated by any certification or degree; our mark is invisible, for it is inscribed into our hearts by the hand of Nature itself. The true herbalist is not just trained by others who heeded the same calling but is instructed by the wisdom of the natural world, a student of the plants themselves.

The work of the herbalist is to understand the intricate patterns of Nature and how they are woven into the architecture of people and plants, to see them as mirror images of the Earth and cosmos, parts that contain the whole. It is the ecological function of the herbalist to bridge the human and botanical kingdoms, the world and the Earth, uniting them in a healing way. The herbalist understands the language of the physiological terrain and its connection to the soul, the medicinal meaning behind the contours of leaves and the colors of flowers. The herbalist sees the plants both as healers and as teachers—each one a school unto itself, with its own unique teachings and medicinal specialty.

The essence of the true art and practice of herbal medicine is rooted in this calling from the plants, this invitation from the untamed places of the Earth. This calling echoes throughout our being, helping us remember that the Nature all around us is also within us and that it has the power to not only heal but to transform life.

My Plant Path

All my life I had wanted to be a doctor. I wasn't raised by hippie parents on organic food, herbal medicine, and in the woods, but rather in conventional middle-class suburbia. I attended public school and thought life was about going to college, getting a job, getting married, buying a home, and living happily ever after. While my childhood was pretty orthodox in many ways, my stepfather used to take me out camping and hiking on the weekends amongst the Western Red Cedars and Douglas-Firs of the Pacific Northwest rainforests. Those times spent in the majesty of the mountains touched something deep inside me, as I've always felt at home in the heart of Nature, more alive, more connected to something that was real and powerful.

Throughout my childhood I always knew I wanted to help and heal others, but I thought the only path to achieving that end was to attend conventional medical school. I was set on becoming a neurosurgeon and following the path of allopathic medicine, because that's all I knew existed. But something inside me felt like that wasn't what I was really meant to do with my life; it never fully sat right in my heart.

When I moved to Venice Beach from suburban Tacoma, Washington, something deep inside me changed, as is common when one finds themselves alone in a strange, new place, far away from everything they once knew. I started to question my cultural upbringing and the status quo as I began to sense that there was much more to life than what the world told me. I gradually began to adopt a more "alternative" lifestyle. My hair grew into dreadlocks, I stopped eating meat, and most importantly, I discovered Earth-based spirituality and mysticism. A spiritual path that was deeply connected to Nature and my own union with the divine source opened up to me. I began questioning the meaning of life and why I was put here on this Earth. I started to realize that the Earth itself was not only beautiful, but alive and intelligent. I started to sense that there was an invisible, spiritual reality behind this physical one.

I also realized that I was carrying a lot of baggage, even at the young age of eighteen, and that if I wanted to grow spiritually, I needed to heal. And as I began to heal, I understood that I needed to grow spiritually. I also started to feel that becoming a neurosurgeon didn't accord with the Earth-centered beliefs and ideals dawning within me. I desperately wanted to become a healer, but didn't know there was any other way until one autumn day.

My plant path began on the patio of a coffee shop where I worked in Santa Monica, California. As I wiped down tables and picked up newspapers, on the front page of the health section I saw two words that changed my life forever: *naturopathic medicine*. The concept of natural medicine had been alien to me until that moment. The idea of using plants instead of pills, of becoming a Nature-based doctor, opened up an entire world of possibility to me. My life trajectory of becoming a neurosurgeon took a major U-turn away from the conventional allopathic route and back into the forest.

A few months later I took my first step on the plant path by packing up everything in my tiny studio apartment in Venice and driving north on I-5 in my 1973 Volkswagen bus to attend the herbal sciences program at Bastyr University in the Seattle area.

My time at Bastyr opened multiple doorways in my life. As the name implied, the herbal *sciences* program focused on the scientific dynamics of plants: pharmacology, anatomy and physiology, biochemistry, pathology, botany, medicine making, and of course the herbs themselves. The science of the botanical kingdom and the dynamic ways they interface with the human organism on a biological level fascinated me. Still, even as my mind enjoyed learning this spectrum of intellectual knowledge, I always had a nagging feeling that something essential was missing.

Before I ever considered myself an herbalist, I thought of myself as a seeker, a soul in search of wisdom and truth. Spirituality was always a critical part of my efforts to understand the world around me. Thus, I began to integrate a spiritual component into my studies of plants. I realized that before universities, before human teachers of plant medicine, traditional peoples understood how to learn about the plants from the plants themselves.

So after my time in the lecture halls and laboratories, I'd leave the pavement behind and enter the forests. I started sitting with the plants, talking to them, making offerings to them, trying to learn how to listen to them. In that process of learning the plants' language, I realized that the science of plants only skimmed the surface of their medicinal potential. As my spirit began to mingle with their consciousness, past traumas were healed, and a new way of seeing the world dawned within me.

This was when I felt the split between my mind and my heart. On the one hand, I was learning all of this incredible science of herbal medicines. On the other, I was having profound spiritual experiences in my secret classroom in the forest. The two didn't seem to fit together. I felt confused, lost, incongruous; two completely different plant languages were all mixed up inside me, and I couldn't translate from one to the other. There had to be some way to integrate the seeming contradictions between the science and the spirituality of the plants.

This led me to explore the many traditional perspectives on plant medicine, spirituality, and healing traditions: Ayurveda, traditional Chinese and Tibetan medicine, indigenous and folk traditions, ancient Greek and Arabic medicine … the list went on. I was seeking a universal model of herbalism that could encompass both their chemistry and their spirit, as well as the human body, mind, and soul. I wanted a *truly holistic* model of plant medicine. I wanted to be able to share the level of healing I was receiving from the plants with the people I wanted to help.

Although elements of these various models helped fill in the gaps, it all came together one day while I was traveling through Tuscany, Italy, where I was introduced to the traditions of alchemy and medical astrology. I attended a lecture on these topics that began with a story of the creation of the universe, a cosmology of the underlying architecture of Nature, and a representation of spiritual principles using chemical terminology. The lecturer discussed the relationship between the part and the whole, the macrocosm and the microcosm—how people and plants contain the whole pattern of creation within them, and how plants can be prepared medicinally in ways that concentrate their chemical, energetic, and spiritual properties, allowing us to use them to heal the body, spirit, and soul. I learned of a tradition that understood that plants can be used to do more than just heal; they can be used to facilitate the evolution of consciousness.

This was a major turning point in my plant path. Since then I have come to understand that universal truths about Nature, plant medicine, and the healing journey have been represented throughout the world's cultural traditions. Each tradition has its own unique way of expressing these truths, but there is a golden thread weaving them together, a perennial philosophy that rests at the heart of Nature and encompasses a universal model of medicine, spirituality, and science. The split between my heart and mind was mended by reconnecting it with the underlying pattern of Nature.

My work has been to unite these truths into a cohesive practice of plant medicine, one that serves to heal the body, clarify the mind, open the heart, and accelerate the evolution of consciousness. This book presents a holistic model of herbalism that recognizes the wholeness of people and plants and acknowledges their connection to the wholeness of Creation. In this model of healing, herbs are not just used like a drug to remove symptoms; they're used to bring people back to their true inner nature, their essential self, and provide healing that contributes to the evolution of humanity so we can create a world in alignment with the Earth. This practice focuses on integrating ancient teachings to create a new paradigm of plant medicine: evolutionary herbalism.

The Evolution of Herbalism

People's interactions with the natural world, and specifically with the plant kingdom, have been instrumental in determining the course of history, the development of culture, and the state of human consciousness.[1] The cross-cultural contacts facilitated by the spice trade, the shift from hunting and gathering to agrarian society, the impact of Tobacco on human health, genetic modifi-cation of food crops, and the growing usage of entheogenic plants and mushrooms have had powerful effects upon humanity and the Earth—some positive, some negative, and others yet to be seen.

Humanity is utterly dependent upon the botanical kingdom. We build our homes from timber, weave our clothes from fibers, and eat plants grown in the soil or animals fed by plants. The very air we breathe is a by-product of plants. Whether we wish to admit it or not, our very existence is contingent on our relationship with plants. I would argue that the current chaos and imbalances in the world are due in part to this relationship having been unconscious for so long because the plant kingdom has been marginalized and seen as inferior to humanity. When we make our relationship to plants conscious and recognize that they are intelligent, conscious beings we can relate to, we become more conscious of life itself. We become more aware of not only our relationship with the natural world and our dependence on it but our unique place within it. Indeed, our relationship to the plant kingdom shapes the world.

One area of human interaction with plants that has maintained this conscious awareness is herbalism, which has been practiced cross-culturally throughout the world, with the oldest recorded systems dating back thousands of years. Of course, plants have been used for food and medicine since far before written records were first created. Today herbalism is often perceived as the use of plants to treat symptoms or as a natural alternative to drugs. What few realize is that plants have traditionally been used to not just heal the body but also to assist in deeper levels of healing the mind, heart, and soul.

The art and practice of herbalism have changed profoundly throughout its history. Our modern practice of this healing art looks quite different even from a hundred years ago. In today's era of rad-ical change, I believe there is a necessity to create a new paradigm of plant medicine that matches the current state of human health and consciousness. To do this, we must observe the human-to-plant relationship, specifically with regard to the practice of herbalism, and learn from its different stages of evolution. We must understand where it has been and where it is now so we can know how to move forward in a good way.

Indigenous Herbalism

The first phase of herbalism could be referred to as indigenous or folk herbalism. If we imagine the very first herbalists, we immediately see they learned about the plants not from universities and obviously not through the internet but directly from the plants themselves. Traditional people have a radically different perceptual orientation from our modern, intellectually driven, reductionist model of the world. They saw things very differently from how we see today, and this led to a very different approach to their herbal art.

Their deep connection to the natural world was not an intellectual exercise; rather, they saw the world through the eyes of the heart. The plant was seen as a living spiritual intelligence, not merely a container for biologically active constituents. This way of seeing evoked a spiritual understanding of health, disease, and the plants they used, connecting the physical world to an invisible, spiritual reality.

Indigenous and folk traditions understood that the natural world is infused with intelligence and that we have an innate ability to communicate with it. In this way, they understood the medicine of plants and the causes of disease spiritually. Their vision enabled them to practice plant medicine to heal beyond the body and into the spirit and soul through prayer, ceremony, and other methods of interweaving the spiritual elements of healing. And yet, these traditional doctors were also well versed in the physical application of medicinal plants to heal acute symptoms and injury. As the primary physicians, they developed an approach to medicine that was exceedingly practical while at the same time spiritual.

These traditions were typically highly localized to specific bioregions, family lineages, and cultures. Medicinal knowledge was passed from generation to generation, teacher to student, elder to child, through direct oral teachings, stories, practical experience, and most importantly, kinship with the plants. Rarely were these practices transcribed, for it was not an intellectually based system of knowledge transferred from mind to mind; it was a bundle of wisdom contained within the heart. It is this wisdom of the heart that we must revive in modern herbalism.

Vitalist Herbalism

Over time, these plant people's direct, heart-centered connection to the living intelligence of the Earth imprinted their mind with the pattern of Nature. Indigenous and folk knowledge gradually became transcribed and developed into systematized, "vitalist" models of medicine.

These are the great systems often referred to when considering herbal traditions—Chinese medicine, Ayurveda, Unani-Tibb, Greek medicine—as well as the later North American traditions such as Thomsonianism, Physiomedicalism, and the Eclectics, among many others. During the vitalist phase, plants were understood to heal through the vital force that expresses itself in the plants' energetic properties, directly influencing the individual constitution of the person. This vital force is the underlying intelligent pattern of Nature directly imprinted in people and plants, determining their unique qualities and characteristics. This model is often summarized through systems of *energetics*.

Energetics is not an esoteric concept; it is rather a holistic description of the relationship between whole plants and whole people. It describes the core properties of medicinal plants that operate *behind* their physiological actions and organ affinities. It understands the root causes of symptoms in the body by looking at the essence of disease. It is an ecological model of medicine, rather than a mechanical one. These systems stress the uniqueness of the individual, outlined through constitutional patterns that are influenced by the energetics of the plants.

In vitalism, the causes of disease are not just spiritual; they can also arise from a misalignment between the organism and its environment. In other words, a person's interactions with the world around them affect them psychologically, emotionally, and physically. Vitalist traditions suggest that people get sick because of how they live every day, including the foods they eat, thoughts they think, people they surround themselves with, the weather, seasonal changes, and a host of other factors. The therapeutic goal is to achieve balance between one's internal constitution and the external environment.

Many of these traditions, born out of indigenous and folk practices, continued to honor the spiritual facets of both people and plants. The primary characteristic of the vitalist phase is that herbalism became systematized and standardized within particular cultural and geographic regions. Vitalism can be seen as striking a dynamic balance between the intuitive faculties of the heart and the rational nature of the mind. Unfortunately, modern medicine has neglected the wisdom of these vitalist models in favor of a strictly biochemical model of medicine, in which our knowledge is solely rooted in the reductionist perspective of the mind while paying no heed to the holistic nature of the heart.

Molecular Herbalism

As Western culture became the world's dominant paradigm, the practice of herbalism changed along with the development of industry and technology. As we moved from the forests and fields and into the city, we distanced ourselves from Nature, and medicine followed suit by becoming mechanized. The standardization of the scientific method, materialism, and analytical and reductionist thinking led the holistic practice of vitalist herbalism to evolve (or devolve) into modern day molecular herbalism.

Whereas indigenous herbalism was born of the heart, and vitalist herbalism was a balance of the heart and mind, molecular herbalism is solely located within the intellect. In this model, which is highly popular in conventional perspectives on herbalism, plants are understood to heal not because of their energetic properties or their impact on the constitution, and certainly not because of their spiritual influence, but rather due to biochemically active constituents that trigger distinct pharmacological processes within the body.

This way of thinking led us down a rabbit hole into the eventual development of isolated compounds—what we typically refer to as drugs. We have taken the holistic nature of medicinal plants, the vast complexity of their intelligence, and reduced them to single active ingredients. Molecular herbalism and drug therapies are results of the desacralization of traditional modes of seeing meaning in the world—alchemy degraded into chemistry, plants into pills. As indigenous and folk traditions became colonized, and as the vitalist systems of medicine became mechanized, there was a gradual shift away from perceiving life through the heart and toward seeing it strictly through the mind. The organic, holistic models became reductionist and linear.

When we attempt to decipher the medicinal properties of a plant strictly through its biochemical constituents—when we try to learn about a plant by studying its parts in isolation—we lose sight of its wholeness. Most research on medicinal plants only studies single compounds injected into mice or petri dishes, and from those results scientists extrapolate conclusions about how the entire plant will operate upon a human. Skewed, diluted information pervades the world of molecular herbalism, ultimately crippling our ability to be effective plant healers.

In molecular herbalism, symptoms are commonly seen as the enemy, and health is defined as the absence of symptoms. Plants are thought to be effective against certain symptoms or diseases, rather than being seen in their specificity for different types of people and patterns of imbalance. Whole plants are not used to treat the whole person; instead, "standardized extracts" or plant isolates are used to treat common ailments.

Although science has made incredible discoveries about medicinal plants, when it becomes the sole method for understanding and using plants, our practice of herbalism becomes divorced from thousands of years of traditional knowledge. Science has its place, although it is relatively new in comparison to the indigenous and vitalist phases and cannot be seen as the only way. Very few practicing herbalists rely on science alone to build an effective therapeutic model, yet we can still honor the profound understanding it offers.

Evolutionary Herbalism

Each phase in the evolution of herbalism provides an essential component of a truly holistic model of plant medicine. I believe a great integration can occur to advance the practice of herbalism for the modern world, a synthesis of the indigenous, vitalist, and molecular models. Through this synergy we can strike a balance between the science and the spirituality of people and plants. This integration is what I refer to as evolutionary herbalism.

The new paradigm of plant medicine encompasses the chemical, energetic, and spiritual qualities of plants and people, allowing us to work with the holistic nature of plants to heal the wholeness of the person, because this is the level of healing that is so desperately needed at this time. Plants are recognized not only as healers but also as teachers. They have the ability to facilitate the healing of our bodies, the clarification of our minds, the opening and strengthening of our hearts, and the evolution of our souls. Their intelligence is vast, their spirits pure, and their chemistry brilliant.

In the new paradigm of plant medicine, healing and evolution are the stamen and pistil of the same flower. To heal ourselves is to facilitate the evolution of our consciousness. And to further our soul's development, we must heal. In this way, we use plants to assist in transformational levels of healing that touch the essence of who we are.

The new paradigm of herbal medicine sees plants not in isolation but in relationship to the wholeness of life. Herbs are not just understood in terms of how they are useful for *us,* not just in the dim light of what they are "good for." They are perceived as intelligent, sentient, conscious beings, embodiments of the universal forces of life, mirror images of the whole.

In the new paradigm of plant medicine, people are not viewed solely through the narrowed lens of their symptoms. Our bodies are not machines; our minds and hearts are not merely constructs of our past. The human organism, like a plant, is a still pond reflecting the totality of life. The body, heart, mind, and soul are not separate, but intricately interwoven in a warp and weft that is the tapestry of our being. And that tapestry is but one thread in the organic unity of Nature.

Evolutionary herbalism sees that plants are not merely plants, and people are not merely people, but both are embodiments of the macrocosm of Nature, designed in accordance with the underlying blueprint of life. By communing with the vital intelligence of plants, we also commune with the powers of Creation that operate through them. As we study plants, we study the self, and as we study the self, we study Creation. The evolutionary herbalist sees that transformational healing doesn't just occur through the plants but also through the archetypal forces of life.

Evolutionary herbalism is a calling for a truly holistic model of plant medicine that can bring about a union of the science and soul of herbalism, an integration of the heart and mind, a wedding between the Earth and sky, a synthesis of the great herbal traditions of the world brought together by a natural language—*a universal model of plant medicine that transforms lives.*

The Five Pillars of Evolutionary Herbalism

I've heard there's a saying in Montana that goes, "The best time to have the map is before you enter the woods." This book maps the landscape of this synergy between the spirit and science of herbalism and shows how to integrate them to facilitate transformational healing. This requires a natural language that relates people, plants, and Nature to the fundamental forces of life by uniting the heart and mind in a way that shows the underlying pattern—the interconnections—woven throughout the natural world. We need a language that shows how each part contains the pattern of the whole.

The five pillars of evolutionary herbalism are the foundations of this natural language. They are certainly not my invention. These principles are reflected throughout cultures and traditions both ancient and modern in the realms of natural medicine, spirituality, religion, and even science. They are guideposts on your plant path, signs to follow when you go astray or when the world pulls you away from the Earth. They deepen your understanding of the natural world, plants, and most importantly, your own self, guiding you to cultivate your healing power and share the fruits of your inner work to heal another.

1. The Light of Nature

To cultivate a model of herbalism that can facilitate the healing and transformation of consciousness, the root of the system must grow within the substratum of the spiritual element of Nature. The Light of Nature is the intelligence and sentience shining throughout the natural world that we have an innate capacity to be in relationship with. This pillar returns us to the root of herbalism as we remember how to learn about plants *from the plants themselves* by perceiving in a way that goes beyond the linear mind. As herbalists, we are first, foremost, and forever students of Nature. Our connection to the

Light of Nature within and without enables us to understand the medicinal properties of plants, their ability to heal us in ways that advance our spiritual development, and it helps us see the archetypal patterns etched into the natural world.

2. Energetic Architecture

As we learn to perceive The Light of Nature, we see that Nature is composed of a living pattern, designed through the interweaving of invisible forces to generate visible forms. Nature is a whole, and each part of Nature contains this pattern of wholeness, which I refer to as *energetic architecture*. This pattern of Nature is at the root of traditional models of medicine and functions as a translation mechanism between spirit and matter and thus relates the physical properties of people and plants to their spiritual attributes. Energetic architecture constitutes the foundation of a natural language that connects the heart and mind. Various energetic patterns are found throughout medical and spiritual traditions around the world, but we will focus on three: the triune pattern, referred to as the Three Principles; the fivefold pattern, referred to as the Five Elements, and the sevenfold pattern, referred to as the Seven Planets. These energetic patterns form the foundational models of many herbal systems. Each layer of energetic architecture will be considered holistically in relationship to medicinal plants and people on the physical, energetic, and spiritual levels, and with regard to their reflections throughout traditional models.

3. Universal Herbalism

All herbal traditions are rooted in the Light of Nature and shaped by their unique embodiment of energetic architecture. While on the surface they appear separate, there are certain golden threads—*universal principles*—that weave them together into a cohesive system that transcends any single traditional model. These synergistic models have greatly enhanced our ability to see herbs in the light of different cultural perspectives, enabling us to understand them more holistically than if we were viewing them through the lens of one tradition. Over the last few decades there has been a great synergy of herbalism as Chinese medicine and Ayurveda have become more integrated into alternative medicine. Evolutionary herbalism extends this synergy by integrating the Western esoteric traditions of medical astrology and alchemy. Universal Herbalism does not merely integrate traditions of plant medicine; it shows how the life force manifests itself uniquely in individual species of plants and people through the model of energetic architecture.

4. Transformational Medicine

This pillar takes our understanding of Universal Herbalism and energetic architecture and applies them in ways that heal people's bodies, spirits, and souls. By learning to see the soul's evolution and the healing process as one and the same, we can assess the wholeness of the person and see how symptoms are a language that communicates deeper meaning about a person's spirit and soul. This pillar reveals that to treat the whole person, we must not only understand the wholeness of plants but create medicines that embody this wholeness. This involves a system of spiritual pharmacy, traditionally known as *spagyrics,* which concentrates a plant's chemical, energetic, and spiritual properties into a single holistic medicine. Such medicines contain both the properties of the plant and its energetic architecture, or the Planet, Element, and Principle the plant corresponds to. Spagyrics focus the *initiatic,* or evolutionary, properties of plants and ultimately catalyze the soul's development by opening one into the archetypal landscape.

5. Know Thyself

The final pillar of evolutionary herbalism is the foundation of the first four, because it's impossible to achieve any of the others without this pillar being solid and unshakable. The only way we can perceive the Light of Nature outside us is if we contact it within us—that is, we must come to know ourselves. We can only understand the energetic architecture of life, plants, and our clients if we see how these forces are represented within ourselves first. We can only discover the synergy of herbal traditions and find our own unique practice of plant medicine when we are deeply connected to our calling and distinct plant path. And the only way we can help other people to heal in a transformational manner is if we ourselves are transformed by the roots, leaves, flowers, and fruits of the medicines we work with.

The level of healing we want to offer to the world will only go as far as we have gone into our own personal healing journey. Our understanding of Nature will only go as far as our understanding of our own inner Nature. To know thyself is to cultivate virtue and your internal healing power. *To know thyself is in fact to heal thyself.*

The path of the plant healer is a path of internal work, of initiation at the hand of Nature, of purifying ourselves bodily, mentally, emotionally, and spiritually. It is a path of letting go of what we are not so that who we truly are can be revealed. It is a path of selfless service, of being an instrument for the healing power of Nature to move through us to help another. It is a path of responsibility, discipline, and commitment to the highest good of humanity and preservation of the Earth. As we walk this plant path and gather medicine from the heart of Nature, it begins to sprout and grow within us into a living inner forest where we ourselves become the medicine.

PART I

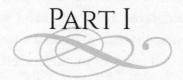

The Light of Nature

The physician does from nature, from nature he is born; only he who receives his experience from nature is a physician, and not he who writes, speaks, and acts with his head and with ratiocinations aimed against nature and her ways. The physician is only the servant of nature, not her master. Therefore it behooves medicine to follow the will of nature. He who would be a good physician must find his faith in the rational light of nature, he must work with it, and not undertake anything without it.

—PARACELSUS[1]

At the center of all life is light. Our solar system orients itself around the Sun, the great distributor of light and giver of life. Each dawn is a renewal, a rebirth, a new day—the pattern of Creation repeating itself every morning as life begins anew. Through the light of the Sun, the cycles and rhythms of the Earth are established: the movements of the seasons, the life cycles of plants, the migration of birds, the progressions of human consciousness.

At the beginning of time, this light divided itself, fractalized, and shined throughout Nature, imbuing itself within everything, connecting each expression of life to its source. As this light emanated from the center of creation, it crafted a pattern within the natural world, impregnating everything with consciousness, intelligence, meaning, purpose, and language. It's as if a small piece of the Sun broke off and planted itself within the deepest recesses of Nature. And just as the Sun is at the center of our solar system, so too is there a light shining forth from the center of every living thing, a secret fire burning within its essence—invisible to the eye, but felt by the heart.

Plants can be thought of as harvesters of light through the miracle of photosynthesis, as they generate energy and substance from the Sun. They are, quite literally, light manifest in material form. The energy that fuels our modern world is based on the combustion of stored sunlight within ancient plants. The processes of the human body are fueled by the energy obtained from cleaving a phosphate bond within the adenosine triphosphate (ATP) molecule, which releases a particle of light called a biophoton. Indeed, the emission of biophotons is integral to the biochemistry of life. Light is central to the molecular communication, to the *intelligence*, that governs the natural world.

Paracelsus (1493–1541), a Swiss physician, astrologer, and alchemist during the Renaissance, coined the term *lumen naturae*, or the "Light of Nature," to refer to the intelligence infused throughout the natural world. This Light is universally distributed and centrally imbued into the inner heart of every living thing. While it cannot be directly perceived, we see its influence within plants, stones, animals, and people, as it shapes their outer form and shines through it. According to most Earth-based cultures and traditions, all things in Nature are seen as alive, as they are a part of life itself, and thus contain consciousness and intelligence within their form. To directly perceive this consciousness and intelligence is what it means to follow the Light of Nature. Paracelsus saw this Light as radiating through all of creation to communicate to us the spiritual origins of everything in Nature; we only need to cultivate the ability to perceive it. He was trying to name and teach a *new way of seeing* that was, at best, unconsciously used in his culture and is mostly atrophied today.

The Light of Nature is the foundational principle for the evolutionary herbalist because it gives us the eyes to perceive the inherent intelligence of Nature. Using plants for transformational healing necessitates cultivating a spiritual awareness that perceives their sentience, merges with their consciousness, and participates in the orchestra of communication within the natural world. *We must remember how to learn about the plants from the plants themselves.*

The Light of Nature teaches us to become acutely aware of patterns within Nature and to see the vital essence of a plant that unifies its parts into a cohesive whole. We learn more than just a plant's peripheral properties, such as its chemistry and what it is "good for," and come to understand the deeper essence of a plant that weaves its seemingly separate attributes together. As we will see, it's not the rational mind that sees this wholeness, but the intuitive heart, which understands through analogies, similarities, correspondences, and patterns. Whereas the intellect divides, the heart perceives unity.

Learning to speak and understand the language of Nature— called the Language of the Birds in the alchemical tradition, or the "green tongue" by esoteric writers—is the first step in the reintegration of the human being back into the natural order of life. As we experience these patterns of wholeness through the intuitive heart, it becomes clear that our standard reductionist language is insufficient to encompass these moments of truth and unity. We need a natural language composed of analogical, metaphorical, and symbolic syntax that adequately describes the patterns of unity the heart perceives. Only by moving beyond the rational intellect can we attain communion with the intelligence of plants through the Light of Nature. We must repattern our minds with the language of the heart.

A central theme of this book is to suggest a set of symbols of widespread provenance that we can use to describe these basic patterns embodied within people and plants, tracing their connection to the archetypal forces of Nature. The reclamation of this natural language reunites us with ecological intelligence, connecting us with the Light of Nature within ourselves and the essence of plants.

The evolutionary herbalist is rooted in his or her capacity to follow this intelligence through *gnosis cardiaca* (heart knowledge) in order to experience spiritual unity with the plants—*synderesis botanica*—and thus understand them holistically. This approach to viewing the world through the Light of Nature and seeing the inner essence within form was named the "Wisdom of Nature," or *natura sophia,* by the followers of Paracelsus, most notably philosopher and theologian Jacob Boehme (1575–1624). Throughout this part of the book we will explore the intelligence of Nature, examine our innate capacity to perceive it through the heart, and discuss how we can return to the plants as the original teachers of herbal medicine.

Natura Sophia

The natural world is not just a collection of material bodies but has an interior, spiritual side as well. The subjective as well as objective faculties must be exercised upon it in order to fully perceive natural phenomena.... Humanity must revert to this natural level of perception in order to have an intuitive understanding of nature.

—MATTHEW WOOD[1]

Most herbal traditions across the globe studied the Light of Nature. Their medical art was not simply informed through trial and error, but through direct observation of the natural world and communication with the intelligence of Nature. The followers of Paracelsus called this intelligence *natura sophia,* referring to wisdom obtained from the Light of Nature. This formed the foundation of their systems and practices of healing, which reflect universal natural truths. Their medical craft was counseled by the plants, guided by the seasons, and revealed by the rhythms and patterns of the Earth and the cosmos. These medical traditions are still applicable to this day because the truths derived from *natura sophia* are not temporally limited knowledge; they are not deciduous facts of the mind but instead constitute a perennial philosophy of wisdom within the heart.

In order to understand Nature as a whole, we must cultivate a new way of perceiving the world around us through what the old alchemists called the "secret fire" of awareness. We must learn to see the world through a mode of perception and cognition entirely different from what is taught in our conventional cultural model, which in fact suppresses the precise way of seeing that perceives the intelligence etched into the natural world. If we are to gather *natura sophia,* we have to let go of what we think we know and change our perceptual orientation to understand the delicate and potent teachings of the plants. For it is only by emptying ourselves that we can be filled with their living language. Though the mind of Nature does not speak to us in words like we are used to, it is far from silent.

To be connected with the wisdom of Nature, we must sensitize ourselves to the subtle patterns of the barks, roots, leaves, and flowers, to the rhythms of the Earth, the cycles of the stars, and the vital spirit that gives them life. For within them lies a profound secret. And that secret is available to all who learn to see anew. The return to communion with the natural world is not a seeking of information or data; it is a seeking of meaning within the world we inhabit. We need only to develop the eyes to see it and the heart to understand it. We must untrain ourselves in the ways of the world to discern the language of the Earth.

Decolonizing Our Perception

When we were born onto this Earth, our consciousness was pure, an unplanted field of potential. As we took our first steps and grew into toddlers, talked back as adolescents, and adopted responsibility as adults, we gradually became adulterated as our teachers, parents, and culture at large sowed their seeds into our field of consciousness. They wanted us to be who *they* wanted us to be, not who we *truly are.* As these seeds sprout, they grow into the conditioned patterns that determine how we think, feel, and perceive the world around us, forming the mask of persona that shades the inner light of our true nature. Thus begins the colonization of the human soul as the concrete shell of the world is poured over the Earth within us.

The same process is taking place on the planet as a whole. Although we typically use the words "Earth" and "world" synonymously, they are as diametrically opposite as day and night. The "world" is manufactured by humans, the mind made manifest, while Earth is the creation of the Source, of something greater than ourselves. "World" is like the conditioned ego, a projection of the human mind stretched over and covering the Earth, just as it covers our internal essential nature. And similar to how our ego not being calibrated to our soul generates internal discord, so too does a world not in accordance with the laws of the Earth create global imbalance.

We are beings of the world—cultivated by industry, conditioned by media culture, shaped by the scientific paradigm, and sculpted by technology, all of which disconnect us from the Earth and our inner nature. In the city, we are surrounded by the artificial fabrications of the human mind made manifest. The current state of the planet is a macrocosmic reflection of a spiritual sickness within human consciousness: our conditioned egos being severed from our souls. This separation between humanity and Nature, the world and the Earth, has created a wound within ourselves that is gradually spreading and infecting the bloodstream of the planet. To perceive *natura sophia*, we must start with ourselves by purifying the programmed conditionings we received from the world. We must recalibrate our egos to the resonance of our souls so the world can be in harmony with the Earth.

One of the deepest falsities we are programmed to believe is that intelligence is nonexistent in Nature, being rather a hallmark of humanity, whose status is at the top of the evolutionary ladder. In our arrogance, we have designated everything in the natural world—everything from which we evolved, according to science—as unaware, unintelligent, and uncommunicative. Science believes that our grand brilliance evolved from unintelligent forms of life, though as we will see, this is far from the truth. It is precisely this conditioning that not only impairs our capacity to learn directly from Nature but also creates a way of living that leads to massive ecological destruction and threatens the self-organization of the very Gaian system that gives us life. It has also created a culture of very unhealthy human beings physically and spiritually.

This perceptual colonization has been occurring for a very long time. The roots of Western philosophy reveal a conceptualization of plants as inferior to humans in a hierarchical model of life. Many religions and spiritual traditions renounce the physical world in favor of a heavenly afterlife or a better rebirth, a perspective that leads to a disconnection from the Earth. And what philosophy and many religions started, science finished. The gradual development of science led to a mechanistic worldview that reduced the meaning and intelligence of natural systems to numbers, measurements, and quantifiable data. When scientists searched for intelligence in Nature, they defined it in terms of human characteristics, so they never saw it.

The combination of traditional Western philosophy, modern science, and conventional religions has led to an unnatural colonization of the human soul. Stephen Harrod Buhner speaks to this when he states:

> The widely disseminated picture of our human exceptionalism is grounded in the assertion that we possess a unique form of intelligence due to our unique, hypertrophic brain. This belief is not true; it has become a kind of intellectual imperialism. It has been, and still is, used to denigrate the orientation that many people still experience, that the world, and the other organisms with which we share this Earth, are alive, intelligent and aware.... This has resulted in the creation of a conceptual monoculture that can't see outside its own limitations. [2]

Conceptual monoculture. This beautiful phrase eloquently describes the modern state of human consciousness that separates us from the natural world, sees it as unintelligent, and denies our ecological function within it. In the same way that agricultural monoculture leads to the collapse of ecological integrity, conceptual monoculture leads to a degradation of the human soul, for it has walled us off from Nature and removed us from the grand council of beings that inhabit this Earth.

In our contemporary worldview, Nature is likened to a machine wherein each facet of the ecosystem is just a gear. We think we can understand the natural world by reducing it to its constituent parts and quantifying it, just as we can learn how a lawnmower works by taking it apart. We separate the part from the whole, study it, and make assumptions about how the whole functions, forgetting that the initial separation completely changes what we're studying. We cannot rely solely on a reductionistic linear model to understand natural systems, for at its root, Nature is a nonlinear phenomenon that cannot be grasped in its wholeness by reducing it to its parts.

Rudolf Steiner wrote, "However great the successes of science in understanding sense-perceptible reality may be, when it takes what is both necessary and beneficial in its own realm as the standard for all human knowledge, it creates a profusion of prejudices that block our access to higher realities."[3] These "higher realities" are not necessarily out-of-body experiences found in some distant dimension; such realities exist here and now in the natural world.

The first step in gathering *natura sophia* from the Light of Nature requires that we decondition worldly belief systems that limit our awareness and cultivate a new mode of awareness that is of the Earth. We must begin with an *unlearning* process, a decolonization of our perception. We must consciously attend to our inner field of consciousness, pull out the weeds and invasives of the conditioned cultural patterns that blind us, and make space for the seed of our true inner nature to grow that sees truth in outer Nature.

This process opens us to a new form of awareness in which, contrary to popular belief, consciousness is not centered strictly in the brain. We begin to understand that consciousness is universally distributed throughout our entire organism and all natural life, because life *is* consciousness, and thus everything of the Earth is imbued with meaning, intelligence, and language. Every cell of our body, every organ system, and subatomic structure, every part of our being contains consciousness because life is flowing through all of it. In this way, consciousness is fluid, mutable, able to pool itself within any part of the body. Where it locates itself is solely dependent upon where we locate our awareness, and most humans have forgotten to locate it anywhere other than the head. Such an approach to life only gets us so far.

The fluid nature of consciousness permits you to perceive through any part of the body as you consciously focus your aware- ness there. As we will see in the next chapter, we have three pri- mary seats of consciousness, each of which enables us to extract and decipher different layers of meaning from the world. These seats of consciousness are the brain, the heart, and the solar plexus, which correlate to the intellectual, intuitive, and instinctual modes of per- ception. Most of us are taught to only reside within the intellect. As we cultivate the capacity to locate our perceptual faculties within these other seats of consciousness, we perceive the world through a different lens and unlock doorways of understanding that the mind cannot open on its own.

Not only can consciousness occupy different locations *within* the body; it also has the capacity to reside *outside* us. As we learn to rest in a state of pure awareness, we cultivate a holistic mode of per- ception that enables us to see that the Earth is conscious and that the Light of Nature within us is the same as the Light of Nature within, say, a plant. As we strengthen our connection to the Light of Nature, we bridge ourselves to where it resides outside of us, within plants and trees, stones and animals, rivers and mountains, even entire ecosystems and other planets. Through the Light of Nature, we are able to communicate with these intelligence forces of life by seeing their unique embodiment of the whole.

The Intelligence of Nature

To consider intelligence within Nature, we must first contemplate how we define both intelligence and Nature. The implied definition of "nature" that most people believe is the phenomenon of the physical world to the exclusion of human beings and their creations. At the same time, most Westerners think intelligence does not pertain to the nonhuman realm. Thus, by our common definitions of these terms, intelligence within Nature is impossible.

Jeremy Narby speaks to this when he says:

> *Nature as an idea implies disengagement with the world. Actually, if one is strict with words, intelligence in nature is a contradiction in terms, because intelligence excludes non-humans and nature excludes humans. But this mainly shows that our concepts which disengage us with other species hamper our thinking. We struggle with words when the slime mold solves the maze because our concepts don't fit the data. It is not that nature lacks intelligence, but that our own concepts do.*[4]

The dictionary defines *intelligence* as "the ability to learn or understand or to deal with new or trying situations; the skilled use of reason; the ability to apply knowledge to manipulate one's environment or to think abstractly as measured by objective criteria."[5] The fact that intelligence is defined as "the use of reason" and "to think abstractly as measured by objective criteria" shows that it's understood as a product of the human mind.

The word *intelligence* derives from the Latin phrase *inter legere,* which means "to choose." Upon a deeper study of the natural world, we find that multiple elements of Nature do indeed learn, understand, deal with new situations, and manipulate their environment—they *make choices*. In this way Nature is, by definition, intelligent.

Intelligence is woven into the very fabric of Nature's formation, which is based upon the ability of life forms to process information from their surroundings, interpret communications, and regulate themselves to maintain a dynamic state of equilibrium with their external environment. This process is referred to as "self-organization," wherein various parts come into synchrony with one another to create new levels of wholeness and complexity. In short, Nature chooses, and it does so with incredible elegance and sophistication, even though it doesn't have a "brain" like ours. This scientific understanding of Nature was brought to the attention of herbalists by the pioneering work of Stephen Harrod Buhner in his revolutionary book *The Secret Teachings of Plants*.

Here's how self-organization works: if you take a bunch of molecules and place them in a closed system, you would notice that each molecule is, in a sense, its own individual self. They act in a random, chaotic fashion, each one displaying individual behaviors and functions. But as the molecules come closer together, they eventually begin to tightly couple and function together as a whole, cohesive unit. Spontaneously, the parts synchronize and create a newly organized system that displays emergent behaviors and characteristics that none of the individual parts had on their own. A new level of complexity—a new organism—is born, and that system is said to be a self-organized unit. Each part plays an integral role in sustaining the ever-changing equilibrium of the whole, and when enough of those parts are removed, the system collapses, losing its self-organization and returning to chaos.[6]

As this new system interfaces with its environment, it encounters fluctuations in temperature, moisture, atmospheric pressure, electromagnetic signals, perhaps a slight breeze—anything that occurs externally might disturb its internal equilibrium. Such environmental fluctuations require the system to respond, which is achieved through communication of the whole to the parts, informing them how to adjust to reestablish the whole's self-organization. Information flows from the outside to the whole, from the whole down to the parts, and from the parts back up to the whole as they reorient themselves, and in turn out to the environment. As this occurs, the new system learns over time and becomes more complex and adaptable. In fact, it becomes more intelligent. This is precisely how bacteria become resistant to antibiotics, plants adapt defense mechanisms to pests, ecosystems adjust to changing seasons, and the immune system reacts to pathogens.

This self-organized system may interact with other self-organized systems and join together in spontaneous synchronization, becoming an entirely new system that displays its own unique behaviors that are newer (and more complex) than those of the parts. Wholes are composed of parts, which are wholes unto themselves composed of subparts, and the subparts of those parts, down and down ad infinitum, with each level displaying self-organization. This process of self-organization is what the Western mystery traditions refer to as the doctrine of sympathy.

This is the essence of how the natural world is organized. Protons, electrons, and neutrons connect to create atoms, which connect to create molecules. In living systems, molecules self-organize to create organelles, which synchronize to create cells. Cells come together to generate tissues, which self-organize to create organs, entraining together into organ systems. Organ systems form organisms, which entrain to create the ecosystems that form the planet itself, which is its own self-organized, intelligent organism composed of billions upon billions of self-organized parts (of which humans are but one type of part). Planets entrain with one another to form the pattern of our solar system, and on and on it goes. This process goes as far up and out into the cosmos as it goes down into the subatomic realm. Each part is its own self-organized system that forms a greater level of wholeness and which is but a smaller part in a larger system. There is one fractal pattern of Nature reflected across all scales of life.

This shows why we cannot understand the whole by studying the parts. The whole is greater than the sum of the parts, and when enough parts are removed, self-organization is fractured. In the same way, we cannot understand a human being by autopsying a cadaver, a plant by putting it under a microscope, or an herb by isolating specific biochemical compounds. We must see them in relationship to the whole, which must be studied directly. Indeed, the herbal healer is a self-organized being whose wholeness extends beyond them to encompass the plants that become a part of who they are.

This entire process of self-organization within Nature is based on intelligent communications and responses between the whole and the parts and between the whole and its environment. Biological systems are incredibly precise and accurate in their capacity to read the language of their surroundings and to craft intelligent responses that maintain their equilibrium through communication with their constituent parts.

One of the most important elements of communication within the natural world, especially for plants, is the electromagnetic spectrum. All biological organisms emit electromagnetic signals, and embedded within those signals are messages—communications within the organism itself as well as to the surrounding environment.

Our own bodies utilize electromagnetic signaling to achieve significant feats of physiology, from the regulation of our heartbeat and intercellular signaling and communication, to the opening and closing of cellular gating channels to allow nutrients and oxygen to enter and to eliminate waste products. All of the natural world uses the electromagnetic dimension, such as the attraction of bees to pollinators, the orientation of birds on ley lines during migration, and plants secreting protective biochemical substances in response to predators. The very self-organization of biological organisms occurs because of electromagnetic communication. Indeed, the electromagnetic spectrum could be seen as the basis for communication on Earth and quite likely beyond. This is direct scientific confirmation of the *natura sophia* spoken of by the philosophers of old.

Much of our modern technology uses electromagnetics as its foundation, such as Wi-Fi, radio, television, and cell phones. Most human advancements stem from a pattern already apparent in Nature but applied in different ways. The internet, for instance, already existed in a different form in the mycorrhiza under the soil, the highly self-organized fungal network of communication throughout ecosystems.

The electromagnetic spectrum expresses itself through waveforms, with peaks and valleys that vary in speed, height, and depth depending upon the particular frequency, or what we might refer to as an oscillatory pattern. The oscillatory pattern of an electromagnetic frequency is determined by the nature of the information encoded within that particular frequency. While electromagnetic variance is as vast as creation, the universal element of the electromagnetic dimension is that *it always contains information* and that all of biological life both transmits and receives electromagnetic signals. In this way, everything has its own particular vibrational quality in the form of the wave that flows through its particles.

An organism's capacity to decipher electromagnetic information is dependent on its ability to be in a state of coherence, in which it synchronizes its field with those it comes into contact with. The greater the organism's ability to be in a state of coherence—that is, the more cells in its body that are entrained with one another, or the more self-organized it is—the more it will have the ability to sense, focus on, and magnify weak signals to extract the meaning contained within them. We can think of this as an organism's capacity to fine-tune its internal dial to become sensitized to specific electromagnetic signals. This strengthens its ability to maintain self-organization, as its capacity to receive a broader spectrum of signals is enhanced, and the system learns and evolves in its complexity. It is thus in greater harmony with its surroundings, cultivating a greater level of intelligence and able to craft more sophisticated and complex responses.*

The dynamics of molecular self-organization and the electro-magnetic dimension form a scientific understanding of what the ancients have said all along—that Nature is intelligent, alive, and interconnected in a vast web of synergistic communication. And we are a part of it.

As we will see, the heart is the largest generator and receiver of electromagnetic frequencies within the body. When your entire body is in a state of coherence with the heart, you become a highly sensitized instrument for decoding information in the electromagnetic dimension of life. Plants also generate and receive electromagnetic information, and we can use this invisible current to engage in conscious communication with them in ways that reach far beyond the linearity of words.

If we are to mend the split between the world and the Earth, we must first heal it within ourselves by stitching together our hearts and minds, the heart of Nature and our own hearts, thus mending the heart of the world. To begin gathering *natura sophia*, we must learn to see beyond the limitations our modern world has placed upon our perception and see the living intelligence of the Earth. And this can only be done through *gnosis cardiaca*—the knowledge of the heart.

---

*For more information on the process of molecular self-organization and electromagnetic communication, I highly recommend reading Buhner's *The Secret Teachings of Plants*.

Gnosis Cardiaca

Is not the core of nature in the heart of man?

—JOHANN WOLFGANG VON GOETHE[1]

Gnosis cardiaca refers to the acquisition of wisdom from Nature through the direct perception of the heart. To truly enter the kingdom of Nature we must suspend our rational thought, let go of our knowledge of botany and chemistry, even dispense with our systems of herbalism—for any potential interference of the mind will get in the way of our capacities to directly perceive the intelligence within the plants. To move beyond herbal knowledge and into herbal wisdom, we must tread the pathway down the mind into the inner temple located just inside our chest.

Ways of Knowing: Instinct, Intellect, and Intuition

The nervous system is one of our most dynamic organ systems. It is universally distributed throughout the body, influencing all other organs and tissues either directly through innervation or indirectly through control of their blood supply. The body contains three primary conglomerations of neural tissue, and these are our largest biological oscillators, generating and receiving strong electromagnetic signals. These neural networks—located in the gut, the heart, and the brain—are the primary seats of consciousness, and each perceives the world through its own unique lens.

Each of these neural seats represents a certain way of knowing, a mode of perceiving the world, and each has its own unique method of extracting and deciphering meaning. These sites could be thought of as three layers of the self: the gut represents the instinctual self, the brain the intellectual self, and the heart the intuitive self. None of these centers is better or worse than the other; they simply perceive and understand the world differently. It is only when they are imbalanced or when one becomes malnourished, weakened, or atrophied that we start to run into problems. That is precisely what has happened in our modern world, with its glorification of the intellect and degradation of the instincts and intuition.

In the gastrointestinal tract, we have our "gut-level" animal instincts. This is our baseline instinctual self rooted in survival, directly encoded into two hundred thousand years of the evolution of our species. The instinctual self is primarily concerned with self-preservation, protecting us from dangers in the environment, and providing impulses for hydration, nourishment, and reproduction. The instinctual self often operates beneath the level of our conscious awareness, especially in our modern world where life has been made so easy (at least according to the instinctual self; the intellectual self seems to figure out many ways to make life difficult). Most people these days don't have to worry about finding clean water, getting enough to eat, having adequate shelter, being safe from animal attacks, or having enough firewood to stay warm on a cold winter night.

Another way of understanding the instinctual self is to think of it as the intelligence of Nature within our body. Luckily for us, a majority of our continued survival is beyond our conscious control and does not require intellectual or even intuitive understanding. Bodily instinct is what keeps our heart beating, our lungs breathing, our digestion secreting, and our cells functioning.

The early evolution of humans was predominantly focused on the instinctual self because life was all about survival. As society became more developed and life became safer, our vital force was able to move up from the gut and into an entirely new dimension of perception: the heart, where we experience our values, emotional truths and falsehoods, relationships and connections, and the meaning in life. Through the heart we perceive the world around us as conscious, intelligent, and communicating. When the heart opened, the human organism stepped out of mere survival and into a depth of communication with Nature.

Over time, human consciousness gradually ascended from the instincts and intuition into the intellect, resulting in the creations of the mind: the advent of science, the industrial and technological revolutions. As we have developed and refined the linear mind, we have effectively disconnected our awareness from the organs of perception that directly bridge us to the Earth. The evolution of the human soul is directly linked to our capacity to consciously shift our perception into the intuitive heart and gut-level instincts to engage with the intelligence of the natural world.

Through the mind, we separate things into their principal components for analysis, seeking to understand the whole by reducing it to its parts. The mind knows nothing of unity. The paradox is that the separation of the part from the whole takes it out of its natural context, causing it to function differently. The core nature of the human being strives for wholeness, but the rational gaze sees pieces and not patterns, parts and not wholes, so we can never find fulfillment through the work of the intellect alone. It will never provide what we seek.

The act of holding a human brain, dissecting a human heart, or mapping out the entire biochemical process of human physiology will not allow us to say, "Now we understand humans." What about art? What about love and beauty and joy? What about struggle, passion, and trauma? What about the *meaning* that makes us human? None of these things can be understood through dissection. To understand what makes us human, we need experience and direct observation of the human being *in life,* not in a laboratory or a petri dish. For this, we must turn to the educated, sensitive, intuitive heart.

The intuitive heart sees life as an integrated and unified pattern, harmonizing the body and the mind together as one. Through the intuitive heart, the sensations of the body are translated into the mind, and thought patterns are turned into tactile sensation. For the heart is the balance point, the center, bridging the volatile elements of the mind and spirit with the fixed elements of sensation and emotion. In this way, it gives birth to a multifaceted mode of perception that is synesthetic in nature—all senses merging into one. Modern culture often associates intuition with an empathetic sensitivity to others' feelings and emotions (which are elements of heart perception, as we will see), but the true intuitive faculty enables us to see patterns and connections beyond the capacity of linear cause-and-effect thought. The intuition awakens as the heart and mind come into a place of entrainment and connection and as understanding dawns within us from a seemingly intangible source.

When we function with an intuitive, heart-centered consciousness, we perceive the Earth as alive. Plants speak to us in secret languages long forgotten. Nature becomes an open book with each of its rivers and mountains, its plants and animals, becoming a unique dialect. An intuitive consciousness is not concerned with the parts of the plant but rather with the patterns of its wholeness. The heart is not just concerned with the symptoms of a person but instead with their whole being, their whole life. In this way, the heart shows us the unity of life. The way of knowing through the heart does not speak in the linearity of words like the intellect or the survival responses of the instinct; it speaks through the vast and subtle spectrum of *feeling*.

To reach a truly holistic state of consciousness in which we use our entire spectrum of awareness, instinct, intellect, and intuition must become congruent with one another. Each perceptual faculty must be recognized and honored for its usefulness, and it must be understood within its limitations. Our way of seeing the world becomes imbalanced when any one faculty becomes dominant and the others become deficient. Therefore, in seeking a universal understanding of plant medicine, we must begin by striking a conscious balance among instinctive sensation, rational thought, and intuitive understanding. When this occurs on a massive scale, we will see a new era where the world is in coherence with the Earth.

Through harmonizing these three ways of knowing, we ultimately perceive them not as separate but as three elements of a trinity of consciousness. To merge these ways of knowing is to learn to sense with our heart, feel with our mind, and think with our body. This synesthetic perception reflects the acuity of awareness necessary to read the book of Nature and the inner world of plants. The only way to perceive harmony in the outer world is to come into perceptual harmony within ourselves.

Of these three ways of knowing, it's the intuitive faculty of the heart that is the bridge to the Light of Nature, to the existential truths inscribed within the Earth. Intellect without intuition, mind without heart, is a dangerous thing indeed—a form of madness that is destroying the Earth. We must open our hearts again and learn to cultivate the ability to locate our consciousness there, for that is the center of our being that connects us to the center of all beings. Through the tremendous silence found in the intuitive heart, we can hear the forgotten language of the Earth.

The Wisdom of the Heart

Our language still preserves some fragments of the truth that the heart does more than merely pump blood throughout the body. We still have idioms that point to the heart as the center of our emotional reality, with an intelligence that surpasses the brain's.

For example, when we believe in ourselves and follow our life purpose, we are said to be "following our heart." When we experience a breakup with a lover or enter the throes of rejection, we feel "brokenhearted." If we become disillusioned by life and pessimistic, we become "hard hearted." We can also eat a "hearty" meal or be an "open-hearted" or "kind-hearted" person. When you do something with full intensity, you "put your whole heart into it." We can also go beyond memorization of facts and come to "know something by heart." And we speak of the "heartwood," the center of the tree. It's no small thing that the heart is equated with some of the highest virtues expressed by humans. The qualities of compassion, kindness, caring, love, appreciation, acknowledgment, and charity are all characteristics that emerge from a place beyond our intellects.

It's unfortunate that modern culture sees the heart as mushy, overly emotional, and thus unintelligent, placing it on a lower rung of importance than the glories of intellectual achievement and the heightened status of higher education. In our society it is considered better to become a doctor or a lawyer, while people who express from the heart—artists, poets, dancers, musicians, the visionaries of the world—are commonly misunderstood and struggle to find their place in a culture of intellectual dominance.

Is it not surprising that heart disease is the number one killer in Western culture? Is it possible that this isn't just because of high cholesterol or a lack of exercise, but that on a deeper level it stems from intellectual dominance and a forgetfulness that the heart holds a specialized role in perception and cognition? Are our hearts sick physically and emotionally because we have forgotten how to live from them spiritually?

Heart Physiology

Much recent research has debunked the myth that the heart is merely a blood pump. The emerging field of neurocardiology has shown that the heart is deeply intertwined with our nervous and endocrine systems and is a critical organ that determines the physiological integrity and balance of the entire body. Buhner's *The Secret Teachings of Plants* sets out the connections between cardiac physiology and the sensory, perceptive, thinking heart. An incredible amount of credit is also due to Doc Childre, Howard Martin, and the researchers at the HeartMath Institute, who have dedicated their work to researching the heart and its influence in regulating physiology and emotions, and who have shown that the heart has its own unique form of intelligence.

The heart is now considered to be the "primary brain," as it is the first to form during embryological development in the womb. The heart even has its own memory, neurological cells, and neuroplasticity, and it directly modifies the functioning of the brain, as proven by the work of neurocardialogist Dr. J. Andrew Armour.[2]

The heart has four primary paths of connection with the brain: neurological, biochemical, biophysical, and electromagnetic. These connections function through nerve impulses, neurotransmitters, hormones, pressure waves, and electrical and magnetic signaling, forming a dynamic orchestra of communication that oversees and regulates our physiological wholeness, with the heart as the central conductor.[3]

The heart is intricately interwoven into the underlying structure of our central nervous system, hardwired directly into the brain. The two are in a constant state of communication, striving to maintain the dynamic equilibrium of our entire being on the physical, emotional, and psychological levels. Direct neural connections relay information from the heart to various parts of the brain, including the medulla, amygdala, cerebral cortex, and frontal lobes. While some of these portions of the brain are responsible for regulating basic physiological functions such as breathing and heart rate—which are also tied into the gut brain—others are related to emotional memory, translating sensory data into meaning, problem solving, spatial orientation, and higher reasoning capabilities. In short, the heart helps control our *perception*. Not only does the heart communicate with the brain through this myriad of neurological signals, but it also makes its own decisions outside of the influence of the brain; it acts *independently* of the head, with its own capacities for memory, sensation, feeling, and cognition. The heart is more in charge than we once thought it to be, and many functional processes in the brain are determined and informed by neurological signaling from the heart first. For these reasons, *the heart is starting to be considered the primary organ of perception and cognition.*

It's rare in the study of anatomy and physiology to see the heart included in the endocrine system, but it does in fact generate its own endogenous hormones, some of which are unique to the heart itself. Hormones produced by the heart—such as dopamine, norepinephrine, oxytocin, brain naturetic factor, c-type naturetic peptide, and atrial naturetic factor—alter physiological processes throughout the entire body and can generate a wide spectrum of psychological and emotional states, from stress to bliss. From the dilation of blood vessels and adjustment of the mineral–fluid balance in the kidneys, to the alteration of blood pressure and stimulation of the autonomic nervous system (also governed by the gut brain), the hormonal secretions of the heart communicate with areas in the brain involved with learning and memory through their influence on the hippocampus.

The heart touches every part of the body through the blood and as such is the primary distributor of life force throughout the system. Traditional systems of medicine in both the East and the West understood this, and they developed diagnostic methods based on reading the pressure waves generated by the rhythmic pulsations of the heart, felt through the pulse—a diagnosis that involved more than just counting heartbeats. These pressure waves affect every cell of the body, carrying nutrients through tiny capillary beds, generating electrical charges throughout the vascular system, and even affecting brain-wave activity. Conversely, the electromagnetic transmissions from the organs affect these pressure waves, creating a conversation between the organs, blood, vasculature, and heart. This constitutes an incredibly dynamic coordinated system that exhibits properties of self-organization, as these pressure waves self-regulate in order to deliver blood where the body needs it to go.

But one of the most important ways the intelligent heart communicates within us, as well as outside the body, is through the exchange of electromagnetic information. The heart has an electromagnetic field five thousand times larger than that of the brain, permeating every cell and extending up to ten feet beyond the physical body (and that's only as far as our current technology can measure it). The electromagnetic field produced by the heart generates a torus shape, like a doughnut, which is the same shape as the Earth's electromagnetic field and of our body's red blood cells (another example of the fractal geometry of Nature). This electromagnetic field generated by the heart is at the root of its capacity to connect to the living language of Nature and botanical intelligence.

A critical point to understand about the physiology and subtle perceptual faculties of the heart is that it brings the entire physiological and perceptual organism into a place of coherence or internal harmony. When the heart becomes the focal point of consciousness, the organ systems come into synchronization, or entrainment, with it. Rather than acting in isolation, they function in coherence with the heart's patterns, becoming a fully self-organized system. This is precisely how random molecules in a closed system spontaneously synchronize, closely couple together, and begin to work in unison as a newly self-organized whole entity. When the intellect is the primary seat of consciousness, the organ systems are left on their own, communication between them decreases, imbalances within the autonomic nervous system develop, and in essence, the entire physiological organism is out of tune with itself. In fact, everything the heart does must be perfectly coordinated, superbly timed, and impeccably synchronized.

This synchronization is expressed in how the blood travels through the heart, as the timing of the beats must move it through the lower ventricles to the rest of the body from the aorta or to the lungs through the pulmonary circuit. The valves that divide the lower ventricles from the upper atria must close at the precise moment of contraction, and the electrical signals generated by the nodes, which trigger these muscular contractions, must be perfectly coordinated to ensure that the blood flows in the correct direction. Because of this, the heart beats in a spiral pattern rather than a singular contraction and relaxation, like making a fist and relaxing it. If there is a malfunction in any of these signals from the nodes, the chambers filling with or expelling blood, or the opening and closing of the valves, the entire circulatory system behaves erratically and won't function properly. Indeed, the *only* way for the heart to function correctly is by being a highly self-organized and coherent system.

Central to the proper functioning of heart cells is their ability to be synchronized with one another. If you separate a heart cell from other cardiac cells, it will fibrillate spontaneously and ultimately die. But if it comes into close proximity to the rest of the heart, it begins to entrain to its rhythm. This is due to the strong oscillatory pattern of the electromagnetic field emitted by heart cells. As the dislocated cell comes into contact with the heart's electromagnetic field, it entrains to the stronger oscillation of the heart and becomes harmonized with it, in exactly the same way that random molecules spontaneously synchronize during self-organization.

This reflects what occurs when our perception and organ systems stray too far from the heart: they start to have their own chaotic pattern, out of tune with what brings them into harmony and

maintains self-organization. Our minds and bodies "fibrillate."
When our perception is located within the heart, our physiological, emotional, and psychological being is attuned to the largest
oscillator of the body, so all of the organs, systems, and cells of the
body begin to entrain to its harmonic pattern. This makes our entire
being a highly coordinated, coherent system, operating in balance,
with the heart leading the way—each part attuned to the whole.

This process is summarized by Rollin McCraty:

> [Coherence] is the harmonious flow of information, cooperation, and order
> among the subsystems of a larger system that allows for the emergence of
> more complex functions. This higher-order cooperation among the physical
> subsystems such as the heart, brain, glands, and organs as well as between
> the cognitive, emotional, and physical systems is an important aspect of
> what we call coherence. It is the rhythm of the heart that sets the beat for
> the entire system. The heart's rhythmic beat influences brain processes that
> control the autonomic nervous system, cognitive function, and emotions,
> thus leading us to propose that it is the primary conductor in the system. [4]

This coherence also extends beyond the heart itself and into the circulation of blood. Contrary to popular belief, the heart actually does
not have the power to move the blood on its own. Luckily, the arteries move in synchronization with the cardiac muscles—both controlled by signals from the sinoatrial node—to push the blood with
their own dilations and contractions. The movement of the blood
in the arterial system is spiralic, like the beating heart, moving like
a tornado. This reduces the amount of energy needed to move the
blood and segregates the heavy and light elements to the inner and
outer portions of the vessels, reducing friction and leakage through
the vasculature.

This constant communication occurring between the heart
and blood vessels is achieved through baroreceptors distributed
throughout the body. They read the circulatory requirements of
certain organ systems, telling the nervous system to relax or to

contract smooth muscles, adjusting how much blood is received. This information is sent back to the heart, which then routes it to the brain—note that in this process, the heart is *primary*—so the body can autoregulate.

Heart cells synchronize with themselves to produce rhythmic pulsations. The heart and vasculature synchronize with each other to regulate the distribution of blood. The brain and the heart synchronize to regulate proper physiological and psychological functioning. Each level of synchronization represents a state of communicative self-organization, an exchange of information internally at the cellular, organ system, and perceptual levels. This is all controlled via neural, hormonal, and biophysical mechanisms, but the electromagnetic transmissions and reception of the heart are at the root of all of it.

Electromagnetic fields not only convey information internally within our bodies; they also extend outward to interact with other electromagnetic fields in the environment. An encounter with another living thing produces an impression upon the heart, a subtle sense, a *feeling* that transcends the logical mind. But the reverse is also true: when another living field comes into contact with ours, it receives *us*. In the same way that the heart synchronizes the body internally, so too does it synchronize with other fields it touches. The interweaving of electromagnetic fields in the outer world with the heart directly affects these physiological processes and generates the feeling-based language that only the heart can speak.

Each point of contact between the heart and an external electromagnetic field that has a stronger oscillation creates a disturbance within our dynamic equilibrium, a ripple in our heart field that shifts our self-organization and requires us to regain coherence. This is the process all organisms experience as they interface with the world and develop intelligence: they experience environmental shifts that perturb their self-organization, requiring the whole to communicate to the parts, which reorient, shift, and adjust in order to maintain balance—and in the process they learn.

Think of a time when you were having a really good day, with everything going just perfectly, until you had an interaction with someone who was really angry—and then you walked away feeling "not right." When you felt really good, you were in a state of coherence, your self-organization stabilized. And then when you had this negative interaction, the other person's electromagnetic field represented a perturbation to your coherence, throwing you off balance and requiring you to reorient yourself to regain equilibrium.

In such a situation, it's easy to get pissed off yourself and stomp away, muttering "What an asshole!" Or you can take the higher road, with the heart being the map. This involves inculcating a certain perspective, a *perceptual reorientation,* that restores your equilibrium and prevents the other person from ruining your day. Heart intelligence sees that person with compassion and without judgment, and it calls you to be strong in your resolve to be happy and not let another person's bad vibes throw you off track. This ultimately requires self-reflection, internal work, and self-determination in your psychology and emotions. You come back to center, regain your internal coherence, and go about your awesome day.

These perturbations to the heart's coherence and its connection to the brain can be measured through heart rate variability (HRV), which assesses the quality of the heart's beating through variances in the peaks and valleys of its rhythm. These patterns engage in a two-way communication with the brain that determines a great deal of our physiological and psychological states. But the prime question here is this: is our HRV being determined by the brain because the heart has entrained to the brain, or is our HRV being consciously generated by the heart itself?

Doc Childre expands on the significance of HRV:

The analysis of HRV enables us to listen in on and interpret ongoing, two-way conversations between the heart and brain. As we perceive and act in the world, messages sent by the brain through the autonomic nervous system affect the heart's beating patterns. At the same time, the heart's rhythmic activity generates neural signals that travel back to the brain, influencing our perceptions, mental processes and feeling states. [5]

What this means is that our specific emotional tones, psychological states, and ways of seeing the world can be measured by using HRV as a proxy to show whether our hearts are in a state of coherence or not.

Childre's work has shown that during states of stress, irritability, or pessimism, HRV patterns are erratic, incoherent, and scattered. When we experience feelings of love, compassion, forgiveness, kindness, and optimism, HRV patterns become smooth and steady, bringing the entire system into coherence. This state of harmony is immediately reflected in a balance of the parasympathetic and sympathetic nervous systems, which literally affects everything in both our bodies and our minds.

The constantly shifting, autoregulating, self-organized, intelligent system known as the heart is in constant communication not only with itself and the rest of the body but also with the inner psyche and the outer environment. Our feeling states are directly reflected in the heart's physiological patterns, and its variability shows our relative level of internal equilibrium. When we learn to orient our consciousness and perception within the intuitive heart, our entire psychological, emotional, and physical organism comes into harmony both internally and externally. Thus we must learn to drop down from the intellect and into the intuition so we can see from the perceiving heart.

The Perceiving Heart

Beyond the physiological facts about the heart lies the truth that it is an organ of perception, with an exquisite sensitivity to electromagnetic fields that generate emotions and feeling tones as a means of communication. When the heart's electromagnetic field comes into contact with an external field with a strong oscillatory pattern, it experiences a disturbance in its constantly shifting balance. It reads the information encoded within the electromagnetic field and routes it up to the brain for analysis, which then redirects it back to the heart in order to find the appropriate response to maintain balance. The primary way we experience these fields is through the vast spectrum of phenomena we refer to as feeling. While this process is constantly occurring from the moment we are born to the moment we die, it often takes place beneath our conscious awareness, because most of us have little or no training in emotional intelligence. To see from the heart requires us to reawaken this faculty and consciously strengthen its perceptual abilities. We have to *work* at it.

When we live from the intellect, our responses to life situations are usually reactions. We re-act based on past experience, with the mind functioning as little more than a highly sophisticated memory storage device. When we live solely within the domain of intellectual perception, we constantly repeat old patterns, habitual psychological and emotional responses based on our past. The heart, on the other hand, responds in the moment. It balances our inner and outer worlds like a person walking a slack line. Because the heart is aware of a deeper order within the world around us, it has a different way of cognizing and understanding life that is more dynamic and intelligent than the cerebral brain.

When we perceive from the heart, the cranial brain and the gut brain entrain with the dynamic field the heart generates and receives from the outer world. The neural cells of the brain and its wave patterns start to oscillate at the heart's frequency, coordinating their activities. This triggers parts of the brain that alter our perception and cognition, specifically within the hippocampus, which is especially sensitive to magnetic fields due to its high concentrations of magnetite. The hippocampus is associated with sensory perceptions, spatial relationships, memory, interpretation of meaning, and shifting physiological responses in association with emotional states. Thus there are specific physiological shifts associated with heart coherence, including activation of the parasympathetic nervous system, physical relaxation, psychological calmness, and slowed breathing. The pupils dilate, triggering soft-focused, peripheral vision and an acute sensitivity to the environment. This enables us to begin to understand the specific sensations associated with entering a state of heart perception so we can enter it more easily.

As the heart comes into entrainment with another electromagnetic field, such as a plant, the heart receives the information embedded within that field, and that interaction generates a particular feeling tone. This information is routed to the brain, where it's processed and meaning is extracted from it. But because the heart is being used as the primary organ of perception from a place of coherence, our brain functioning is altered, so we open up a new way of understanding the world around us. We aren't actively thinking about the plant; we are feeling our way through the plant, passively allowing the meaning contained within those feelings to dawn within us.

As we have seen, the heart's physiology is based on synchronization or entrainment. This is the function that allows the heart to perceive information flowing through the electromagnetic spectrum. Imagine the heart emanating a certain electromagnetic field, with its own unique frequency of peaks and valleys, and a plant emanating its own unique frequency. Those two fields interweave when you are walking through a forest. They overlap and synchronize when you sit before the plant and consciously attune yourself to your heart, extend your heart field outward from your chest, and wrap it around the plant's leaves and stems and flowers. You touch the plant, but not with your hand; you touch it with the living field of your heart.

As you deepen this connection with the plant through your heart and senses, you tune your whole being like a dial to match the electromagnetic frequency emanated by the plant. Rather than two overlapping waveforms with totally different patterns, your heart entrains, attuned to the electromagnetic frequency of the plant. You and the plant ride the same wave. At this moment of synchronization a vast amount of information is exchanged; an invisible, unheard feeling-based language is spoken between yourself and another kingdom of life. This is how traditional people all across the world learn about plants *from* the plants, which we will explore further in the next chapter.

This synchronization with another electromagnetic field is not uncommon in our daily experience. If you've ever gone for a walk with a friend and noticed that you're walking in unison, or in the midst of a deep conversation you have an inner knowing of what your friend will say next, then you've experienced coherence with another being. Unfortunately these experiences often occur beneath the level of our conscious awareness. Cultivating heart perception necessitates bringing this process into our conscious awareness, moving through the world with our heart field extended, feeling its way through life, and becoming highly sensitized to the feeling dimension of the world. This not only opens us to perceive the Light of Nature; it also makes our lives incredibly rich as we experience a deep intimacy with the world around us. We touch the Earth, and in return, the Earth touches us, as we allow what is "out there" to enter "in here."

Gateways into the Heart

There are four primary ways to access the perceptual heart. The first is simply by locating our consciousness within the heart itself. This is achieved by feeling the beating of our heart, placing a steady flame of awareness within our chest, and consciously redirecting our perceptual focal point from head to heart. We become receptive, which requires a balance between relaxation and highly attentive focus. This can take some practice, because most of us have little or no training in how to perceive the world through our hearts and have a habit of strictly residing in the intellect.

The second gateway is more engaged with the outer world and is activated through attunement to our senses. Whenever we become aware of our sensory perceptions, we lose track of our thoughts. Anyone who has become immersed in artistic or creative activities knows this: time slows down when you are fully submerged in painting, playing a musical instrument, singing, or dancing. All of these acts require not thinking about what we are doing, just simply doing it, fully engaged in our sensory mechanisms.

Most of us go through our lives taking our senses for granted; we don't fully engage with them. When we consciously infuse a particular sensory faculty with the flame of our awareness, it transmutes that sense's capacity to engage with deeper levels of meaning. When we are oriented in the intellectual mode of perception, we go through our lives *looking* at things, but we don't really *see* them. We *hear* the sounds around us but we don't really *listen* to them. We might *eat* foods but we do not *taste* them. We might *touch* objects but we do not *feel* them. The difference is subtle and is primarily determined by our level of presence.

The senses are associated with the animal or wild self, the gut brain, so they are coming from the opposite direction from the mind. As such, they form the foundation of heart perception, bringing us into the present moment and connecting us to the outer world.

When we pay attention to the troubles our client is sharing with us, we are not thinking about our past. When we are fully sensing the plant we are sitting with, we are not daydreaming about our future. There is no room for mind during conscious sensory attunement, no space for interpretation of what is entering our senses. The moment the mind comes in and tries to "figure out" what it's sensing, we immediately move from the heart to the head.

Because the heart is a place of unity, it is the melting point of the senses. When we enter a profound state of heart perception, so deep that it's like a trance, we start to experience synesthesia, or sensory crossover. In the heart, the boundaries between seeing, listening, feeling, smelling, and tasting begin to dissolve. In this state, what we see transforms into auditory experiences, what we listen to becomes what we feel, and what we feel becomes what we see. Synesthesia is a multidimensional form of awareness that can extract deep levels of meaning expressed by the nonlinear electromagnetic pulses of natural organisms. Synesthetic perception is like having 360-degree vision. We open our awareness to the heart of the world, the meaning infused within it, and the signatures etched upon it.

The third gateway into the heart is physical relaxation. One of the hallmark signs of entering heart coherence is activation of the parasympathetic nervous system, which directly relaxes the muscles of the body. When consciousness is located in the intellect, it generates tension in the body. The word *tension* comes from the same root as the word *tense* in a temporal sense, as in past or future tense. The only way we can be in the past or the future is through the memories and projections of the intellect. Tenses of time are tenses of mind, and locating awareness within the mind produces tension in the body, a common response of the sympathetic nervous system. When we are relaxed, the survival-based, gut-level instincts are able to calm because we are safe. This frees them to move up into the heart, opening our receptivity to the living language of the Earth.

The final gateway into the heart is entered by conscious attunement to the breath. On a physiological level, the respiratory system is the shortest pathway into the heart. Each inhalation reoxygenates the blood, which is immediately routed to the heart for systemic distribution. The breath is a bridge not only into the heart but between the mind and the body. When we enter a state of psychological or physical relaxation, we often sigh. Conversely, when we try to calm ourselves down we usually do it by attending to the breath. This is why breathwork is always an essential part of meditation practices; slow, conscious breathing immediately stills the mind. Breathing replaces thinking because the two activities are connected by the Air Element (see chapter 10, "The Elemental Human").

Because breathing is governed both by the autonomic nervous system (beyond our conscious control) and the somatic nervous system (within conscious control), we can use it to consciously control our minds, hearts, and bodies.

When you see a friend who is having a really bad day, all stressed out, nervous, and anxious, what's one of the first things you tell them to do? *Take a deep breath.* When we're stressed, our breathing becomes shallow and rapid, immediately triggering the sympathetic nervous system and severing heart coherence. When we are calm and relaxed, our breathing is deep, slow, and rhythmic. Our mind is at peace, the space between thoughts widens, and we are more consciously aware. An experienced pulse diagnostician once commented that when a person meditates, the space between the diastole and the systole actually lengthens, showing both that the heart is resting more between beats and that there is more spaciousness between thoughts.

It's interesting that one of the first physiological responses after entering natural environments is sighing, a sign that the linear mind is slowing down, the sympathetic tone is relaxed, and our awareness is on its way down from the intellect to the heart. Buhner notes that the Greeks had a word for this: *aisthesis,* which literally means "to breathe in." It derives from the same root as our word *aesthetic,* illustrating our capacity to perceive and appreciate beauty, a quality associated with the heart. The Greeks understood that when we come into contact with *natura sophia* through the heart, the living vitality of the world reaches inside and touches a place deep within us. At that moment there is a sigh, a gasp, a deepening of the breath as we feel connected to someone beyond ourselves.

As we learn to understand the meanings embedded within the forms we perceive by harmonizing our whole being with them, we establish a feeling connection that is the essence of *gnosis cardiaca.* Through this perceptual reorientation, the intellect ever so slowly becomes restructured with the symbolic, pattern-based language of the natural world received by the heart. And this is the language spoken by herbalists who listened to the plants and followed the Light of Nature for a very long time, a language we must remember.

Synderesis Botanica

Although it is true that the secrets of the outer world disclose them-
selves inside us, in the spirit we step outside of ourselves and let the
things themselves tell us what is significant for them, rather than
for us.

—RUDOLF STEINER[1]

There is a term in Christian mysticism, *synderesis*, that refers to the essence of the soul that is directly united with God. Typically this term is only used to refer to the human soul, but from the perspective of many herbal and spiritual traditions, this element of the soul is present within all of creation: as the Light of Nature shimmers from the heart of the Source, it shines through the center of every living thing. In this way, everything reflects that Source energy, embodies the divine intelligence, and is connected to God through its own soul.

The botanical kingdom thus contains synderesis, characterized by a quality of soul presence. Plants evince a unique expression of consciousness and intelligence, and they have their own distinct purposes, sentience, and functions outside the sphere of human benefit. A great deal of scientific research has shown that plants display dynamic communications within themselves and with their environments, as well as memory, sensory capacity, and incredibly sophisticated responses to the flux of life flowing through the ecosystem.

Far too often when we study or work with plants, we approach them through the narrow lens of how we can use them only for our benefit. Industries look for natural resources, farmers aim to yield higher crops, pharmaceutical companies search for new alkaloids. Even herbalists fall prey to this trap, studying what types of symptoms and diseases plants are "good for." By only looking at what plants can do for *us,* we limit our understanding of them. When we change our orientation to directly perceive their synderesis without ignoring their bodies, when we equally recognize their chemistry and their spirit, our practice of herbalism drastically changes.

To create an evolutionary paradigm of plant medicine, we must deeply honor the plants by recognizing that they are conscious and sentient, and we need to acknowledge that there is a living soul within them that surpasses what we can understand through science or intellectual reductionism. If we want herbalism to address the souls and spirits of people, we must address the souls and spirits of the plants first.

A profound truth found within the body of philosophy known as Hermeticism (one of the sources of the *natura sophia* tradition) is that the macrocosm and microcosm are united in a complex web of interconnectivity, expressed in the axiom "as above, so below." This principle states that the precise pattern of the cosmos is imprinted within each and every living organism—*and this includes plants.* They are as much an embodiment of the totality of life as we are; they contain all of the elemental and celestial forces, the entire holistic pattern of life, embodied within their soul.

Plants display intelligent behaviors, communicating both internally and externally throughout the ecosystem and with other species, including humans. The ability to communicate with them is crucially important on the plant path because it shows the herbalist how to develop relationships with plants in ways that reveal not only how they benefit us but also *who they are* and their unique expressions of synderesis. I learned how to communicate and commune with plants from the work of Stephen Harrod Buhner, who eloquently explains the process of gathering knowledge from the heart of the world,[2] and from Pam Montgomery, author of *Plant Spirit Healing*.[3] Much credit is due to these two pioneering herbalists for disseminating teachings on how we can learn directly from the plants.

Evolutionary Emergence

During the earliest evolutionary phases of life on Earth, a radical transformational process occurred when bacterial life forms spontaneously self-organized into a more advanced system and evolved one of the most important emergent behaviors in evolutionary history: photosynthesis. Small organelles called plastids formed when single-celled eukaryotic organisms self-organized by engulfing photosynthetic cyanobacteria, thus enabling a light-mediated transformation of carbon dioxide and water to produce oxygen and sugars. Earth became oxygenated, supporting the evolution of all subsequent life forms and forever changing the planet.

Over time, these plastid organelles evolved into chloroplasts (similar to the mitochondria of our own cells), whose genetic makeup encodes the ability to generate oxygen and carbohydrates from light. Chloroplasts contain the pigment chlorophyll, giving plants their green coloration. Our red blood cells are built upon the same molecular pattern as chlorophyll, which contains magnesium at its center, whereas red blood cells contain iron. When a photon of light hits a chloroplast, chlorophyll releases an electron that passes through an electron transport chain to generate the two primary forms of cellular energy: ATP and a molecule called nicotinamide adenine dinucleotide + hydrogen, or NADH. The empty space where the chlorophyll electron used to be is filled by an electron split off from a water molecule, which is then separated into hydrogen and oxygen. This released oxygen makes our atmosphere habitable for most of the animal kingdom. To complete the cycle of photosynthesis, the plant pulls carbon dioxide from the air and combines it with water, driven by the power of ATP and NADH, to form carbohydrates.

Thus photosynthesis creates oxygen and produces sugars from no more than light, carbon dioxide, and water. In this way, we can see the primal Fire, Air, and Water Elemental forces combining within plants to create the Earth—a process described by the alchemical tradition long before the discovery of photosynthesis. Plants harvest light and thus are materializations of the Light of Nature.

Plant Sensory Mechanisms

If we think of ourselves as intelligent, it only makes sense to consider the possibility that other forms of life may also contain intelligence. Often we define intelligence only in terms applicable to humans. But if intelligence is an awareness of one's environment and the ability to take in communication, process information, and craft an appropriate response, then it is apparent that plants exhibit intelligent characteristics.

We often limit intelligence strictly to humanity and animals in part because of the divergent evolutionary paths taken by these different kingdoms of life. Whereas animals developed locomotion, vegetable life opted for a different evolutionary pathway—stillness. Animal life thus evolved different survival capacities based on their nomadic nature and necessitated by their need to feed on other living organisms, such as the abilities to run, jump, fly, and swim.

Plants, on the other hand, are autotrophic, meaning they sustain themselves from what is immediately available in their environment: water, soil, air, and sunlight (i.e., the Elements). A unique aspect of plant life is that their anatomy and physiology are not located in individual organs, like animals; rather, their basic structures are equally distributed throughout the entire organism. This is why, if you remove the heart of an animal, it will die, because each organ performs a specific function not performed elsewhere in the body. But if you clip the stem off of a plant, it does not die—in fact, it will often grow back more robustly! The stationary nature of plants required them to equally distribute their vital functions throughout their entire being to ensure their survival.

This makes perfect sense, if you think of how many animals eat plants to sustain themselves. If a plant had centrally located organs like animals do, it might die as soon as one of its leaves was eaten. But because a plant's physiological functions are modular and are thus disseminated throughout every part of it, a plant can get munched down to the roots and still survive. This evolutionary strategy for self-preservation ensured plants' survival and required them to evolve highly intelligent methods of being aware of and responding to their surroundings.[4]

Plants have sensory awareness.[5] We think that only animals have senses because we associate sense perception with specific animal sense organs, but if we redefine sensory perception outside the context of animal anatomy, focusing on the *function* of the sense, we find that plants are indeed sensory beings. For instance, plants don't have eyes like we do, but if we define sight in terms of the physiological function of eyes—the perception of light—plants definitely see. They don't have two eyes like we do; instead they have *billions* of eyes in the form of chloroplasts, which are acutely aware of light through photosynthetic activity. When deciduous trees sense the change in light resulting from the advent of autumn, they drop their leaves, closing their eyes to sleep and returning to their roots throughout the cold of winter before they grow once again in the spring.

Certain plants are highly sensitive to and aware of light. California Poppy *(Eschscholzia californica)* closes its bright orange flowers when it's in the shade and at night, but when the sun shines the petals open in all their glory. Evening Primrose *(Oenothera biennis),* on the other hand, is sensitive to moonlight; its flowers suddenly pop open when touched by the silvery light of the moon. Anyone who has kept house plants knows they possess the property of phototropism, as they reorient themselves in space to grow toward windows and get the maximum amount of light.

But plants are not only sensitive to the light of the sun or moon; they have multiple other types of photoreceptors, such as phytochromes, cryptochromes, and phototropins, that detect various wavelengths of light, even into the ultraviolet spectrum. A plant's ability to "see" determines its entire growth process. Sprouting, leafing, flowering, and fruiting are all based on plants' sensitivity to light and the way it changes, as the orientation of the Earth to the Sun changes throughout the seasons.

Plants also smell. They have a variety of specific receptors for volatile chemicals encountered within the environment, and many release their own smells to communicate with their neighbors about particular dangers or stressors, such as pests or fluctuations in temperature or moisture. Most aromatic compounds form a component of a plant's innate immunity, manufactured and secreted when they sense a pest nibbling on their leaves. Plants can't run or fly away, but they can make their common pests flee instead. As herbalists, we know that when a plant is aromatic, that often indicates that it can convey its immune-stimulating properties to us; what helps a plant's immunity helps our immunity. They are the greatest biochemists of Nature.

If the sense of taste is defined as the perception of food, flavor, and nutrients required for nourishment, then plants have this capacity as well. Roots have the ability to detect specific nutrients in the soil, determine where greater amounts of water are located, and begin to grow in that direction. They direct their growth to seek out the most optimal mineral content in the soil, even planning for the future by sensing distant nutrients that cannot be utilized until later. And let's not forget the carnivorous plants, like the Venus Flytrap *(Dionaea muscipula)*, which senses the presence of an insect on the surface of its leaves, closes down on it like jaws, and secretes enzymes to digest it.

Plants are also aware of touch. Roots growing through the soil can feel rocks and tell the difference between stone and soil, and they will grow in a pattern that traces the rocks' periphery. The Venus Flytrap has such a sensitive sense of touch that its mouthlike leaf will only close if a fly touches two of the three little hairs on the leaf within a twenty-second period of time. The fly must also be in the middle of the plant's "mouth" for the leaf to close, ensuring that the plant gets its meal. It would be a waste of energy if every little touch, like a drop of water, made its mouth close. If it's going to close, it makes sure dinner is there first.

Vines and climbing plants also have a distinct sense of touch. They have the ability to sense the location of other physical objects in space and will grow in that direction to grab on and start climbing. This is noticeable in plants like Ground Ivy *(Hedera helix)*, Jasmine *(Jasminum* spp.), Hops *(Humulus lupulus)*, and Passionflower *(Passiflora incarnata)*.

If we conceptualize hearing as the perception of vibrational wavelengths moving through space, then plants do indeed hear. They are particularly aware of vibrational qualities; plants that are exposed to classical music tend to grow faster and produce more abundant fruits with greater nutritional quality. Anyone who grows a garden or tends household plants knows that plants are healthier when the gardener talks or sings to them. There are recent theories that roots produce small clicking sounds when their cells split in order to communicate with themselves and with other life forms in the soil.

I find it quite interesting that many traditional cultures that are deeply engaged with the intelligence of plants sing specific songs to them, many of which they say are taught to them by the plants themselves. There are songs for harvesting, making medicine, and awakening the spirit of the plant to heal the spirit of a sick patient. This has been highly refined throughout Amazonian herbalism, where it is said that to receive the song of a plant is the highest honor and a sign that you carry the spiritual medicine of the plant within your own heart.

Plant Communication

Plants contain dynamic systems that enable their various parts to communicate with one another. They possess their own unique form of a nervous system that conducts electrical signals through the plasmodesmata, or tiny openings within the cell walls. These are quite similar to the gap junctions used in neural signaling within animal nervous systems. Longer-distance electrical signaling occurs through a plant's vascular system, called the xylem and phloem. This system connects the roots with the aerial parts to transmit fluids and nutrients back and forth, because roots collect nutrients that leaves cannot and vice versa. These messaging highways enable the various parts of the plant to assess the surrounding environment, communicate with one another, and autoregulate themselves to maintain the equilibrium and self-organization of the whole plant.

Chemical messaging systems form their own sort of hormonal or endocrine system. Photosynthesis is a prime example of chemical communication occurring within plants, governed by the stomata, which are similar to our skin pores. When the stomata open, more light is allowed into the chloroplasts, and photosynthesis occurs; but this can also lead to dehydration as water evaporates (as if the plant is sweating). When the stomata close, photosynthesis stops (as if it has closed its eyes), but the plant conserves water. A constant conversation is conducted between the roots and the leaves via chemistry, determining what takes greater priority—conservation of water, or production of sugars and energy through photosynthesis.

One astounding aspect of plants is the brilliance of their roots. Charles Darwin, in his treatise *The Power of Movement in Plants,* revealed the incredible sensitivity of root tips, likening them to the plant "brain."[6] The root tips constantly survey the substratum of the Earth, measuring multiple qualitative factors such as gravity, temperature, moisture, light, pressure, electrical fields, mineral composition, chemical gradients, the presence of toxins, and vibrations. An incredible number of variables determine the decisions made by root tips—whether to grow in the direction of one or another nutrient, search for water, grow upward for aeration, or exchange nutrients with mycelium. They must also consider the needs of the aboveground portions of the plant. When we consider that a single plant has literally millions upon millions of root tips all working together as a self-organized system, we see that the root tips literally function like a neural network, thus validating Darwin's description of them as the plant's brain.[7]

It's also been shown that plants communicate with their neighbors. Plants of different species growing near each other form significantly larger roots as they compete for water and nutrients, whereas plants of the same species don't display this sort of competition. In a sense, they recognize their relatives. Intimate mycorrhizal relationships with the fungal kingdom initiate synergistic communication whereby fungi provide the plants with specific nutrients (primarily minerals like phosphorous), and in return the plants' ability to photosynthesize offers carbohydrates to the fungi. In a beautiful, harmonious relationship, plants use the mychorrhiza to plug in to the grand nervous system resting beneath the soil.

But not all of these interspecies relations are positive. Plants discern which types of relationships will prove beneficial and which ones will be parasitic, and they develop specific biochemical defense mechanisms to ward off these undesirable neighbors. When insects start eating certain plants, they manufacture customized aromatic or bitter biochemical compounds to deter that pest. Some have the ability to "read" the type of attacker and develop a biochemical deterrent specific for that pest. Many of these compounds volatilize into the air, bind to the receptors of nearby plants, and warn them of the attack so they can start strengthening their own innate immunity. Some of these volatile compounds will even summon reinforcements by signaling other insects that predate on the insect eating the plant, letting them know that dinner is here.

Plants also communicate with the world through their reproduction methods. The bright colors of showy flowers, the beauty of their fragrance, the sweetness of their nectar—all are responsible for attracting the right pollinators that reinforce their reproductive capacity. From hummingbirds and bats to bees and other insects, flowering plants evolved highly strategic methods for calling upon the aid of the animal kingdom to work in synergistic ways to ensure pollination. Fascinatingly, plants induce a kind of trance in most pollinators, which botanists refer to as "site fidelity." In order for a plant to properly reproduce, pollinators must transfer its pollen to the same species of plant; it would do no good if pollinators simply went flying from Rosemary to Thyme to Oregano. So plants enchant their pollinators to be true to the species they chose to work with at the beginning of the day. Without this mechanism there would be significantly less plant diversity.

After pollination and producing fruits and seeds, plants further ensure their survival by enticing a wide range of animals to spread their future generations far and wide. The fruits' bright colors, sweet flavors, and enticing aromas are all tactics to attract animals to eat them and spread their seeds to new locations via excretion. Most fruits taste really bad when they're unripe, and the plants have a reason for this. From the plants' perspective, it's not the fruit that they're ripening but the seeds. Most fruits don't develop their delectable flavors until the seeds within are mature enough to grow a new plant, ensuring that animals will be attracted by the fruit at the precise time when the seeds are fertile.

One of the most important dimensions of plant communication is the electromagnetic field. This invisible informational field permeating space underlies all of these different messaging systems within the plant and in the environment beyond it. From the tips of the roots to the edges of the flowers, plants constantly communicate through the electromagnetic spectrum. This in turn translates into specific chemical messages that lead to a wide range of behavioral responses. Plants are complex electromagnetic generators and receivers, sensitive to the smallest signals in the air and Earth, even those emitted by the human heart. As plants communicate within themselves and with other plant and animal species, is it too much to assume that they communicate with us as well—but we have forgotten how to listen?

Sensing Plant Intelligence

If we are to learn from the intelligence of plants, we must see that everything about them is a living language, and every element of their being is a communication. Herbalists cultivate a certain sharpness of the senses and humble willingness to set aside prior knowledge of what they *think* they know about a plant, whether they learned it from a book, their own research, or what an expert has told them. That way they are always willing to learn something new about plants. They are open to the mysteries of plants that only the heart can comprehend. To cultivate this perspective, we have to see that *everything about a plant is a communication,* purposeful in its syntax, precise in its diction, rich in its descriptions, vast in its meaning. Plants are composed of language beyond words.

Purpose, intelligence, and meaning are everywhere in Nature. There's a *meaning* behind the fact that St. John's Wort *(Hypericum perforatum)* likes to grow on southern-facing slopes in open fields and not in the deep, dark woods. There's a *reason* why Devil's Club *(Oplopanax horridus)* doesn't grow in the open fields and prefers the moist, hidden places in the forest. There's an expression behind the color and smell of the Rose, a communication behind the prickles and sharp sting of Nettles. As we learn to decipher the communications embedded within the forms of a plant, we start to translate its messages and understand its deeper meaning instead of just thinking about it.

Sensing plant intelligence begins by consciously infusing our awareness into each sensory faculty, shifting our orientation from looking into seeing, tasting into savoring, hearing into listening, touching into feeling. We must learn to trust our senses as much as we trust our thinking, for they are the bridges that unite the inner and outer worlds, the gateways through which the living language of Nature reaches into us and touches our hearts.

When you come across a plant in the forest, stop and become highly aware of what you perceive with your eyes. Allow your vision to soften, pulling your awareness to the backs of your eyes, becoming a receptivity, a passivity through which the plant flows into you. Pay attention to the habitat where the plant prefers to grow. Is it in the shade or full light? Is it growing by itself, around other plants of its own species, or around plants of a different species? What is the nature of the soil? Rocky? Hard? Soft? Damp? Dry? Plants have preferences just as people do, and if we pay attention to where a plant prefers to grow, we can learn about the unique ecological state that the plant heals within a person's physiology. Medicinal plants often grow in a habitat similar to the one they treat therapeutically in the body's ecosystem. Conversely, they can generate that type of ecosystem within the body.

Then approach the living plant and sit in front of it. Use your capacity for seeing to become acutely aware of its shape. Is it tall? Short? Thin? Stout? Observe the color of its leaves, its unique spectrum of green, its texture and overall pattern. Is it smooth or rough? Soft and silky? Thick and waxy? Without labeling, without allowing words to dam the river of your seeing, just allow the plant to wash over your visual field, flow into you, and touch the stillness inside you. How does what you *see* make you *feel?*

Next, touch the plant—or, rather, *feel* the plant. As if your only sense was touch, place the leaves between your fingers and rub them together. Run your hands through the foliage, touch the delicacy of the flower, cup the fruits in your hands, move your fingers along the stems. Become fully engaged and alive in the act of physical feeling.

As you rub some of the leaves or flowers between your fingers, lean in closely and breathe the plant in, allowing its aroma to enter you. The moment you smell the aromatic property, the plant has physically entered your body and begins to communicate biochemically. The sense of smell is intimately connected to the limbic system of the brain, which is deeply associated with emotional memory. When we pay close attention to the act of inhaling the plant, subtle spectrums of feeling can be generated. Take time to sit and breathe with the plant, knowing that your outbreath becomes its inhalation, and its exhalation becomes your next breath. Through this exchange you are profoundly interwoven.

From here, deepen your awareness of the plant by placing it in your mouth, holding it on your tongue—not passively tasting the plant but infusing your consciousness into your tongue and *savoring* it, allowing the entirety of your being to become what you taste. Is it bitter? Astringent? Sour? Pungent? As you savor the plant, a vast amount of information is conveyed to your body, causing instantaneous physiological changes to occur. At the point of contact with your sense of taste, an orchestra of biochemical communication is initiated as your body deciphers the messages encoded within the plant's chemistry.

As you take this time to "come back to your senses" with the plant, you enter an entirely new level of awareness that you wouldn't reach by just looking at it, analyzing it with your mind, or thinking about its properties. This practice involves replacing your thinking with your sensing, which permits you to see the plant's unique signatures—the meaning behind its form—and to connect its physical structure and habitat to the properties you learn about in the books. Sensory observation opens your capacity to read a plant's unique language and perceive its deeper underlying patterns, as it is one of the primary gateways into the heart.

Learning Plants by Heart

After consciously engaging in sensory awareness, we move into the next layer of our plant communication by attuning ourselves to the heart of the plant. To do this, we must first attune ourselves to our own heart.

Allow your physical body to relax and be held by the Earth, slow and deepen your breathing, and reorient your perception into your chest to directly activate a state of heart coherence. Then, from your internal coherence, consciously engage your heart with the plant. Radiate outward, stretching yourself out from your chest, reaching toward the plant to nonphysically touch it. Wrap your heart field around the plant and trace its contours with your feeling. Breathe it into your center, and in turn, breathe your center into it. Each inhalation brings the plant closer to you, and each exhalation brings you closer to the plant. Focusing on the plant in this way, from a place of internal coherence, begins the process of entrainment as you fine-tune your heart field like a dial on a radio, moving through the static until you find the right "station."

In this attunement process, there comes a point where you feel a certain "click," a distinct sensation that you and the plant are synchronized with each other. You notice this arrival by a sigh, a warmth in the chest, a softening of the gaze, and a subtle but noticeable shift in consciousness. An etheric bridge is established between you and the plant as you enter a sort of waking dream. This moment of initial harmonization with the plant is accompanied by a distinct tonal hue of feeling. This subtle feeling—always difficult to put into words—must become the focus of your perception. The more you are aware of these feelings, the stronger they become, as your heart takes a weak electromagnetic signal and strengthens it. When you focus on this feeling, you are watering this inner sensation so it can grow. You pour the totality of your awareness into it, allowing it to wash over your entire being, bathing every cell in your body. As this feeling received from the plant grows, it becomes all that you are aware of.

These delicate feeling tones, the subtle impressions made upon your heart, are the nonlinear semantics received from the plant's electromagnetic field. They are living forms of meaning, the unique syntax and diction of the plant. Yet they are merely your first impressions, the beginnings of your relationship. You can't expect to reach the essence of the plant the first time you do this, just as it's rare to meet a person and have her reveal her deepest secrets in the first hour of conversation. As with any relationship, this process takes time and commitment.

With your heart radiating outward from your chest and wrapped around the plant, you maintain the connection by nonphysically embracing it, tracing the edges of its morphology with your heart, feeling its colors, becoming its environment. The deeper you wade into the invisible territory of the plant, the more deeply it enters into you. As you learn about its nature through this very different way of perceiving, it's learning about you as well.

Vitally important to this process is the nonverbal communication *you send to the plant*. Consciously imprint your care, gratitude, and commitment to learning its medicine into your heart field, and breathe this communication out into the plant's essence. You're not communicating through words but through a feeling-based language extended from your heart to the heart of the plant. Like water poured into a cup, allow your pure intent to understand its medicine to flow into and touch the essence of the plant. Communication is always a two-way street, and we must express as well as listen.

The next step is achieved through a short-lived disconnection with the plant, which allows the electromagnetic communications taken in by the heart to be routed up into the brain, where they are deciphered and analyzed for meaning. Because the brain is in coherence with the heart in this scenario, the brain's physiological functioning is altered, primarily through heightened activity of the hippocampus. This part of the brain is associated with the interpretation of meaning. From the heart, the brain decodes the meaning embedded within the feelings received from the plant and displays it to your consciousness in a way that you can understand, although sometimes it takes awhile to fully unravel every dimension of this meaning.

Because the heart is the primary receiver of plant language, these communications are always nonlinear, irrational, beyond comprehension of the intellect alone, even though the brain plays a central role in unraveling the meaning. As the brain deciphers the message, your emerging understanding of the meaning can take the form of a vision, audible words, or physical sensations within the body, such as tingling, pressure, heat, or cold. Emotional hues or memories buried within the subconscious may surface. Intuitive flashes of understanding may burst into your awareness. The form of this communication varies from person to person based on whether their learning style is primarily tactile/sensory, audible or visual.

Whatever form the message takes, *everything you experience in this state of entrainment with the plant conveys meaning.* This is not a rational, cause-and-effect process; rather, meaning spontaneously emerges within you, obtained from a place beyond the self. There's a distinct sense of such meaning not being internally generated. The plant will use whatever means necessary to translate its message into a meaningful and understandable form, searching for something in our life that is resonant with its electromagnetic field to *show*—not tell—us what it means.

During your time sitting with a plant, you must become aware of everything happening internally and externally, for you are entering a particular kind of dreaming where *everything has meaning.* You become attuned to the spectrum of feelings and emotions that arise within your heart. You are acutely conscious of physiological shifts inside your body. You're aware of the random thoughts that enter your mind, the memories that surface, the songs that spontaneously pop into your head, the shapes, symbols, and images that emerge in your imaginal vision. All of these are subtle messages from the plant, unique ways its language is translating from your heart to your brain so you can understand its semantics. It requires a high degree of sensitivity to attune yourself to these subtleties. Otherwise, you'll miss them.

The form these communications take differs from plant to plant, person to person. It also depends on each person's primary sensory constitution, or your main "psychic function." There are three sensory constitutions: clairvoyance (clear seeing), clairaudience (clear hearing), and clairsentience (clear sensing). Thus, the meaning of a plant's communication can take visual, auditory, or tactile forms. Knowing how you learn from the invisible world is very helpful in understanding how messages are translated from the plant to your consciousness. To me, all three of these modes of receiving nonlinear communications are different facets of a *vision,* which is something far greater than mere fantasy, for vision comes from beyond the self. A vision involves intentionally exercising our imaginal faculty in a form of conscious dreaming, where seeing, feeling, and hearing blend together.

To the evolutionary herbalist, *every plant is a visionary plant,* not just those with psychoactive constituents like DMT, mescaline, or other compounds that alter perception by adjusting sensory gating channels. *Every* plant has a spirit; *every* plant generates visions. We only need to sensitize ourselves to them by internally generating a nonordinary state of consciousness. This is possible without putting anything into your body. Anyone can do it at will through the heart, which takes practice and habituation.

As people learn to communicate with plants, confusion commonly arises, and people ask: "How do I know I'm not just making it all up?" This is an important question, for people often sit with plants without really being present with them. They just sit within their own minds and mistake their own thoughts for "getting a download."

Whenever you question whether you've received something from the plant or if you just made it up, the essential question to ask is, "Was I authentically connected to the plant through my heart at that moment, or was I thinking?" If you answer this question honestly, you usually have a good idea of where the communication came from.

We must become highly cautious of confusing our interpretation of what we receive from a plant with what we internally generate within the mind. Remember, this form of communication is *beyond thinking.* It is a message administered through feeling that transforms into sensation, vision, and understanding that spontaneously emerges from beyond ourselves. Thinking is secondary; feeling is primary.

Awareness of the mind is critically important in this process. The mind will sneak up on you in a moment of carelessness; words will tempt you, pull you off track, and try to get your attention. When your connection with a plant evokes subtle feelings, sensations, and impressions, your mind will immediately want to bring them into the sphere of the intellect by labeling and classifying them. Although the brain is important in the interpretation of what the heart receives, *the heart is central.* The heart takes center stage in this process. As Henry David Thoreau put it, "Your mind must not perspire."[8]

After the momentary pause when you retract your heart field and give your brain a moment to interpret the meaning of the communication you've received from the plant, you reengage with the plant by expressing your heartfelt prayer to understand its medicine. Allow your felt sense of the plant to gradually fill the emptiness of your receptivity to its brim. As you reach the point of fullness, disengage again to allow your brain to interpret the meaning of what you've received. From there you reengage with the plant again. You repeat this process over and over again, each time taking it to deeper levels, each time encountering new layers of understanding transmitted to you from the plant. You are gradually building an experiential library of understanding that you have directly received from the plant.

This is precisely the same process all natural systems undergo in maintaining their self-organization. We are simply mirroring what Nature already does. However, because most of us are not habituated to this mode of perception and cognition—because it is in fact strongly discouraged in our culture—many find it difficult to maintain it. Heart perception and cognition is like an atrophied muscle; we must exercise it, *work it,* and nourish it so it can become strong again. Like any skill, it requires practice.

In addition to time and practice, this process requires your perceptions and insights into the plant to be refined, clarified, and tested for accuracy. You do this by holding within you both the initial felt sensation of the plant and the interpreted meaning you received from it. Then you blend them together within your heart, testing whether they are coherent with one another. You are essentially comparing the initial feeling received from the plant with the burst of understanding achieved through the teamwork of your heart and mind. As these two domains overlap within your heart, you pull your awareness back again and allow this testing to be routed up to the brain in the same way as before. This allows any inaccuracies or discrepancies between the plant and the interpreted

communications you've received to be weeded out of your understanding. This refinement and clarification of your understanding
take time, patience, and no small amount of focus. *We must make
sure that what we receive, and our interpretation of it, is indeed true to
the plant itself.*

Through this intimate communication, you form a deep bond
with the medicinal plants you work with, awakening an ancient
form of communication with the natural world that is the root of
herbalism. As you progressively connect to the deeper sentience
of the plant, gathering parts of the whole through sensations,
feelings, visions, and audible phrases, you ultimately come to an
edge—a moment where you feel as though you are standing on the
brink of a chasm. Your own consciousness and the consciousness
of the plant are but a millimeter away from one another. At this
threshold you may pass through the doorway from communication to communion, thus entering into the archetypal landscape
of the plant.

Conscious Dreaming in the Forest

Communication between you and the plant gives you pieces of a
puzzle. Each feeling, bodily sensation, memory, or insight that surfaces during entrainment is like one facet of a crystal, each one a
window into the plant's interiority; yet they are still fragments,
parts of its essence. It is our job to assemble these parts to see the
pattern of wholeness within the plant. With patience and persever-
ance, we can move beyond communication and into the depths of
communion by consciously dreaming in the forest.

Communion is a beautiful term. It's composed of two words:
common and *union*. Our commonality with a plant indicates a certain similarity between us, and when union enters the picture, the
division between our self and the plant dissolves. You see the plant
as a part of yourself. To enter a state of communion is to be in deep

intimacy with the world around you—to see into it and allow it to see into you.

This requires becoming vulnerable and receptive, opening ourselves in ways that our wounding resists with all its strength. As a result of our trauma, we pour a concrete shell around our hearts to protect ourselves from fear of future hurt. But over time the plants break through the shell, just as weeds grow in the cracks of the sidewalk. You must undefend yourself to let the plants in, till the soil of the soul of invasive conditionings to give them space to sprout and grow. You become so open, so receptive, that you let the plant weave itself into your innermost core.

Within this dreamy, trancelike process, as we enter deeper levels of heart perception and approach that millimeter distance from the plant's essence, we also enter deeper levels of synchronization. We are synchronized unto ourselves as our physiological and psychological being entrains with the heart's oscillations. Another layer of unification occurs as we entrain ourselves to the plant. And yet another occurs within our sensory perceptions as we enter synesthesia. There comes a point when the senses begin to cross-pollinate, blending together in a state of synesthetic perception. The feelings sensed in your heart anchor themselves in your body as sensations. Those physical sensations then take on an auditory quality of pulsations, dynamic rhythms, harmonic melodies, or bursts of meaningful phrases. These sounds, which were physical sensations, which were themselves feelings, then transform into colors, shapes, textures, or full-blown visions. As your senses become synergized into a singular perceptual whole, a quintessence of awareness, you are able to perceive the singular essence of the plant, which is its wholeness. Synesthetic perception is a hallmark sign that you are treading the delicate edge between communication and communion.

The wholeness of your being is infused with the consciousness of the plant, its intelligence interfacing with every dimension of your awareness—a 360-degree mode of perception. Each facet reveals the wholeness of the plant from a different perspective, yielding significantly richer layers of meaning as your sensory faculties are merged into a cohesive, nonlinear state of perception.

The final level of unification, beyond internal coherence, beyond synesthesia, beyond entrainment with the plant, is when you unify with its pure consciousness. At this point of opening, you step across the chasm and hollow yourself completely, becoming an emptiness that's filled by the plant. It enters, merges with your essence, and becomes a part of who you are, like two ice cubes melting into a pool. *Unio mystica.* As you and the plant become a single being, you have the capacity to know and understand every facet of it, including its medicinal properties, ecological functions, psychological and spiritual properties, and much more.

Buhner describes this unification beautifully:

> *It occurs after sensory focus, after feelings, after you have connected with the living reality of the plant, and after its wholeness bursts into awareness and you are at the pregnant point. In a sense, what you have inside you now is the living phenomenon itself, held in the multidimensional, imaginal field of your heart. That whole, meaning-imbued image you are now holding within you is a living reality.... You can, in this tiny instant of suspended time, view the living, meaning-filled image from multiple points of view, rotate it to see it from any perspective you wish.* [9]

When a plant stands before you, *within you,* revealed in this way, you understand the totality of its being, its wholeness disclosed to your holistic perception. Moving beyond knowledge of the plant, you cultivate wisdom by seeing its underlying pattern—not the *what* of the plant, but the *who* of the plant. Every individual thread of its characteristics is woven together into a tapestry of being that is stitched into your heart. From this place you understand the wholeness of the plant—how it relates to the wholeness of the person, as well as how it embodies the wholeness of life. You receive the vision of its unique reflection of the macrocosmic pattern, its connection to the energetic architecture of Nature. The spiritual seed of the plant is sown in your heart, and you carry the wholeness of its divine medicine, its living language, inside you. An inner forest begins to grow.

PART II

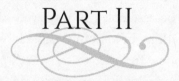

Energetic Architecture

*Man is a microcosm, or a little world, because he is an extract from
all the stars and planets of the whole firmament, from the earth and
the elements; and so he is their quintessence.*

—PARACELSUS[1]

Energetic architecture is the underlying blueprint or map of the
macrocosm, present within every living thing in the microcosm. It
is the core fractal pattern of Nature that exists at every scale of life,
from the smallest subatomic level up to the largest astronomical level
and at all points in between. This pattern informs the great herbal,
spiritual, and esoteric traditions of the world and is even reflected in
modern science (although most don't see it there). Energetic architecture allows you to perceive the invisible forces that influence all forms
and thus understand the relationships between substance, energy, and
consciousness. As a universal, natural language, energetic architecture
repatterns the mind with the intelligence the heart perceives as it connects to the Light of Nature. It is the pattern that binds and connects
the parts to the whole and forms the foundation of *natura sophia*.

Energetic architecture can be likened to the blueprint for a house. If you observe the room you are sitting in, you only see the surface level of the structure: walls, electrical outlets, lights, sinks, faucets, etc. But in order for these elements to serve their functions, they must be assembled in ways you can't see on the surface. There's something beyond the visible form that facilitates the underlying functions. In order to see what's *behind* the walls and understand how and why the house functions the way it does, you need to consult a blueprint. With a blueprint, you can see into the underlying pattern of the house: where the electrical lines, pipes, and studs are. A blueprint allows you to understand how and why the house has the forms and functions it provides, because it allows you to see what is invisible—what is hidden behind the surfaces.

This is what energetic architecture does for your understanding of herbalism, but instead of peering behind the walls of a house, you see into the invisible structure of a plant and a person, as well as the foundation of herbal traditions. You see the formative powers that give rise to a plant's unique form and function. You perceive a person's unique composition of the forces of life, its specific embodiment of the macrocosmic pattern, revealing how each part contains the whole.

With regard to medicinal plants, energetic architecture moves you beyond studying the mere surfaces of the plant, such as botanical characteristics, chemistry, or even clinical properties. By perceiving the energetic architecture of a plant, you see the binding forces that unite all of its properties, and you understand how each quality and characteristic is interrelated in a greater pattern of wholeness.

This blueprint, this pattern of energetic architecture, is the map that guides you in your explorations of the invisible landscape of plants and the archetypal forces that operate through them. It's a translation mechanism, a natural language that encompasses the wholeness of plants, showing how their physical attributes, chemistry, and medicinal properties are related to their psychological, emotional, and evolutionary properties. Energetic architecture also allows you to see the relationships between physiological imbalances in organ systems and their underlying psychological and emotional dynamics, as well as the lessons the soul needs to integrate to advance its evolution. This model ultimately equips you with the knowledge of how to apply medicinal plants in a transformational context that facilitates the evolution of the soul. This holistic framework shows how the wholenesses of both people and plants are, in their essence, embodiments of the wholeness of Creation.

4

The Cosmology of Nature

*The material universe is an insoluble riddle to the materialist
because he insists on trying to explain it in terms of its own plane.
This is a thing that can never be done at any sphere of thought.
Nothing can ever be explained in terms of itself, but only by being
resumed in a greater whole.*

—DION FORTUNE[1]

Many modern herbalists experience a nebulous feeling that something essential is missing from our approach to herbalism. They feel a vague sense that we're overlooking something vitally important for us to use plants to their fullest capacity. I believe this is due to Western herbalism lacking a spiritual backbone, a metaphysical structure behind it that relates people, plants, and healing to the greater order of life. There's an absence of cosmology.

Many texts on Western herbalism begin by talking about herbal actions, chemical constituents, physiology, or the symptoms and conditions plants are used for. Yet when we study texts from the East, the first few chapters often begin with a big-picture discussion of Nature as a whole and its spiritual context. They describe the formative patterns of creation, situating people and plants within a cosmological framework and the wholeness of life. The foundations for these systems of medicine are rooted in a metaphysical understanding of the world, weaving together the spiritual and practical aspects of plants and human health.

The Western esoteric tradition of Hermeticism, and specifically the alchemical lineage, holds keys to unlock the Western cosmology that once stood behind our medical and herbal traditions. In fact, what we know of the Western mystery teachings about the cosmology of Nature accords very closely to what is said elsewhere. East or West, North or South, those who followed the Light of Nature saw the exact same patterns within natural phenomena, the same energetic architecture of life.

To understand the energetic architecture of herbalism, we must go back to the primal themes of creation. In attempting to explain where life, spirit, matter, and humanity come from, traditional cosmologies provide a holistic context for the study of Nature and the practice of medicine. In order to perceive the wholeness of a plant or of a person, we must start from the whole, and cosmology—which is based on the grand themes of life—is therefore intrinsic to the holistic perspective. The patterns we observe in cosmological systems correspond directly to the foundational principles of many traditions of energetic medicine, such as the concepts of yin and yang, the Three Alchemical Substances, the Five Elements, and the Seven Planets.

The Doctrine of Emanations

"In the beginning God created the heaven and the earth. And the earth was without form, and void; and darkness was upon the face of the deep."[2]

All of existence emanated from a single source. Before time or space, there was a creative void, a nothingness that contained the potential of all things. This singularity existed before all of existence. It is beyond duality and intellectual comprehension. It is formless, yet it contains all forms; empty, yet full; everything, and yet nothing. It is the One and only One.

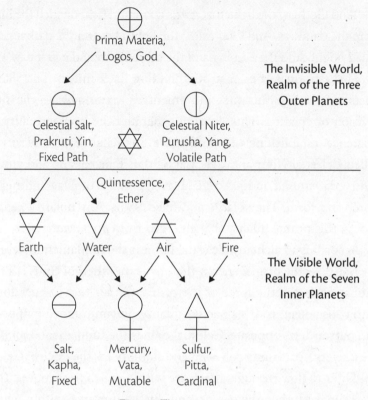

Figure 1. The ten emanations

This transcendent force has been known by many names throughout time: God, Allah, the Creator, the Great Spirit, and countless other names for the One that cannot truly be named. Whatever word we choose, this is the essence of life and the Source of all creation. It is the unknowable mystery.

In alchemy, this source is referred to as the *prima materia* or the "first matter." Paracelsus called it the *Yliaster*.[3] If you were to imagine every single thing in the entirety of the universe—all past, present, and future, everything that was, is, and could be, condensed into a single point that exists outside of time and space—that is the *prima materia*. This is impossible to comprehend, of course, which is why it is referred to as chaos.

"And God saw the light, that it was good: and God divided the light from the darkness. And God called the light Day, and the darkness he called Night. And the evening and the morning were the first day."[4]

This emptiness began to stir, dividing itself in two. The alchemists referred to this first movement as *prima mobile*—the first division of creation. This division generated the primal duality of existence, establishing time and space. In alchemy, this polarity is called Celestial Niter and Celestial Salt; in Taoism yang and yin; in Ayurveda *purusha* and *prakruti*. Heaven and Earth. Day and night. Force and form. The volatile and fixed Paths. Any polarity has its root in this primal duality that emerged from *prima materia*.

According to alchemy, Celestial Niter is the fundamental *force* of the universe, the primal energy that turns the wheel of time. It's the animating factor, the force of the primal Father that imbues form with consciousness. It's an active quality, dynamic, moving upward and outward. Its opposite, Celestial Salt, is the fundamental *form* of the universe, providing cohesion and stability for the force of Celestial Niter to flow through; the space within which time moves. It is the primal Mother, the great womb of the universe, within which the seed of Celestial Niter is planted. It's a passive quality, receptive, downward and inward in its movement, magnetic in its property. The interactions between force and form generate life, which contains these inherent qualities, as do all things that exist within time and space. The dynamic equilibrium of the world rests upon the axis of Celestial Niter and Celestial Salt.

These two principles underwent their own division to generate four fundamental forces universally recognized in every culture and tradition around the world: the Four Elements.

Celestial Niter divided into the two volatile Elements, Fire and Air, seen in the way Fire burns up and out, constantly moving, emanating light and heat, and sending smoke into the atmosphere. We see the volatility of Air as it moves with a dynamic yet invisible quality, the way everything breathes the invisible life-giving force.

Celestial Salt divided into the fixed Elements, Earth and Water. Just as yin moves down and in, so too does Water fall from the sky, flow downstream, moisten, and cool. Earth provides the structure and boundaries necessary for the material realm to exist. The Four Elements born from the division of Celestial Niter and Celestial Salt generate a new organizational level of creation, as the vital spirit gradually condenses into physical form.

As we have seen, life generates itself through a process of self-organization, with everything in a constant process of interaction and relationship, and the Elements are not exempt from this natural law. Each of the Elements came together in particular patterns to generate a new level of organization. According to alchemy, Fire and Air recombined to form what is called Sulfur, Air and Water merge to form what is called Mercury, and Earth and Water synergize to form what is called Salt. These primal substances are referred to as the Three Philosophical Principles, or *tria prima*. In Ayurveda, they are called the three *doshas*†. All things in creation—mineral, vegetable, animal, and human—are made of the Four Elements and the Three Principles.

While Paracelsus used chemical terminology here, it's important to remember that the chemicals are physical expressions of greater archetypal forces, their most basic definition being the Soul, Spirit, and Body of something. There are multiple triune patterns in various traditions around the world, and most have their place within this scheme, which we will explore in the coming chapters. This is the primal trinity of life and thus forms the three-dimensional reality where we reside. When we reach the level of the Three Principles, we have materialized in this physical world.

Each layer of energetic architecture, from Source to duality to the Elements and the Principles, represents a gradual descent from

---

† Although the three *doshas* of Ayurveda have slightly different Elemental configurations, when we study their primal characteristics and properties, we see they are synonymous to the Three Principles of alchemy. These correspondences will be further delineated in chapter 6, "The Three Principles."

the invisible, spiritual world down into the visible, material world. They are the specific steps the vital force takes in the process of creation. Yet as we stand upon the Earth and look up, we see another layer of architecture in the cosmos, represented by the Planets.

Whereas the Four Elements correspond to the four directions, the Three Principles correspond to above, below, and middle, forming the horizontal and vertical axes of the world. In Native American cosmology, these seven directions form all that we know in the world. In the same way, the Three Principles and the Four Elements add up to seven powers, represented in prescientific Western cosmology by the seven Planets: Sun, Moon, Mars, Venus, Jupiter, Saturn, and Mercury. These are the "ancient planets" that existed before the invention of the telescope.

Each Element and Principle corresponds to one of these seven planetary bodies, thus representing the visible dimensions of the world. On the other hand, Celestial Niter, Celestial Salt, and the *prima materia* correspond to the three outer Planets of Uranus, Neptune, and Pluto, respectively, representing the invisible world. Between the Elements and the celestial realm of duality, there exists a boundary between the seen and the unseen, which can only be accessed through the Quintessence. Astrologically this can be correlated to the asteroid Chiron, which moves between the unseen world of the outer Planets and the seen world of the inner Planets.

While the Three Principles each formed through the merging of two Elements, the fifth Element formed as Earth, Water, Air, and Fire came into perfect balance, fusing into something greater than the sum of the parts. This is known in the East as Ether, Wood, or Wind; in the West, it is called the Quintessence. This fifth Element is the balance point, the center of the above, the below, and the four directions. It is thus capable of connecting all levels, elements, and emanations. For this reason, it is the access point between the invisible and visible domains of existence.

Thus we can see the primary patterns of energetic architecture: the Three Principles, the Five Elements, and the Seven Planets. This map reveals the underlying order and structure of the macrocosm, and it is also the blueprint of the microcosm, because each force is present within every living thing. Nothing can exist if it doesn't contain each facet of this cosmological pattern, though everything embodies each force in varying ratios and degrees, which determines its constitution and temperament.

The pattern of this cosmological framework is present in a majority of cultures and traditions across the world, represented within their spiritual traditions, medical systems, mythologies, traditional stories, pantheons, and philosophies. When studying herbal medicine, it's quite common to come across these patterns repeatedly in traditions from every point of the globe because they are *universal life principles* revealed to those who perceived the Light of Nature.

The Doctrine of Correspondences

Perceiving the Light of Nature through the heart reveals the underlying order of energetic architecture as it expresses through the natural world. Because the heart functions on the principle of entrainment and the perception of unity, it sees how each facet of Nature is in relationship with the pattern of energetic architecture. You can see how Earth, Water, Air, and Fire are embodied within a particular plant, how the unique constellation of the Planets is imprinted within a person's form and psyche. Heart perception opens a holistic mode of perception that allows you to become aware of how each part *corresponds* to the pattern of the whole.

This is summarized in the Hermetic doctrine of correspondences. This principle states that all expressions of life are interrelated with one another and that nothing exists in isolation. Instead, everything resides within a vast web of relationships. The unique form and function of any particular being can be understood in its totality by seeing these layers of relationship, as each part is subsumed within the greater whole, which grasps its essence. Matthew Wood eloquently notes that "every created thing has an archetype from which its outward manifestation springs. The creation as a whole is in correspondence with the primordial archetype which stands behind the universe."[5]

The doctrine of correspondence is congruent with what modern science has discovered about the self-organization and nonlinearity of Nature. Each organism is formed by various subparts entering spontaneous synchronization, in which they self-organize and exhibit new and distinct behaviors not shown by any of the subparts. The stability of the new system is further anchored as it interacts with its environment: being thrown slightly off balance requires the organism to craft new responses and behaviors to maintain equilibrium. Everything exists on the border between self-organization and collapse (i.e., chaos and disintegration). The nature of every being is formed based on dynamic interactions and responses to the environment within which it is embedded. Ecosystems are a prime example of this vast web of relationships and correspondences. As Luther Burbank succinctly stated, "Heredity is nothing but stored environment."[6]

The doctrine of correspondences shows that each and every being is in dynamic connection not only with its immediate environment but with *everything in creation,* expressed through the pattern of the macrocosm. Through acute perception, we can see patterns of relationship and spectrums of similarity between the part and the whole. The pattern of energetic architecture, as demonstrated through the doctrine of emanations, reveals the essential archetypal forces imbued into all life forms, and everything corresponds to various layers of architecture. These relationships between the part and the whole are based on a state of resonance that exists between them. To use an older term, they are *sympathetic* with one another;

hence it is the heart that perceives these patterns. In this way we are able to see chains of correspondence, or patterns of relationship, throughout the natural world.

An example of a chain of correspondence would be: the summer season, flames, the Sun, a lion, the heart and cardiovascular system, carnelian, willpower, St. John's Wort. Among each of these aspects of Nature there is a certain similarity: they are all in a state of entrainment with the specific frequency of the Fire Element. A good way to think of it is that each force of energetic architecture emanates certain qualities encoded within a particular frequency. As that force emanates its frequency, specific expressions of Nature will fall under its influence and express its qualities more prominently. Through this vibrational resonance, each facet of the natural world has primary correspondences with the various archetypes of energetic architecture.

It's a lot like the color spectrum or notes on a musical scale. We can look at one of the primary colors, say yellow, and then look at the Sun and agree that it is yellow. But we can also look at St. John's Wort flowers and say they are yellow, and that a shaft of wheat is yellow, and that mustard is yellow. There is a vast spectrum of colors we might refer to as "yellow." Each shade could be thought of as having its own individual frequency, its unique expression within the larger dominion of the greater frequency of "yellow." In the same way, there is a vast spectrum of how the Fire Element, the Moon, or any aspect of energetic architecture will manifest within Nature. And just as the different spectrums of color convey different meanings, so too do different natural beings express different layers of meaning of an archetypal force.

In the sphere of plants, we can observe two very different medicines that contain the same overall energetic correspondence—for instance, Nettles *(Urtica dioica)* and Echinacea *(Echinacea angustifolia)*. Both of these plants embody qualities that correspond to the planet Mars, such as their intense and sharp morphological characteristics, actions upon the blood, inflammatory processes, and immunity. Yet at the same time they are incredibly distinct medicinal agents. Both embody the celestial force of Mars in different ways, and thus they bring about that energetic quality differently.

Another example of correspondence is Marshmallow root *(Althea officinalis)* and the Water Element. The roots are used to hydrate the mucosal membranes of the lungs, urinary tract, and digestive system because they soothe, cool, and moisten dried, irritated tissues with a deficiency of water. In esoteric physiology the mucosa are ruled by the Water Element. Marshmallow roots are incredibly moist, and the active constituents (mucilaginous polysaccharides) can only be extracted in water. We can see through these simple observations that Marshmallow embodies the archetype of the Water Element more strongly than any other Element; thus, Water is Marshmallow's strongest Elemental correspondence.

The process of determining correspondences between a plant and the energetic architecture of Nature is the foundation of the practice of herbal alchemy, or spagyrics, a system of spiritual pharmacy that extracts the chemical, energetic, and spiritual properties of a plant as represented by its unique energetic architecture. These forces are directly concentrated within alchemically prepared medicines, enabling them to act upon the corresponding patterns within our organ systems, psychology, and soul. Because the medicines embody and act upon these archetypal patterns, they trigger an evolutionary healing process. From this perspective, the plants are seen as channels that connect the microcosm of our being to macrocosmic forces. Thus, it is important to perceive these correspondences not only within plants but within people as well, giving us a single universal language that unites both to the wholeness of life.

Evolutionary herbalism is rooted in this process of seeing correspondences between people, plants, and energetic architecture. To do this we must observe with a distinct acuity of perception, attuning ourselves to see these patterns of relationship and decipher their unique language. This language is not composed of words but of richly symbolic *signatures*.

The Doctrine of Signatures

Everything in the natural world has its own unique signature, just as you sign your name in a way that's distinct to you. The word *signature* is a combination of two words, *sign* and *nature;* thus, the signature of something can be thought of as the signs of nature directly imprinted upon it. It's commonly defined as a distinctive pattern, product, or characteristic by which someone or something can be identified. Signatures are the living language through which we read the energetic architecture of life as it is inscribed within matter, and they communicate a being's particular function and character.

Paracelsus states:

> *This signatum (or signature) is a certain organic vital activity, giving to each natural object (in contradistinction to artificially made objects) a certain similarity with a certain condition produced by disease, and through which health may be restored in specific diseases in the diseased part. This signatum is often expressed even in the exterior form of things, and by observing that form we may learn something in regard to their interior qualities, even without using our interior sight. We see that the internal character of a man is often expressed in his exterior appearance, even in the manner of his walking and in the sound of his voice. Likewise the hidden character of things is to a certain extent expressed in their outward forms.* [7]

A signature is what connects the inner and outer nature of something and reveals its connection to the macrocosm, enabling us to see its energetic architecture. Signatures, in their essence, are patterns perceived by the heart. As humanity has strayed away from the perceptual heart, we have lost touch with this innate capacity to see patterns of wholeness through intuition. Paracelsus continues, "As long as man remained in a natural state, he recognized the signatures of things and knew their true character; but the more he diverged from the path of Nature, and the more his mind became captivated by illusive external appearances the more this power became lost."[8]

The doctrine of signatures explains the particular way we perceive the pattern of energetic architecture within a plant, revealing how its functions are intricately interwoven into its form. Indeed, form and function are merely two sides of the same leaf and are directly influenced by the forces of life that correspond to it. Signatures reveal correspondences, and correspondences reveal the emanations within life. The doctrine of signatures shows us how the macrocosm and microcosm—the above and below—are intimately connected. This is what Paracelsus referred to as *anatomia,* whereby the invisible forces of life can be seen imprinted within visible forms. An excellent and beautiful book that goes into detail on patterns of signatures is *The Language of Plants: A Guide to the Doctrine of Signatures* by Julia Graves.[9]

Modern herbalism commonly defines the doctrine of signatures as the way in which a plant's morphological characteristics (its overall shape, texture, color, and other physical qualities) or its habitat will somehow reflect the particular organ system, tissue, or disease for which the plant is remedial. For instance, Eyebright *(Euphrasia officinalis)* flowers look like eyes and are therefore good for treating the eyes; Greater Celandine *(Chelidonium majus)* exudes a bitter yellow sap that resembles bile and is therefore a liver/gallbladder remedy; a Walnut *(Juglans regia)* looks like a brain and is therefore good for brain health. Each of these remedies is indeed beneficial for the parts of the body that their signatures point toward. This is about as deep as many herbalists go with regard to the doctrine of signatures, but this is merely its most superficial aspect.

The problem with this perspective is that it's a primarily anthropocentric approach. It observes plants and asks, "How are you reflecting me?" as if plants were only concerned with people.

According to esoteric traditions, plants are not only reflective of people but are microcosms of the greater forces of Nature. For this reason, the doctrine of signatures reveals a great deal more about a plant than simply what organ systems and diseases it treats.

This is a critically important point, because there are many plants whose morphology does not necessarily look like the parts of the body they treat. For example, Nettle leaf is commonly used to treat the blood, the urinary tract, and the liver. But Nettles don't exactly look like any of these parts of the body. Therefore, with the old perspective on the doctrine of signatures, we may conclude that Nettle does not appear to contain any particular signatures that point to its affinities and properties (although we do see a kidney signature in that it grows near water; I have yet to find distinct human-based signatures that point toward Nettle's strong affinity for the blood). But when we broaden our definition of signatures beyond humans and look at the patterns of energetic architecture, we see a deeper level of communication and connection.

The form of Nettle is particularly sharp and prickly, with small formic acid crystals that look like little needles covering the entire plant. The margins of the leaves are sharply serrated, and upon touching the skin they immediately give a sharp sting and provoke an inflammatory process. With just this small amount of information, we can see that all of these morphological characteristics are signatures for the planet Mars. The red planet is commonly associated with intensity, sharpness, redness, the blood, heat, and inflammation, all of which we can immediately experience with nettles rather quickly. Nettle has a unique embodiment of the warrior spirit of Mars, and these signatures point to its medicinal properties and virtue. On a deeper level, we also see that the seeds of Nettle have an affinity for the adrenal glands and that the roots operate upon the male prostate gland, two organs classically ruled by Mars. Its leaf distinctly modulates inflammation, cleanses and builds the blood, and contains high amounts of iron, all of which also correspond to

Mars. Thus the "star signatures" within the form of Nettles reveal many of its physiological functions.

When we tap into our ability to perceive signatures, we see that the botanical kingdom is composed of a language of symbols. The esoteric writer Dion Fortune states, "What words are to thought, symbols are to intuition."[10] Because symbols are the words that speak directly to the intuition, they are not simply figured out or rationally deduced; they can only be perceived through the intuitive heart, which perceives unity. And yet the true accuracy of a signature shines when it is in alignment with the intellect, when function and form connect in a way that actually makes logical sense.

Because the composition of a plant is a language, we must learn to trace the outlines of its morphology with our heart field, to breathe in its color and allow it to move us and touch the deepest parts of the self, so we can see that the living texture of the plant is a communication. William Gass put it succinctly when he said, "We inhabit a forest of symbols."[11] The heart is the perceptual mode that enables us to see the patterns of relationship between the inner function and outer form of the plant, connected to the human organism and the macrocosm as a whole. I like to think of symbols as the universal language that function as a bridge that connects the invisible and visible worlds.

Just as we can cultivate the awareness to see signatures of the Elements, Principles, and Planets within plants, we can also see them within people. We can do this by observing everything about a person: the shape of the body, posture, skin color, organ system imbalances, disease predispositions, tone of the voice, psychological dynamics—everything about a person, just like a plant, is a language. Jacob Boehme explains:

And now observe, as it stands in the power and predominance of the quality, so it is signed and marked externally in its outward form, signature, or figure; man in his speech, will, and behavior, also with the form of the

members which he has, and must use to that signature, his inward form
is noted in the form of his face; and thus also is a beast, an herb, and the
trees; everything as it is inwardly (in its innate virtue and quality) so it is
outwardly signed.[12]

Everything is stamped with particular signatures that indicate the primary energetic forces that influence it physically, energetically, and spiritually; we only need to learn to decipher them.

Perceiving signatures and correspondences for ourselves is central in the development of the evolutionary herbalist, because they reveal to us how the macrocosm is imprinted within people and plants. For the alchemist, these correspondences determine how that plant will be used within the context of spagyric pharmacy. For the clinician, correspondences determine the course of their therapeutic strategies. Unfortunately, it's all too common for people to look up Planetary or Elemental correspondences in a book. Not only are many of these correlations inaccurate, but they don't explain the reasoning behind them. In addition, many plants aren't even on those lists. If our goal is to deepen our understanding of Nature internally and externally, we must learn to perceive signatures and correspondences for ourselves, making the Light of Nature our primary reference material, not books.

It reminds me of the age-old adage that if you give a man a fish he eats for a day, but if you teach him how to fish he feeds his family for life. That's why this text doesn't provide lists of plant correspondences. Instead, it reveals the fundamental signatures that point toward a plant's relationship to each facet of energetic architecture. I'd rather teach you how to fish. That way you don't just memorize correspondences and signatures; you learn them by heart.

A correspondence between a plant and a force of energetic architecture must be established by considering the wholeness of a plant, as opposed to a single quality, such as a yellow flower corresponding to the Sun. *Every aspect of the plant must be considered.* Generally speaking, we can observe seven primary qualities that contain signatures that point toward correspondences:

1. Habitat

2. Morphology

3. Taste

4. Affinities to organ systems

5. Medicinal actions

6. Energetics

7. Unique properties or spiritual qualities

As you'll note, some of these involve observing the plant on its own in Nature, while others relate to its properties within the human organism. I highly recommend *The Language of Plants* by Julia Graves and Matthew Wood's essay "The Doctrine of Signatures" for more details.[13]

Part III of this work will explore the physical, energetic, and spiritual signatures and correspondences of plants and people through the lens of the Seven Planets, Five Elements, and Three Principles, drawing upon a variety of traditional perspectives to further clarify these qualities and characteristics.

The Doctrine of Sympathetic Medicine

The doctrines of emanations, correspondences, and signatures are ultimately brought together in the doctrine of sympathetic medicine. All derive from alchemical theory and the work of Paracelsus (especially his major source, *Hermetic Writings*), yet these themes are, of course, universal. The principle of sympathetic medicine was further developed and refined by Samuel Hahnemann in his "law of similars," the core guiding principle of homeopathy, which denied any connection or reference to Paracelsian medicine.

In the practice of traditional and natural medicine there are two primary approaches. The first is "antipathetic" medicine, which is how a majority of traditions practiced for a very long time, such as Ayurveda, Chinese medicine, the Greeks, and the Arabs. This approach uses medicines that have an opposite quality to the symptom or disease, to guide the body back to balance. Thus we use heat to treat cold, damp to treat dry, relaxants to treat tension, etc. Antipathetic medicine is, at its root, rational and makes logical sense. Paracelsus, who was one of the first to adopt a sympathetic model of medicine, strongly rejected treatment by antipathy, claiming it was quite simply false and against Nature in the way it suppresses the intelligence of the vital force.

Sympathetic medicine takes a quite different approach. Here we use a remedy that is similar to the disease, symptom, or afflicted part of the body. The plant either looks like the part of the body or disease (doctrine of signatures) or causes the symptoms (the homeopathic model). On a deeper level, sympathetic medicine is based on understanding the essence of a plant and how it matches the essence of a disease, afflicted organ system, or constitution of the person. The sympathetic doctor sees patterns of relationship within the essences of people and medicines, and uses resonant forces to achieve balance. These essences, according to Paracelsus, were best reflected in the qualities of the Seven Planets.

In its most ancient form, the concept of sympathetic medicine was taken quite literally, based on signatures. So if you had a problem with your liver, you eat liver; if there's a problem with your left eye, then the left eye of a certain beast will be your medicine. Many of these approaches to sympathetic medicine are commonly regarded as superstitious, though I am hesitant to judge them as such, because I believe traditional medicine practitioners understood things in ways that we do not today. Paracelsus, on the other hand, didn't agree with this literal interpretation of similars. He wanted the similar to be *like*—but not *identical*—to the disease process. Hahnemann followed the same principle.

Paracelsus's perspective on medicine was deeply rooted in cosmology and the inherent correspondence between microcosm and macrocosm. He saw a certain three-way connection between person, plant (or metal/mineral), and planet, all of which were seen in sympathetic correspondence to one another. Thus, when a person displays symptoms of heat, irritation, inflammation, and sharp, burning pain, the disease is best treated through sympathy by a medicine corresponding to Mars, which governs these pathological patterns. In his model, every Planet is said to cure its own disease.

Whereas antipathetic medicine is rational, appealing to the spectrum of duality (e.g., hot/cold, wet/dry), sympathetic medicine is paradoxical—even transcendental—rising above the linearity of cause and effect. This is why I consider a sympathetic approach to touch closer to the level of the soul, which is beyond duality, whereas antipathetic medicine focuses more directly on the body.

Matthew Wood comments on sympathetic and antipathetic medicine in the writings of Nicholas Culpeper, the great astrological herbalist:

> Culpeper noted that using the "physical" properties of a plant—hot to cold—did not get to the core of the problem, but only palliated. He warned, in fact, that such cures based on "antipathy" (opposition) would weaken the system by working against it in a forceful manner. On the other hand, the "hidden" properties of the plant would radically cure. They acted in a "sympathetic" manner (by similarity). The essence of the problem would be addressed by the essence of the plant.[14]

Paracelsus, Culpeper, and Hahnemann all oppose the use of antipathetic or contrary therapy. As we will see, however, this method is also related to the essence, though by opposition. Therefore, antipathetic medicine can also touch the essence as long as it is used in a gentle, supportive way, not forcing the organism into submission.

If we think of using Mars plants to treat a Mars condition, the rational mind gets confused. When I teach this concept, people always ask, "If you have an excess of Mars and take a Mars plant, won't it excessively build Mars in the system?" Each planet cures its own disease by adjusting the flow of the vital force through the astral body, working in an amphoteric manner—meaning that it can lower excesses and strengthen deficiencies. It must be understood that alchemically prepared medicines function quite differently from standard herbal preparations because they embody the essence of the plant *and* of the planet it relates to, thus operating upon the essence of the person. In this way, alchemical medicines teach the archetypal force within the person how to express in a healthier way, as the medicine establishes a sympathetic connection to the corresponding archetypal force in the macrocosm and helps it evolve into its most virtuous manifestation.

According to this perspective, the sympathy between say, an organ system, a planet, and a plant, is based on coherence, or what is classically called "sympathetic resonance." Different facets of Nature possess a similar vibrational resonance to one another, and they *correspond* through that resonance. Indeed, the entire process discussed in chapters 2 and 3 with regard to the heart is a perfect example of sympathetic resonance, whereby we come into a place of entrainment with the electromagnetic field of a plant. It is interesting to note that this can only be achieved by using the heart as an organ of perception. I love that the old doctors used the term "sympathy" to describe these relational connections, showing an underlying cardiac connection. After all, when we are sympathizing with a friend having a difficult time, are we not approaching them directly from our hearts?

Samuel Hahnemann's law of similars is basically identical to Paracelsian doctrine, with the emphasis placed on the action of the substance (causing symptoms, then curing them in a smaller dosage) rather than the doctrine of signatures and macrocosmic correspondences. Hahnemann's law was founded upon the principle that poisons or agents cause symptoms that the body then responds to by self-generated healing. This is a fact admitted in modern pharmacology, which calls the response the "rebound effect."

In addition, Hahnemann discovered that small and large doses can have opposite reactions. This principle is called *hormesis* in modern pharmacology, though it is presented as a principle that *sometimes* occurs, rather than as a universal law, as Hahnemann taught. In his model, everything has both a medicinal and a poisonous effect. The difference rests in dosage, which was also a notably Paracelsian concept. When you take a medicine in large, toxic dosages, it will generate the symptoms that it remedies in smaller dosages. The toxic reaction of the organism is called the primary response; in homeopathy, the self-healing reaction against this (the rebound) is called the secondary response. The primary reaction is overstimulating and toxic (the substance working directly on the body) while the secondary response is counteractive or the body reacting against the remedy. Similar to the Paracelsian concept that every planet cures its own disease, Hahnemann found that every medicine cures its own disease. In this perspective, each medicinal plant has both a therapeutic expression and a disease expression. In short, the practice of homeopathy is based upon using remedies at very small doses for constellations of symptoms that they generate in very large doses, forming an axis of medicinal influence based on sympathy.

Another axis useful for studying medicinal plants (as well as people) is distinguishing short-term effects from long-term effects. For example, bitter plants may increase secretions in the digestive system with a short-term moistening effect, but as these fluids leave the body over the long term the effect can be excessively drying. Another axis present within people is acute versus chronic symptoms, or local versus constitutional imbalances, which commonly have different therapeutic approaches.

Another polarity looks at the difference between the local and systemic actions of a plant, showing how they can be seemingly paradoxical. This was brought to my attention by Michigan herbalist jim mcdonald in a class on astringents. He notes how astringents are often considered drying, as they dry the mouth and fluid secretions. However, consider someone with relaxed kidneys who urinates too frequently or whose sweat pores are stuck open, leading to excessive sweating. These fluids leaving the body will ultimately lead to dryness, a result of overly relaxed tissues, which is our primary indication for using astringents. By tightening up the kidneys and pores to reduce sweating and urination, an astringent can conserve fluids. So we can think of astringents as *locally* drying and potentially *systemically* moistening. The primary effect is drying but the secondary effect is moistening. This spectrum is important to consider when studying medicinal plants.

I mention these polarities because they represent the opposite (and legitimate) kinds of influence an herbal medicine can have, and they often indicate both sympathetic and antipathetic correspondences. In Nettle's relationship to Mars, we can see both sympathetic and antipathetic signatures. The needles, serrated leaf margins, and sharp sting of a Nettle leaf are all sympathetic to the red planet, as are its affinity for the blood, prostate, and adrenals; whereas its cooling, anti-inflammatory property is distinctly antipathetic to Mars.

We can also see the spectrum of sympathy and antipathy in the habitats of plants. Aloe *(Aloe vera)* grows in hot and dry landscapes, yet it produces a soothing, cooling, moistening gel that treats a hot, dry landscape in the body. In this way, the plant embodies an antidote to the environment outside of itself and inside us and is thus antipathetic. Nettles and Horsetail *(Equisetum arvense)* are often found growing near waterways, and they just happen to operate upon the inner waterways of the body through the kidneys and urinary tract, showing a sympathetic signature. Where the plant grows in Nature often reflects the aspect of the body for which it is remedial, which would be a sympathetic quality. Herbs work both ways: counteracting the environment or adapting to it.

From a therapeutic standpoint, we can use sympathetic and antipathetic qualities at the same time, because they do not necessarily have to be opposing models of medicine. For example, when treating the lungs, we obviously want to use a remedy that is sympathetic to this organ system. And yet, if there is excess moisture we do not want a plant sympathetic to moisture; instead, we want an opposite that will return the tissue back to balance. Thus, the principles of sympathy and antipathy can be used together harmoniously.

In the alchemical model, sympathetic medicine focuses on the archetypal level. When working with a person, we observe the archetypal essence of the organ system, tissue, or disease by seeing the signatures and correspondences to the forces of the macrocosm—the Planetary, Elemental, or Principle essence of the disease. We then select a remedy that is sympathetic to these macrocosmic forces, prepare it according to the principles of spagyric alchemy (which concentrates these forces), and administer it to the person. The medicine will then act sympathetically upon the corresponding forces within the microcosm of the person, through the astral and physical bodies, and bringing the archetypal pattern back into balance, whether it was in excess or deficiency.

The doctrines of emanations, correspondences, signatures, and sympathetic medicine form a cosmological understanding of the world, reinforcing a pattern of intuitive thinking that represents what the heart perceives. They are the basis of the *natura sophia* tradition. These principles give us a metaphysical backbone that connects our model of herbalism to the larger forces of the universe present within all life. This is central to an alchemical model that always seeks to connect the microcosm with the macrocosm and see the whole within the part. It also provides a way of understanding how traditional people came into direct relationship with these fundamental forces of Nature and saw their reflections in the patterns of people and plants. Matthew Wood says:

> *These primal classification schemes relate to basic functions within the body-psyche continuum, and are therefore important in bringing about healing, although they are not used in conventional medical practice. Such symbols strike us at a deep level as intuitively real, though they may not be real in a strictly materialistic or rational sense. That is not their prime function. They are a part of the mythopoetic universe which is essential to our wholeness.* [15]

The following chapters will briefly introduce the primary layers of energetic architecture—the Five Elements, Three Principles, and Seven Planets—revealing different ways they are expressed throughout herbal traditions. In part III, the specific signatures and correspondences of these patterns will be explored within the holistic person and the holistic plant in significant detail. When we see the macrocosm within people and plants, we hold a key that enables us to magnify these archetypal forces within the medicines we prepare and trigger a process of transformational healing.

The Five Elements

The elements in nature concretely represent a subtler and more fundamental discrimination of five aspects of the primordial energy of existence. There is nothing in any dimension that is not composed wholly of the interactions of these five aspects of energy. The elemental processes create the universe, sustain it, and ultimately destroy it. This is also true for individual beings: at birth the play of the elements creates the body, mind, and personality. At death these dissolve as the elements collapse into one another. And during the whole life, the individual's relationship to the elements determines the quality of experience.

—TENZIN WANGYAL RINPOCHE[1]

The Elements—Earth, Water, Air, Fire, and Ether—are at the very foundations of life. They represent the energetic forces that exist behind all forms, the primal clays shaping creation. The Elements were the foundation of many cultural, medical, and spiritual traditions of medicine from all over the world. Indeed, it is likely one of the most universally accepted models that encompasses a holistic understanding of Nature.

When speaking of the Elements I'm not referring to the water you drink or the fire in your fireplace; these are merely physical reflections of greater archetypal powers pervading all life. The Elemental forces are *intelligent spiritual beings*. Just as we can commune with plants, so too we can commune with the Elemental beings.

The Elements were formed through the mitosis of the polarity of creation, the splitting of Celestial Salt and Celestial Niter. As primal force and form were generated through the first movements of Creation, the Ether Element was established as the space within which all manifestation takes place. These first movements blew the first wind that generated friction, creating a spark that ignited the Fire Element—the Light of Creation.

As this light shined throughout space, it was contained and held, and light and darkness divided, and the Air Element was generated through its movements—the Movement of Creation. As heat radiated from the primal Fire held within the Air, there was a coolness in the distance that gradually congealed into a liquid, poured downward and pooled, generating the Water Element—the Womb of Creation.

As this Water continued to cool, it solidified to form matter, the physical receptacle for the other Elements to manifest, and generated the Earth Element—the Land of Creation. Earth contains Water, Air, Fire, and Ether, uniting them to generate the world as we know it, implanting themselves within everything. This is the alchemical understanding of the cosmology of the Elements.

Below is a general description of each Element, though for the practical purposes of herbalists, we will go into significantly more depth to outline their relationship to people and plants on the physical, energetic, and spiritual levels in part III. We will also consider some of the ways in which the Elements are reflected throughout different traditional models to show their universality.

▽ The Earth Element

The Earth Element is the most material Element, representing the stability, cohesion, and form of the physical world. It is generated by the merging of Ether, Fire, Air, and Water, and thus contains all four of these Elements in varying ratios and patterns. Earth is the principle of separation, dividing life into various manifestations of physical bodies. Without Earth, everything would lack boundaries in a constant merging and melting of etheric and liquid forms. It's through the density, heaviness, and fixed quality of Earth that the other Elemental forces are able to manifest within this world. Earth is considered the most yin or fixed Element—the container or vessel for all of life. This is why the Earth Element represents our physical bodies and the roots of plants, as well as the solid state of matter, which we perceive through the sense of touch. It is generally related to the winter, when plants return to their roots, life slows down, and animals hibernate. The mineral kingdom, being the most condensed form of the Earth, relates to this Element.

▽ The Water Element

The Water Element is the second of the fixed Elements. Also generated from Celestial Salt, it is considered more volatile, or lighter, than Earth, as it is more mobile. Water is the vehicle through which Air and Fire descend from the Ether and are implanted into Earth; in this way, Water is the bringer of life. Hence we are all gestated within Water. In fact, many mythological stories (and modern biology) speak of life emerging from a primordial ocean. Earth on its own is fixed, rigid, unyielding, and unmoving. Only through Water being infused into Earth does life become ensouled, enlivened, fluid, and mobile. This is why Water relates to our emotions and feelings, which we can *feel* in our bodies and the stems of plants that conduct fluids and connect the above- and below-ground parts. It's commonly associated with autumn, when the rains come in many parts of the world, as well as the liquid state of matter and the fungal kingdom, which is highly dependent upon moisture and typically grows in the fall.

△ The Air Element

Formed from the active Celestial Niter, Air embodies the principle of movement, the space where the Fire shines its light, what Water evaporates into, what holds the Earth. The Air Element imbues Earth and Water with the principles of intelligence, communication, and language, representing the mind of Nature. This is why Air relates to our intellectual faculty, as well as the leaves of plants where gaseous exchange occurs. Air is associated with the gaseous state of matter and our sense of smell, which perceives subtle compounds floating through space and is connected to our respiratory system. It generally corresponds to the spring season, as plants begin to grow up and out, the birds start singing, the bees start pollinating, and life starts moving from the depths of winter. In this way it relates to the botanical kingdom as a whole, which is central to the communication and self-regulation of the planet itself.

△ The Fire Element

Moving upward from Air, we enter the second volatile force: Fire, the primary power of transformation. Fire exists at the center of every living thing, a reflection of the Sun residing at the center of the solar system. Many traditions maintain that a Fire has been burning at the center of creation since the beginning of time, commonly seen as our Grandfather witnessing all of life. The Air Element is the carrier of Fire into the Water and the Earth, for it is through the Air that light shines and heat is felt. As the most volatile force, Fire is the primary agent able to take the fixed Elements of Water and Earth and volatilize them into the Ether of the spiritual realm. Hence, Fire is of critical importance in the work of the laboratory and inner alchemy. Fire correlates to our intuitive faculty, which unites the Air of our minds with the spirit of Ether, enabling us to perceive wholeness within parts and develop a deeper level of cognition. Its association with light relates it to our sense of sight, as well as the summer season, when the Sun is at its peak, and the flowers of plants. The animal kingdom relates to Fire because animals hold a different level of consciousness from the plant, fungal, or mineral kingdoms.

The Ether Element

The Ether, or Quintessence, is formed through the harmonization of the other Four Elements as they enter coherence and self-organize. Whereas Earth, Water, Air, and Fire are the warp and weft in the web of life, Ether is the weaver of the web, the invisible, spiritual source that gives birth to all things. Through Ether we can understand all of the Elements, for it is their Mother and Father. It is pure consciousness, the power that imbues all of life with purpose and meaning. Ether is perfect balance, the union of Celestial Niter (electric) and Celestial Salt (magnetic), and thus can be likened to the electromagnetic spectrum, that invisible communication network central to maintaining ecological self-organization. These waveforms are how we perceive vibrations and sound, relating Ether to our sense of hearing. Within people, Ether is the "watcher on the hill," the pure consciousness within which intuition, thought, feeling, and sensation arise. It's the consciousness that permeates every cell of the body. We can relate it to humanity as a whole and to the transitional periods between the seasons, when the winds blow one season out and the next season in. Within plants it relates to the seeds and fruits, which contain the entire pattern of roots, stems, leaves, and flowers for the next generation.

Figure 2 shows a table of Elemental correspondences throughout various aspects of Nature and traditions from around the world. Many of these relationships will be further explored in chapters 10 and 14.

	EARTH	WATER	AIR	FIRE	ETHER
Ayurveda	Prithvi	Ap	Vayu	Tej	Akasha
Platonic Solid	Cube	Icosahedron	Octahedron	Tetrahedron	Dodecahedron
Molecular	Carbon	Oxygen	Hydrogen	Nitrogen	Quantum
Season	Winter	Autumn	Spring	Summer	Transitions
Four Worlds of Qabalah	Assiah	Yetzirah	Briah	Atziluth	
Astrological Signs	Taurus Virgo Capricorn	Scorpio Cancer Pisces	Gemini Aquarius Libra	Aries Sagittarius Leo	
State of Matter	Solid	Liquid	Gaseous	Combustion	Ethereal
Kingdom	Mineral	Fungal	Botanical	Animal	Human
Dual Nature	Yin	Yin	Yang	Yang	Balance
Steiner's Elements	Physical Body	Etheric Body	Astral Body	I-Consciousness	
Jung's Psychic Functions	Sensation	Feeling	Thinking	Intuition	Imagination
Sense	Touch	Taste	Smell	Sight	Hearing
Constitution	Melancholic	Phlegmatic	Sanguine	Choleric	

	EARTH	WATER	AIR	FIRE	ETHER
Dosha	Kapha	Kapha/Pitta	Vata	Pitta	Vata
Humor	Black Bile	White Bile (Phlegm)	Red Bile (Blood)	Yellow Bile	
Organs	Liver, Bones, Connective Tissue	Kidneys, Lymph, Stomach	Lungs, Large Intestine	Heart, Blood, Small intestine	Nerves, Brain, Consciousness
Tissue State	Cold Depression	Damp Relaxation, Damp Stagnation	Dry Atrophy	Heat Excitation	Wind Tension
Plant Morphology	Root	Stems	Leaves	Flower	Seed, Fruit
Plant Constitution	Stout, thick, oily, broad	Lush, moist, flowing	Thin spindly, dry, "feathered"	Sharp, prickly, intense, red	Similar to Air
Herbal Action	Tonic, Astringent, Alterative, Bitter	Diuretic, Lymphatic, Demulcent	Expectorant, Nervine, Carminative	Diaphoretic, Stimulant, Adaptogen	Entheogenic, Nervine, Spasmolytic
Energetics	Cold	Wet	Dry	Hot	Balance
Taste	Sweet, Astringent	Sweet, Salty	Pungent, Bitter, Astringent	Sour, Salty, Pungent	Bitter

The energetics of the Elements here is based on the astrological tradition, as opposed to the Aristotelian tradition, which relegates 2 energetic qualities to each Element, such as Air being damp and hot, and Fire being hot and dry. Further detail on the concept of Elemental energetics will be explored in chapters 9, 10, and 14

Note: The correspondences between tastes and the Elements are based on traditional Ayurvedic classification.

Figure 2. Table of Elemental correspondences

The Elements in Alchemy

In alchemy there is an important division among the Elemental forces: Fire and Air are considered the volatile, yang Elements born of Celestial Niter, and Water and Earth are the fixed, yin Elements born of Celestial Salt. Fire is the most volatile Element, followed in volatility by Air, then Water, and finally Earth as the least volatile Element. The relative volatile and fixed qualities of the Elements form a critical aspect of the alchemical philosophy of Nature, for every being must pass through each Elemental force sequentially during its process of transformation, gradually progressing from one to the next. This forms the basis of laboratory spagyrics.

There are two "vital currents," according to alchemy: the volatile path, governing the movement of Earth up into Water, Air, and Fire; and the fixed path, governing the vital force moving down from Fire into Air, Water, and Earth. These are also referred to as the manifestation and liberation currents. The volatilizing of a fixed form up into the Heavens and the fixing of volatile forms down into the Earth constitute the great circulations of alchemy as well as the cycles of transformation we go through as people. This is why the ouroboros—the snake eating its own tail—is a classic alchemical symbol for regeneration, rejuvenation, and circulating between Heaven and Earth.

The Elements are the forces used to extract the Three Philosophical Principles (Sulfur, Mercury, and Salt) from plants in alchemy. The premise of this tradition is to "volatilize what is fixed, and fix what is volatile" by using the powers of Fire and Water. It is only through Fire's ability to send substances up into the Air that they can collect the celestial energies of the Heavens, and only through Water can they return to the Earth. Medical alchemy stressed the importance of seeing the unique ways each Element manifests within people and plants, which is also central in many constitutional systems of natural medicine.

The Elements in Ayurveda

In Ayurvedic medicine the Elements form an essential part of their cosmology of the world. They are said to spring forth from the three *gunas: sattva, rajas,* and *tamas.* These are three primal qualities of existence, or life attributes, relating to the properties of inertia *(tamas),* movement *(rajas),* and equilibrium *(sattva).* These are similar to Celestial Niter *(rajas),* Celestial Salt *(tamas),* and the *prima materia (sattva).* The Five Elements emerged from these three primal qualities: *sattva* generates Ether; *rajas* generates Fire; *tamas* generates Earth; between *rajas* and *sattva* comes Air (movement and invisibility); and between *rajas* and *tamas* emerges Water (movement and stability).[2]

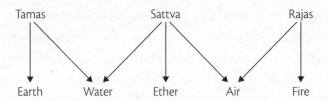

Figure 3. Ayurvedic cosmology of the Elements

Ayurvedic medicine is rooted in a threefold pattern of energetics, based on the *doshas,* which are formed through particular combinations of the Elements. Air and Ether form the *vata dosha,* Fire and Air create the *pitta dosha,* and Earth and Water generate the *kapha dosha.* Although the Elemental derivations of the three *doshas* are slightly different from the Three Principles of Alchemy (because of a difference between a Four- and Five-Element model), their core characteristics are essentially the same. The Elements in Ayurveda are used to classify the tastes of medicinal substances and the qualities of the seasons, as well as to delineate the anatomy, physiology, and psychology of the human being. While the terminology is often relegated to the three *doshas,* remembering their Elemental composition is helpful in understanding these delineations. We will look into this threefold pattern in the next chapter and in part III.

The Elements in Chinese Medicine

Whereas India has a Five-Element model consisting of Earth, Water, Fire, Air, and Ether, the Chinese have a slightly different approach. While their system still consists of Earth, Water, and Fire, the differences rest in the last two Elements: Wood and Metal. These latter Elements generally correlate Metal with Air (lungs) and Wood with Ether (as the principle of growth and change).

Whereas Western Elemental models relate the Elements to different states of matter (solid, liquid, gas, combustion), the Chinese see them as phases of transformation. This was commonly symbolized by a five-pointed star that showed how each Element transformed into another according to particular patterns. This is referred to as *Wu Xing.* These cycles of transformation formed the foundation for Chinese knowledge of seasonal rhythms, anatomy, physiology, psychology, and constitutional patterns, as well as an overall cosmological scheme of Nature.

The Chinese also classified herbal remedies through the Elements and their connection to tastes: Earth (sweet), Water (salty), Fire (bitter), Metal (acrid/pungent), and Wood/Wind (sour). They also relied on their understanding of the "four natures" (energetics) of herbs (hot, cold, wet, dry) for herbal classification. Together these systems enabled them to determine the organ systems and bodily cycles of transformation that a remedy would influence. We also see the Five Elements as a central part of *Qi Gong,* or the Chinese model of internal alchemy.

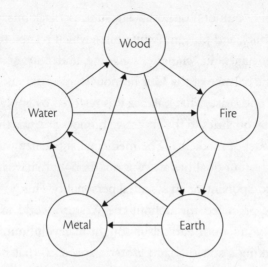

Figure 4. The Chinese Five Elements, or Wu Xing

The Elements in Western Medicine

The foundation of Western philosophy comes to us from the ancient Greeks, whose philosophers contemplated the original and primal constituents of the world. As Matthew Wood explains:

> *The origins of the four elements lie far back in the mists of time, but it was Empedocles who introduced them into Greek philosophy and argued for them as the basis of the world. Plato lent his weight to this view but Aristotle felt that the four elements were derivative. He postulated the four qualities from which they were derived.... The four elements subsequently became more of a philosophical or mythological system, while the four qualities were used in the science and medicine of antiquity to describe the attributes of stones, plants, animals and people.[3]*

The model of medicine established by the Greeks was based upon the four qualities of hot, cold, wet, and dry, from which the Elements derive (as per Aristotle). This is typically referred to as "Galenic" medicine, established by Galen of Pergamon (129–210 AD) based on Hippocratic teachings. Galenic medicine was primarily founded upon the four "humors" or bodily substances: black bile, yellow bile, blood (red bile), and phlegm (white bile), which related to four constitutions: melancholic, choleric, sanguine, and phlegmatic. Disturbances in the balance of the four humors were understood to be the root causes of disease. That balance was restored by applying opposing medicinal qualities to the excessive humors and was thus an antipathetic model of medicine. The medicinal substance was seen as a vehicle for the four qualities and was not thought to have intelligence, a spiritual component, or an essential personality. This was the model of medicine practiced throughout the Western world for well over a thousand years, until Paracelsus sought to revolutionize medicine by reintegrating a spiritual and esoteric approach that honored the essential intelligence of both the body and the remedy.

The Elements in Hermeticism

Hermeticism is a term used to denote a particular philosophical orientation based on the teachings of Hermes Trismegistus, or Thrice-Great Hermes, the patron saint of alchemy. This body of knowledge is at the root of alchemy but also encompasses astrology, qabalah, and theurgy (ceremonial magic), with the intention of divine union with God. Hermeticism is the foundation of many esoteric schools, including Rosicrucianism and the Order of the Golden Dawn, among many others.

The Elements play a highly important role within these sister sciences of alchemy. They are attributed to the four worlds of the qabalah, forming a primal organizational pattern on the glyph known as the Tree of Life, as well as the basis of the tarot, expressed through the four suits of the minor arcana: wands, swords, cups, and discs/pentacles along with the sixteen royalty cards. Many rites of initiation and the practice of ceremonial magic incorporate corresponding symbols and attributes that relate to the Elements and alignment with the cardinal directions.

The Elements are central in astrology, as they are one of the constituents of the twelve signs of the zodiac, along with the "three modes." Thus, there are three signs placed under each Element:

Earth: Taurus, Virgo, Capricorn

Water: Cancer, Scorpio, Pisces

Air: Gemini, Libra, Aquarius

Fire: Aries, Leo, Sagittarius

While modern astrology is commonly oriented around psychology, personality type, or the soul's evolution, the astrologers of old also placed strong emphasis upon the physiological and anatomical expressions of the signs, Planets, and Elements. They traced these archetypal patterns into organ systems and disease patterns, enabling a translation between body, psychology, and soul. These forces also formed constitutional patterns delineated through the natal birth chart, based on excesses and deficiencies of certain Elements or Planets.

The Elements in First Nations Traditions

The Four Elements also appear throughout traditions of many First Nations peoples in both North and South America, and quite likely elsewhere in the world. In the Americas, there's a strong orientation towards the four directions: east, south, west, and north. It's impossible to give universal correlations between the directions and the Elements because each culture and tradition has different perspectives on this, based primarily upon their cosmological models and on environmental differences. Some say the east relates to Air, others to Fire, etc. Yet we see the Elements as a universal component in their understanding of the world. Each of these directions is home to spiritual intelligences that become guides for life, healing, and prayer. It's common in these traditions for particular attributes to be associated with each direction and Element, such as colors, stones, plants, animals, and seasons.

These directional intelligences are not seen as nebulous forces of Nature but as living, intelligent *spirits*. Thus, traditional peoples speak to them directly, orienting their prayers in ways that address the essence of these spiritual beings to bring about healing, guidance, support, and protection. These spiritual forces are integrated in a wide variety of ceremonies and prayers to create relationships with them and bring about miraculous healing and a deeper understanding of life itself.

The Elements in People and Plants

The Elements form multiple organizational patterns within both people and plants. One of the basic ways we can approach this understanding is through basic anatomical structures. All humans have a physical body (Earth), an emotional body (Water), an intellectual body (Air), an intuitive self (Fire), and consciousness or imagination (Quintessence). These are based on the four psychic functions proposed by Carl Jung, who was an adept student of alchemy. He said we perceive the world through four primary means: sensation, feeling, thinking, and intuition, which were related to Earth, Water, Air, and Fire, respectively. He connected the fifth Element, the Quintessence, with the imaginal faculty. The Elements also correlate to specific organ systems and tissues of the body and to pathological patterns afflicting the body or psyche.

The Elements also relate to the overall anatomy of a plant. One day when I was wildcrafting *Angelica arguta* roots in the Cascade Mountains in Washington, I was contemplating the Elements and how *everything* contains them; nothing can exist if it doesn't incorporate all of them. I thought that was pretty interesting, and I was trying to understand what that fact really meant with regard to plants. Digging *Angelica*'s roots, I noticed how perfectly poised between Heaven and Earth she was, with her aromatic roots, hollow stem, and umbrella-shaped inflorescence opening up to the sky … and then it dawned on me. Simply by looking at the whole plant dug from the Earth, I realized that the basic morphological structures of a plant directly relate to the Elements: they all have roots (Earth), stems (Water), leaves (Air), flowers (Fire), and fruits or seeds (Quintessence). The Quintessence contains all Four Elements in the exact same way that the seed contains the roots, stems, leaves, flowers, and seeds of the next generation. It was one of those intuitive flashes of insight that only truly comes when my heart is connected to the Light of Nature.

A few months later, I read this passage in David Frawley and Vasant Lad's *The Yoga of Herbs:*

> *The five parts of plants in Ayurveda, pancangam, show how plant structure is related to the five elements. The root corresponds to earth, as the densest and lowest part, connected to the earth. The stem and branches correspond to water, as they convey the water or sap of the plant. The flowers correspond to fire, which manifests light and color. The leaves correspond to air, since through them the wind moves the plant. The fruit corresponds to ether, the subtle essence of the plant. The seed contains all five elements, containing the entire potential plant within itself.*[4]

I was stunned when I read this, as it stated precisely what I'd learned up in the mountains with *Angelica* when a glimmer of *natura sophia* touched my heart.

Rudolf Steiner also correlated plant parts to the Elements, though his model used Four Elements instead of five, so it's slightly different. For him, roots relate to Earth, the leaf and stem relate to Water, flowers correspond to Air, and fruits and seeds to Fire. The Elements also represent everything a plant needs to be sustained: they grow in the Earth, drink Water, absorb carbon dioxide from the Air, photosynthesize the Fire of the sun, and require the space of Ether.

The Elements form a fundamental pattern for understanding how the vital force of Nature expresses itself throughout people and plants. They are a foundational pattern of energetic architecture and begin to reveal the underlying language of life itself, as well as the patterns revealed to the student of the Light of Nature. These patterns rest at the root of the great herbal traditions of the world and connect their system of healing to the archetypal forces of life. The above descriptions are meant to give a brief introduction to how the Elements are reflected in some of these traditions, to reveal their universality. Understanding the full depth of these traditions would require a lifetime of study and is beyond the scope of this work, although deeper correlations between the Elements within people, plants, and herbal traditions will be explored in more detail in part III.

The Elements are but one layer of this language, one dialect of the larger linguistics of Nature. The Elemental forces are what exist just behind the physical world and are thus a translation mechanism between the physical and spiritual realities. They never exist in isolation, but only in their synergy. Life only occurs through the interweaving of Earth, Water, Air, Fire, and Ether. These Elements combine with one another in very specific ways to generate the three-dimensional world that is our abode; thus, they synergize to form our next pattern of energetic architecture: the Three Philosophical Principles.

The Three Principles

The Taoist masters reasoned that to become connected to the outer universe, they first needed to gain control of their own inner universe. They experienced this inner universe as a flow of energy, or chi, through their bodies. The Microcosmic Orbit, running up the spine and down the front of the body, was uncovered as the pathway through which the distilled essence of this energy flows. They perceived that the Microcosmic Orbit connects three bodies—physical, soul, and spirit—within each individual and ultimately fuses them into one immortal body. It was with this perception that the study of Internal Alchemy began.

—MANTAK CHIA[1]

The Three Philosophical Principles are the basis of alchemical chemistry, philosophy, and metaphysics. They resemble a variety of other threefold systems of energetic architecture. Anywhere we see a threefold division of life, it often corresponds to these universal principles, which can be seen scattered throughout religious symbolism, mythologies, pantheons, and a variety of medical and herbal traditions. Just like the Elements, this pattern was directly observed by following the Light of Nature. It was integral to traditional systems, though they each one understood them in unique ways based on differences of culture, tradition, and ecological context. By studying the various reflections of these principles across different systems, we see their multidimensional, universal nature.

Cosmology of the Three Principles

The Three Principles represent the functional patterns formed through Elemental interactions, achieved through their entrainment and the subsequent formation of new levels of self-organization. Each Element is a part that recombines with another in specific ways to create new wholes, the same way all of Nature generates new levels of complexity. The Principles are the vehicles through which the Elements physically manifest. While they are born of the Elements, they also contain distinct qualities greater than the sum of their parts.

It is worth briefly mentioning the slight differences in the cosmology of both the Elements and the Principles within Eastern and Western traditions. In Ayurveda, the Elements descend from the most volatile to fixed in the order of Ether, Air, Fire, Water, and Earth, whereas in the West the progression moves from Quintessence to Fire, Air, Water, and Earth. In the West, there's a stronger orientation around Four Elements, whereas the East preferred to use a Five-Element model. This changes their relative perspectives on the formation of the Three Principles.

According to Ayurveda, the Three Principles (called *doshas*) are generated as follows: Ether and Air combine to form the *vata dosha,* Fire and Water fuse to create the *pitta dosha,* and Water and Earth synergize to generate the *kapha dosha.* In alchemy, the formation of the Three Philosophical Principles occurs by Fire and Air combining to form the Sulfur Principle, Air and Water conjoining to generate the Mercury Principle, and Water and Earth coming together to manifest the Salt Principle. While we see these basic differences in their Elemental configurations between the East and West, the importance rests in understanding how the three *doshas* of Ayurveda and the Three Principles of alchemy are, at their cores, the same energetic patterns.

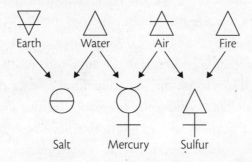

Figure 5. Cosmology of the Three Principles of alchemy

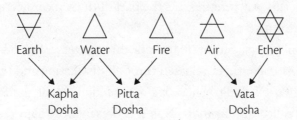

Figure 6. Cosmology of the three doshas of Ayurveda

The Three Principles of Alchemy

The Three Philosophical Principles of alchemy are Sulfur, Mercury, and Salt. As mentioned, these are not *chemical* but *philosophical,* representing greater archetypal life forces of which the three substances are merely physical expressions. Their archetypal representation is the soul, spirit, and body of any living thing, yet they also have particular physical manifestations—that is, material substances you can directly work with. In plants, the physical expressions of Sulfur, Mercury, and Salt form the foundation for spagyrics, which uses

them in crafting medicine. Each Principle within a plant is separated, purified, and recombined to form a holistic form of medicine
that operates upon the whole person—body, spirit, and soul.

🜍 **Sulfur:** Chemical sulfur has a distinctly pungent smell (like
rotten eggs) and a bright yellow color. The alchemists saw these
characteristics as a signature for the light of the soul (yellow color)
and its relationship to the Fire and Air Elements, represented by the
pungent smell that volatilizes into the air. Sulfur relates to the soul
of any living thing, its unique, individualized essence that's particular to itself, unlike anything else in creation. Within people, Sulfur
represents the purpose we carry into this life, the growth process
needed for the soul to evolve. Sulfur is the conscious self experiencing life. It's also considered the most volatile part of anything,
the first component released by the Fire Element to evaporate into
the air. In this way, it represents the part of the self connected to the
celestial realm.

Within plants, Sulfur manifests through essential oils, which
are the first constituent released through distillation and the application of Fire. I don't believe it's a coincidence that the Sulfur of
plants is called an *essential* oil, as it represents the soul essence of
the plant, highly volatile in nature. While not all plants have essential oils, they all contain Sulfur, albeit in a more fixed form that
is extracted as a resin called the Salt of Sulfur. In the same way
that Sulfur relates to our unique, individualized soul, so too are the
essential oils of plants completely distinct unto themselves. Sulfur
generally corresponds to the *pitta dosha*.

☿ **Mercury:** Chemical mercury is unique, as it's a liquid metal
with a highly volatile nature, meaning that it easily transforms
into gas. Mercury has the capacity to transition swiftly and easily
between the three states of matter—solid, liquid, and gas. This is
why the glyph of Mercury contains the crescent, circle, and cross,
symbolic of its ability to move between these states of matter,
classically represented by the upper, lower, and middle worlds. The

harmony of the Air and Water Elements reveals a specialized function of Mercury: to bridge the volatile and fixed realms of Sulfur and Salt, which is why it is correlated to the spirit.

In Western culture the words "soul" and "spirit" are often used interchangeably, seen as representing the same component of the self, but the alchemical tradition understands them as distinct. Whereas the soul is defined as the unique individual essence, the spirit is the universal essence that infuses all of life with intelligence. A simple way to differentiate these essences is to say that soul is individual, whereas spirit is universal. The universal essence of Mercury is the one vital life force stitched into the fabric of every living thing, whereas the Sulfur essence is our individualized expression of consciousness.

Mercury manifests in people in several ways. The first is the invisible vital force that suffuses our entire organism with intelligence, organizing and informing the functioning (or malfunctioning) of the body. The second is the overall architecture of our psychology, expressed through our thinking and feeling. The quality of our thoughts and feelings is directly influenced by the patterns encoded within Sulfur, or the soul, of which Mercury is the messenger. This is revealed by Mercury being an amalgam of the Air (thought) and Water (feeling) Elements. As the bridge between Sulfur and Salt, Mercury unites the impulses from the soul and manifests them directly in the physical organ systems and tissues through psychological and emotional patterns.

In their explorations of Nature, the alchemists stumbled upon an interesting truth within the plant kingdom. When a plant is drowned in a vat of water and allowed to putrefy and decompose—i.e., to ferment—it always yields ethyl alcohol. Bark or seed, root or leaf, flower or fruit, any plant submitted to fermentation generates alcohol. In their understanding of the meaning behind form, the alchemists determined alcohol to be the manifestation of the Mercury Principle within plants, representing the universal spirit of the entire botanical kingdom, just as there is a universal spirit that unites us all. This is why distilled alcohols are referred to as "spirits." Mercury is commonly extracted through fermentation and distillation, although in modern herbal pharmacy this is usually done through maceration or percolation with an alcohol menstruum. The Mercury Principle generally corresponds to the *vata dosha*.

⊖ **Salt:** This final Principle represents the essential form through which Sulfur and Mercury materialize in the physical world. The Salt Principle is represented by common salt, or sodium chloride, and is the union of Earth and Water; indeed, the evaporation of seawater results in salt. Many cosmologies, mythologies, and creation stories speak of a primordial ocean and how all physical life emerged from the Water Element. The Salt Principle could be thought of as Earth contained in Water, an embodiment of the first physical matter and the coagulation of material forms.

Salt relates to the body of any living thing, the vehicle through which the soul and spirit operate in this tangible reality, enabling the volatile forces of Air, Fire, and Ether to condense into the world. Without this Principle, all of existence would simply be a boundaryless, unformed world with no distinction, separation, or beauty to perceive. It's only through Salt that the Elemental and celestial forces of Mercury and Sulfur actually manifest; thus, it is the most fixed component of the energetic architecture model.

Within people, this Principle constitutes our physical bodies, from the organelles and cells, to the tissues and organs, to the interweaving of our organ systems to form a cohesive, self-organized, optimally functioning body. As with the Elements, none of these Three Principles exist in isolation from one another; they are inextricably linked in a cohesive state of wholeness. Our bodies without Mercury and Sulfur would be completely immobile, lacking the intelligence and purpose that maintain our self-organization. Mercury directly enters into Salt, permeating every cell, tissue, and organ with its own unique intelligence that communicates with the rest of the body. Because

Mercury is suffused with Sulfur, every part of Salt contains a unique expression of consciousness, its own particular purpose and function within the physical ecosystem, its own archetypal form.

The Three Principles can be seen as a fractal pattern applied to the whole human being as soul, spirit, and body but also to the individual organs, systems, and tissues. For instance, the liver has a physical form (Salt) that possesses a particular type of intelligence (Mercury), such as the production of bile, metabolism of nutrients and waste products, and dynamic relationship with the blood, kidneys, gallbladder, and digestive system. These traits fulfill the liver's purpose (Sulfur) of maintaining the dynamic homeostasis of the body, being the seat of metabolism, sending nutrition throughout the body, building and cleansing the blood, and so on, as well as its archetypal relationship to Jupiter. This is an important reflection of the doctrine of correspondence because each part contains the pattern of the whole and thus contains a specific form (Salt), a particular intelligence (Mercury), and a unique purposeful function and archetypal relationship (Sulfur).

The Salt Principle in plants relates to the alkali minerals, which are separated and purified from the plant's body through incineration by Fire and further purification with Water. This yields a wide range of crystalline structures that resemble quartz crystals. Just as our physical bodies are the vehicle through which our consciousness and intelligence become embodied, so too are these crystalline mineral salts—the purified body of the plant—the physical delivery mechanism for the plant's intelligence and consciousness. They are the grounding rod for Mercury and Sulfur. The Salt Principle generally corresponds to the *kapha* dosha.

Although the tradition of alchemy doesn't appear to go as deep into constitutional and organ system dynamics as the Ayurvedic *doshas* do, it does provide methods of herbal preparation not seen in Ayurveda. Both systems developed different aspects of these same Principles, so bringing them together allows us to understand them in more depth.

The Three Doshas of Ayurveda

The foundation of Ayurvedic medicine is rooted in Ayurveda's Three Principles, called *doshas,* which translates to "that which goes out of balance" or "that which contaminates."[2] This definition shows how *vata, pitta,* and *kapha* relate to disease and states of imbalance. Todd Caldecott defines *doshas* in his text *Inside Ayurveda:*

> *These three principles of function are called dosah (plural of dosa) because they are subject to influences from both within and without. The term dosa literally means "blemish" because it is the increase, decrease and distur- bance of one, two or all three of the dosah that are responsible for all patho- logical changes in the body.*[3]

Vata, pitta, and *kapha* are three primary modes through which matter and energy express themselves, representing core constitutional types, psychological temperaments, and the governing of vital organ and system functions. At the heart of Ayurveda rests an under- standing of the specific reflections of the *doshas* within all things: people, plants, seasons, foods, tissues, ecosystems, thoughts, etc.

Plants are related to the *doshas* through their morphological pat- terns, habitat, organ system affinities, and especially their energetic actions upon the *doshas* within a person. This is demonstrated by their effects upon the body, mind, and consciousness. The *dosha* qualities of medicinal plants form the crux of Ayurvedic herbalism and represent a core pattern of herbal classification, properties, and energetics.

While the *doshas* primarily represent physiological-energetic imbalances within the organism that require balancing (i.e., they are pathological), they also have a "transformed" state that imbues health within the body, mind, and spirit. These rarified essences of each *dosha,* called *tejas, prana,* and *ojas,* form a primary goal of rejuvena- tive therapies in Ayurveda, whereby the body is cleansed of impuri- ties and the *doshas* are transformed into a refined level of expression, bestowing our consciousness with particular beneficial qualities and characteristics. *Pitta* is said to become rarefied in the form of *tejas,* the flame of pure perception; *vata* transmutes into *prana,* the pure air of consciousness; and the essence of *kapha* is *ojas,* the refined pearl of physiological essence and rejuvenation. By alchemically transforming each *dosha* into its corresponding essence, the body and psyche reach new levels of clarity, courage, and vitality.[4]

Pitta is formed through the Fire and Water Elements and is associated with the qualities of heat, lightness, oiliness, and dynamic energy. Constitutionally, it creates a medium build, prominent muscular tissue, red coloration to the skin, and freckles. As the primary *dosha* with the Fire Element, *pitta* is the digestive fire of the small intestine and regulates the blood and circulation. *Pitta* tends towards excess heat, physical and psychological irritation, immune excess, inflammation, and high metabolism, lending a strong appetite and digestion. This excess energy is a strength, but it's also a weakness, as people with primarily *pitta* constitutions can "burn the candle at both ends" until they burn out. Psychologically they embody qualities of leadership, empowerment, confidence, and courage, but in excess they can be domineering, irritable, and easily angered.

This *dosha* is typically associated with the summer and late spring seasons, when it accumulates the most. Plants that increase *pitta* are typically hot, pungent, oily remedies that stimulate circulation, digestion, and sweating. In its highest manifestation, *pitta* transforms into *tejas,* which is the pure flame of awareness and perception that instills self-confidence and courage.

Vata is formed through Air and Ether and is associated with qualities of lightness, movement, dryness, and tension. *Vata* constitutions are often tall, thin, and wiry, with prominent veins, connective tissues, and joints. Because they are often cold, the skin may be pale and dry, and they may have brittle nails and thin body hair. Air and Ether are volatile Elements, so they manifest constitutionally as a less "material" body. Through Air, *vata* relates to the lungs and the colon, which is prone to gaseous accumulation. The nervous system is also prominently associated, as *vata* is often nervous, anxious, and prone to tension and spasm. This is a highly active constitution, exemplified by dynamic, quick movements of both body and mind. They are often creative and visionary, but when imbalanced they become nervous, timid, restless, and fearful, with scattered thoughts and a feeling of being "ungrounded." It's common for them to learn (and forget) quickly.

This *dosha* typically accumulates in the autumn season and is aggravated by plants that are cooling, drying, bitter, and astringent in nature. In its highest manifestation, *vata* transmutes into *prana,* the pure Air of thought and higher mental faculties, instilling creativity and adaptability.

Kapha is formed through Earth and Water and is thus the most fixed of the *doshas,* associated with heaviness, slowness, dampness, and cold. *Kapha* constitutions are typically thicker in stature, with broad shoulders, large chests and abdomens, and a prominence of adipose tissue. They generally have well-developed bodies, whereas *vata* is slightly underdeveloped, and *pitta* is in the middle. The hair is often thick, lustrous, and oily, the skin moist and cold. *Kapha* relates to the stomach, mucus production, the kidneys, and bodily fluids. Therefore it has a tendency toward damp accumulation, slowed metabolic functions, heaviness, and sluggishness. Psychologically *kapha* is calm, even-tempered, sweet, forgiving, and gentle, though in excess it can be mentally foggy, depressed, greedy, and possessive. Their life is often highly structured, steady, and consistent, but once a *kapha*'s habits are in place they can be hard to break.

Kapha accumulates in the winter and early spring months, though it should be noted that the seasonal qualities attributed to the *doshas* may differ in varying ecosystems. It is aggravated by plants that are cold, moistening, heavy, and sweet. Its highest manifestation is *ojas,* the refined essence of the tissues of the body that promotes health, longevity, endurance, and vitality. We will explore the three *doshas* in more detail in part III as they specifically relate to people and plants.

Another correlation with the Three Principles of the East is represented by the three primary *nadis,* or energetic circuits, that govern the vital force of the body: *ida, pingala,* and *sushumna.* These are the magnetic, dynamic, and balanced aspects of energy, which spin the *chakras* as the vital force moves up and down these channels. This centralized axis of Ayurveda's energetic anatomy is strikingly similar to the caduceus of Western alchemy.

The Three Modes of Astrology

The Western astrological equivalent of the Three Principles is the three modes: cardinal, mutable, and fixed. Judith Hill describes the modes as "the rate of matter in motion."[5] These are three particular ways the Four Elements manifest, taking the cosmological pattern to a new level of specificity as they interweave to generate the twelve signs of the zodiac. Thus, we see cardinal-Fire (Aries), mutable-Fire (Sagittarius), and fixed-Fire (Leo); cardinal-Air (Libra), mutable-Air (Gemini), and fixed-Air (Aquarius); and so on. This takes our understanding of how the Elements manifest to a greater degree of precision.

Cardinal represents an active and dynamic quality, the energy required to initiate force into form and instill it with the vital principles of life. This fiery quality is quite reminiscent of *pitta* and Sulfur[‡] and is best thought of as *energy.* There are four primary reflections of the cardinal mode through the four Elements. Cardinal-Fire is the spark, represented by Aries. Cardinal-Water could be seen as the turbulent ocean, represented by Cancer. Cardinal-Air could be seen as active winds, embodied in Libra. Cardinal-Earth could be seen as power within form, represented by Capricorn.

---

‡ It's important to note that not all of the cardinal signs will tend to manifest as *pitta,* nor the mutable signs as *vata* or fixed signs as *kapha.* Considering constitutional characteristics from the astrological perspective is complex, requiring assessment of the entire astrological chart to see particularly dominant modes, elements, planets, or signs that generate the constitution.

As the great initiator, the cardinal mode is found at the beginning of each of the four seasons, providing the energy required to
catalyze a new seasonal quality. The cardinal signs rest directly on
the equinox and solstice axes: Aries at the spring equinox, Cancer
at the summer solstice, Libra at the autumn equinox, and Capricorn at the winter solstice. This reflects the Sulfur Principle as the
primal force of Nature that brings energy into action within the
physical world as a new season.

Mutable is the quality of changeability, movement, and variability, quite similar to the *vata dosha* and the Mercury Principle. The
mutable mode governs the signs of the zodiac at the end of each
season, before the cardinal signs. They bring about the change or
transition between the seasons, the winds that blow one seasonal
quality out and the new one in.

Gemini is composed of mutable-Air, the whirling winds at the
end of spring. Virgo is mutable-Earth, the end of summer, when
the plants change the directional flow of their vital force down into
the Earth. Sagittarius is mutable-Fire, the flickering flames we gaze
into for warmth and comfort during the shift into winter. Pisces
is mutable-Water, the deep emotional reflections and transformations that occur as the cycle ends and is renewed during the shift
from winter into spring. These seasonal patterns are precisely how
Ayurveda denotes seasonal transitions being governed by *vata,*
which brings the necessary movement of wind in order to dispel
one seasonal influence and spark the cardinal flame that initiates
the next.

Fixed is the quality of stability, coercion, and solidity, and corresponds with *kapha* and Salt. I find it interesting that the name
of this mode is the same word used in alchemy to denote qualities
of the Earth Element and the materializing current moving from
the spiritual world down into the material world. The fixed mode
strengthens an Elemental force, anchoring it more deeply in the
world, restricting its dynamic movements and creating a greater

degree of structure and boundaries around it. It's a binding and holding quality, whereas cardinal is *pitta,* the force of energy, and mutable is *vata,* the movement of change.

The four fixed signs of the zodiac are: Taurus, fixed-Earth, which governs the middle of spring and the bountiful growth of nature; Leo, fixed-Fire, ruling the heat of the summer and creative expression; Scorpio, fixed-Water, the middle of autumn and the return of Nature to the roots and the lower world, death, and letting go; and Aquarius, fixed-Air, the frozen depths of winter, when the air is so cold it touches your bones. The fixed signs of the zodiac reside in the middle of the seasons, when that seasonal force is in its peak expression. In the study of Western astrology, paying attention to the attributes of the seasons and their internal reflections of our evolutionary journey is critically important to understanding the archetypes of the zodiac.

The Three Treasures of Chinese Medicine

In Chinese medicine, the principle of *san jiao,* or the "triple burner," and the "three treasures" are both representations of the threefold pattern. The triple burner is a basic understanding of human anatomy and physiology revealing the flow and distribution of heat, fluids, and energy throughout the body. It's essentially the traditional Chinese understanding of our modern concept of metabolism. It divides the body into upper, middle, and lower portions, segmented by fascial compartments via connective tissues in the thoracic, abdominal, and pelvic cavities. The primary function of *san jiao* is the overall regulation and metabolism of the body as a whole. Thus, it relates to a variety of organs, such as the Kidneys, Spleen, and Heart (note that these are traditional Chinese "organs," which are slightly different from our Western equivalents; hence they are capitalized for distinction). This basic threefold division of the body shows the vertical-axis orientation of the Three Principles, similar to how Sulfur, Mercury, and Salt have relative volatile and fixed qualities. Indeed, the anatomy and physiology of *san jiao* is quite similar to the process of distillation in alchemy.

Another threefold pattern in Chinese medicine is the "three treasures" or the "three precious substances," called *shen, chi,* and *jing.* These are considered vital essences that sustain and support human life, quite similar to *tejas, ojas,* and *prana* in Ayurveda and the Three Principles of alchemy; all refer back to fundamental substances at the roots of all life. The three treasures are related to physiological essence *(jing),* energy or vital force *(chi),* and spirit *(shen),* moving from the most fixed to the subtlest.

Shen is the most volatile of the Three Treasures, related to the realm of deity and the spiritual forces of life. It's similar to Sulfur in that it correlates to the perceptual consciousness of a person that transcends the limitations of the analytical mind. To quote Ted Kaptchuk in his excellent introduction to Chinese medicine, *The Web That Has No Weaver:* "Spirit depends on more than mind-consciousness. Spirit is self-awareness that fosters the human experience of authenticity and personal meaning. Spirit allows self-reflection, art, morality, purpose and values. It depends on self-relationship."[6] This points to the aspect of Sulfur that relates to our individualized expression of consciousness, which can only be developed by strengthening our connection to our essential nature that dwells within the heart. While *shen* is stored in the heart, it is interesting to note that it is commonly associated with psychological disturbances when imbalanced, showing how the Chinese understood that the heart does indeed think.

Chi refers to the energy of movement, just like *vata* and Mercury. It's the all-pervading, global vital force that permeates every aspect of our physiological and psychological being—invisible unto itself, but physically seen through its influence. There is a wide variety of manifestations of *chi* within the body, including the unique functions of organs, the qualities we inherit from our parents, our constitution, and the energy we derive from the digestion of food and respiration. *Chi* is said to be the balance of yin and yang on a more generic, cosmological level. It is stored in the chest, aiding in the rhythmic pulsations of the heart and governing respiration as well as communication and self-expression through the voice. These are also notably Mercurial attributes.

As Ted Kaptchuk explains (using the alternative spelling of *chi* as *Qi*):

> *Qi is not some primordial, immutable material, nor is it merely vital energy, although the word is occasionally so translated. Chinese thought does not easily distinguish between matter and energy. We might think that Qi is somewhere in between, a kind of matter on the verge of becoming energy, or energy at the point of materializing.*[7]

This definition speaks to the bridging quality of Mercury and how it unites the volatile realm of Sulfur and the fixed realm of Salt, or the balance of yin and yang, showing the similarity amongst these Principles.

Jing is commonly referred to as "essence." This confused me for a long time because I used to think of *jing* as similar to Sulfur, because it is the soul essence. In the Chinese system, *jing* is instead an expression of the *physical essence* of the human organism, the most vital part of the body, stored in the kidneys. *Jing* governs the functions of birth, growth and development, maturation, and ultimate decline and death. It's primarily concerned with the cycles and rhythms of the body associated with proper development and maintenance. We have *jing* inherited from our parents at the moment of conception and birth, as well as the *jing* we either maintain or deplete through our diets and mental, emotional, and physical exertion. It is generally suggested to adopt a lifestyle that maintains our *jing* in order to preserve our physiological essence and promote longevity. Thus, this vital essence of the body corresponds almost precisely with our understanding of the *kapha dosha,* its transmuted form of *ojas,* and the Salt Principle.

Mantak Chia speaks to the connections of the trinity in Chinese philosophy:

Traditionally, the Three Pure Ones were visualized as three emperors residing in the three palaces or centers of the body called the upper, middle, and lower tan tiens. They govern the development of the three bodies—physical, soul (or energy), and spirit—within an individual by cultivating three forces manifest in the human body as ching, chi, and shen, respectively. [8]

The Three Miasms of Homeopathy

Samuel Hahnemann (1755–1843), the founder of homeopathy, introduced the concept of three primary miasms at the roots of chronic disease. These were seen as pathological patterns with deeply seated, inherited, or chronic tendencies, under which a multitude of specific symptoms and diseases are categorized. These patterns of predisposition are referred to as syphilis, sycosis, and psora, which were, interestingly enough, treated with homeopathically prepared mercury, salt (nat mur, in homeopathic terms)[§], and sulfur, respectively. These are of course our Three Alchemical Principles. The miasms were named after common chronic diseases of Hahnemann's time: syphilis, scabies (psora), and gonorrhea (sycosis). Given that they are considered constellations of symptoms rooted on a constitutional level, they are in a way similar to the *doshas,* which are also seen as primary patterns of constitutional imbalance.

Hahnemann's concept of miasms came under much criticism, but homeopaths took his ideas to heart and further developed them into a model of practice that ultimately turned into a valid clinical model. Although the original concept was not particularly

---

[§] The other primary remedy used in the treatment of sycosis was *Thuja occidentalis.*

metaphysical in nature, Hahnemann's followers did notice those implications, as explained by Matthew Wood:

> Like the law of similars, from the doctrine of the chronic miasms came the basis for the generation of much commentary of a theological and theosophical nature. The idea that psora was the primordial disease, going back to the very beginning of human existence, offered ample scope for imaginative dilation. Psora was identified with the primal human contagion, contracted in the fall from Paradise. This connection was made both by writers who were critical of Hahnemann and those that supported him. [9]

Psora generally relates to symptomatic patterns associated with irritation, inflammation, and overall hypersensitivities of the body. These are notably *pitta* dynamics. It adversely affects the digestive and eliminative organs and thus can lead to overall states of toxicity and inflammations associated with it. Like Sulfur, people with the psora temperament are often focused on philosophical and religious concepts, high in their ideals but not necessarily practical. Psora was classically treated with homeopathic Sulfur.

Syphilis generally relates to diseases of the nervous system, blood, skeletal system, degeneration and ulceration of the tissues, and congenital defects. Many psychological disorders, such as depression, addiction, and insanity, are considered syphilitic. These all point to the vital force not being correctly anchored in the body to generate proper formation. Temperamentally they are similar to *vata* and Mercury in that they consistently change from one mental state to another. It was classically treated with homeopathic Mercury.

Sycosis generally produces hardened masses, overgrowths, and infiltrations. It often leads to water retention and slowed metabolism, sexual and urinary tract disorders, and afflictions of the joints and mucosal membranes, all which are usually worse in damp weather. These characteristics are quite similar to the *kapha dosha* and relate directly to Salt. This correspondence is also shown in their temperament, which is commonly pessimistic and jealous and has fixed ideals that are difficult to change. It was classically treated with homeopathic Salt and *Thuja*.

Other Threefold Patterns

Other reflections of this threefold pattern include William Sheldon's "three types," which is a simple constitutional system of thin, thick, and medium, shown to be quite compatible with the three *doshas* of Ayurveda in Wood's *The Practice of Traditional Western Herbalism*. The types are the ectomorph (*vata,* thin), mesomorph (*pitta,* medium), and endomorph (*kapha,* thick), their terminology being based on the three main layers of development within the embryo (mesoderm, endoderm, and ectoderm). Sheldon attributed specific physical, psychological, and disease predisposition tendencies to each type. Wood notes the connection of these constitutional patterns to other threefold models, such as the motive, visceral, and nervous types of nineteenth-century Western constitutional analysis, Ayurvedic *doshas,* and primary neuroendocrine pathways.[10]

Wood also points out the derivation of the triadic system of nineteenth-century Physiomedical botanical medicine from the threefold pattern that modern neuroscience calls the ECR cycle (excitation-constriction-relaxation). The ECR cycle describes the physiological connection between the nervous system and muscles via the process of a nerve being excited or stimulated, followed by muscular contraction, and then muscular relaxation after the nerve impulse stops. The same triune pattern formed the basis of the Physiomedicalists' primary threefold energetic understanding of medicinal plants: stimulants (excitation), astringents/tonics (constriction), and relaxants (relaxation). We will explore these dynamics in more detail in chapter 13.

Outside the territory of medical traditions, we see the triune pattern in a wide variety of mythological, religious, and spiritual traditions, as well as modern science. From the Holy Trinity of the Father, Son, and Holy Spirit in Christianity, to Thor, Loki, and Odin in Norse mythology, to the upper, lower, and middle worlds of Greek mythology, and even the neutron, proton, and electron of science—everywhere we look we find a triune pattern. As we study what each of these patterns represents, we often find that they have at least a loose connection to this fundamental trinity.

Figure 7 outlines some of the general correspondences that various traditions have with the Three Philosophical Principles. Their universality is revealed as we see their similarities throughout these traditions. This Holy Trinity is the primary layer of energetic architecture that most directly relates to this physical world as three distinct yet integrated components of every aspect of life. And while they have their material representations, they are also reflected on an energetic and spiritual level. It's only through these Three Principles that the Elemental forces are able to weave together to generate the grandeur of the natural world. They form the foundation for a holistic perspective that enables us to see cohesive patterns within the people we heal and the plants we work with, which we will explore in more detail in part III.

ALCHEMY	SALT	MERCURY	SULFUR
Ayurveda	Kapha, Ojas	Vata, Prana	Pitta, Tejas
Astrology	Fixed Mode: Scorpio, Taurus, Leo, Aquarius	Mutable Mode: Gemini, Virgo, Sagittarius, Pisces	Cardinal Mode: Aries, Cancer, Libra, Capricorn
Chinese Medicine	Jing	Chi	Shen
Homeopathy	Sycosis	Syphilis	Psora
Plants	Minerals	Alcohol/Water soluble chemistry	Essential Oils
Vital Signs	Motion	Respiration	Circulation

ALCHEMY	SALT	MERCURY	SULFUR
Constitution	Endomorph	Mesomorph	Ectomorph
	Visceral	Nervous	Motive
Nutrition	Fats	Carbohydrates	Protein
Molecular	Neutron	Electron	Proton
The 3 Worlds	Lower World	Middle World	Upper World
People	Body	Spirit	Soul
Kingdoms	Mineral	Botanical	Animal
Christianity	Son	Holy Spirit	Father
Hinduism	Vishnu	Shiva	Brahma
Taoism	Taiqing- Grand Pure One	Shangqing- Supreme Pure One	Yuqing- Jade Pure One
Buddhism	Nirmāṇakāya	Sambhogakāya	Dharmakāya

Note: It's important to remember that these are general correspondences and correlations among various traditions. Each tradition elucidates different aspects of the Principles. The purpose of the table is to show the universality of the threefold model and the underlying archetypal expressions of the Three Principles, which span the realms of medicine, physiology, science, spirituality, and myth.

Figure 7. The Three Principles table of correspondences

But there is a much greater pattern, a larger aspect of this cosmological framework that moves up and out beyond the Earth and reaches into the Heavens, coming into contact with the archetypal structure of reality itself. Here we move into the celestial spiritual forces that are channeled down through the Elements and into the Principles. For us to have a complete understanding of the underlying structure of Nature, we must shift our gaze up into the sky to glimpse the eternal light shining through the stars, to see the Sulfur, or soul, of the universe, which is organized according to the pattern of the Seven Planets.

The Seven Planets

*The Principles of Truth are Seven; he who knows these, under-
standingly, possesses the Magic Key before whose touch all the
Doors of the Temple fly open.*

—THE KYBALION[1]

The Seven Planets bring us to a new organizational level of energetic architecture, moving further into the cosmos and at the same
time deeper into the recesses of people and plants. The Sun, Moon,
Mars, Venus, Jupiter, Saturn, and Mercury constitute the pattern of
Nature that reflects our essential self or soul—the Sulfur of people
and plants. They're an essential aspect of energetic architecture in the
art of alchemy and the practice of evolutionary herbalism, for they
allow us to practically apply the ancient axiom of "as above, so below."
Central to Paracelsian medicine is the ability to directly see the Heavens within the Earth.

The Seven Planets of the visible solar system represent the harmonic pattern of creation. It's no coincidence that the visible light
spectrum is divided into seven primary colors, the auditory range has
seven notes on the musical scale, there are seven days of the week,
seven electron rings surrounding atoms, seven *chakras* in the Vedic
tradition, and seven days of creation in the Bible. The pattern of

seven is incredibly rich with mythological, religious, and metaphysical symbolism, as well as practical applications in the sphere of medicine.

Ancient cultures across the globe recognized that celestial bodies directly affect life on Earth, influencing the nature of reality itself. Just as sailors used the stars to navigate through vast oceans to reach new lands, so did the ancient astrologers use them to navigate not only the physical world but also the archetypal landscape. Astrology doesn't just tell you who you are; it helps you see the universe uniquely imprinted in the architecture of your being, with a wide range of practical and esoteric applications. Astrology was not just the concern of mystics, natural philosophers, artists, visionaries, and political leaders, but also of physicians. In the older days of medicine, it was standard procedure for university-trained physicians to be well versed in astrology. Nicholas Culpeper summarized the importance of astrology when he said, "To such as study astrology, who are the only men I know that are fit to study physick [medicine], physick without astrology being like a lamp without oil."[2]

The astrological pattern was seen as the Light of Nature shining throughout the physical world, illuminating the path of the ancient physicians. A common analogy that helps us understand what astrology does for a physician notes that we use telescopes to see things far away and microscopes to see the miniature world, whereas astrologers use horoscopes to see the underlying influences affecting the human body, spirit, and soul. Astrology forms a critical element of diagnostics, assessment, classification of medicines, therapeutic principles, formulation, and pharmacy. This long-forgotten element of the practice of medicine offers precise, indispensable tools for understanding people and plants holistically. This medical application of "as above, so below" takes holistic medicine to entirely new levels, as we not only understand the whole plant and the whole person, but their relationship to the *whole cosmos.*

It's important to understand that the Seven Planets not only refer to the bodies orbiting the Sun in our solar system. Just as the Elements and the Principles have specific physical manifestations, the planets are material representations of greater archetypal forces. They are an organizational pattern of the natural world and thus are embodied within all things in varying amounts and ratios. While I am using the terminology of the Planets here to maintain the language of alchemy, it's important to recognize that they also generally correlate to other sevenfold patterns, such as the *chakras* of the Vedic tradition and the *dhatus* of Ayurveda.

The astrological model provides a new lens for seeing into Nature, functioning as a translation mechanism that correlates the physical, energetic, and spiritual characteristics of people and plants. While it's common in medical astrology to see physical correspondences and in general astrology to focus on psychological or spiritual attributes, my goal here is to show how they are reflections of one another and are intricately interwoven. *They are the same pattern applied on different scales of being.* Here we will briefly introduce each Planet and some of their general correspondences, with further detail on their specific signatures and correlations in people and plants in part III.

☉ The Sun

The Sun, resting at the center of our solar system, is the physical embodiment of the pure energy of Creation that provides, sustains, and distributes life. Its traditional glyph—a circle with a dot in the center—signifies its central location at the heart of the cosmos and the vital spirit at the center of all things. Within us, it's the spiritual essence of the heart that nourishes every part of our being. The Sun exists at the center of any living thing, so all peripheral properties and attributes orbit around the solar essence. As the center of the wheel of time, it regulates the four seasons, plant growth, migration patterns, and the cycles of Gaia. In its most simple definition, the Sun represents Life itself.

Classically, the solar archetype is represented by the King, the leader of the world, the central hub that governs all the parts. It represents power and thus displays similarities to the *manipura chakra,* located in the "solar" plexus. The Sun represents our inner life force that imbues the body with vitality and instills personal power in the psyche. The astrological sign of Leo—present during the summer, from June 21 to July 21, when the Sun is at its peak—is ruled by the Sun. Leo represents the expressive nature of the individual and is often related to people who like to be the center of attention, much like the Sun is at the center of all the Planets. The alchemists saw gold and recognized it as a metallic reflection of the Sun, or rather, a material embodiment of light. Thus, the value of gold was not originally based upon any particular material value, but rather its spiritual virtue.

The Sun has an orbital period—the length of time it takes to circulate the entire birth chart—of one year. This means our birthday is our solar return because that's when the Sun returns to the precise place in our chart where it was at the time of our birth. Wherever the Sun is located within the chart represents our core identity, the gravitational center of our psyche around which our entire being orbits. Its evolutionary function is to develop our essential spirit and unite it with our persona, teaching us to shine outward from the heart and live in accordance with our truth.

☾ The Moon

Whereas the Sun is the dynamic yang, the radiant force of life, the Moon is its opposite: the receptive yin, the magnetic form of existence, ruling the night as the Sun rules the day. In alchemical cosmology, the Sun is sometimes related to Celestial Niter, and the Moon to Celestial Salt. Together they are the King and Queen, rulers of the Heavens. As the Sun is the outward personality and spirit, the Moon is the inner nature, represented by our emotions and feelings. This is signified by her glyph, the crescent, which symbolizes the chalice, a universal symbol for the Water Element. We can consider the essential function of the lunar force as being the inward, receptive quality that receives impressions from the outside world to generate feeling. The Moon doesn't have its own light; it only reflects the light of the Sun, which further indicates her governance of our interiority.

The Moon's nature can be understood by observing her cycles through the sky and their correlation to the feminine archetype. The waxing and waning patterns govern the female reproductive cycle and possess the power to raise the oceans; hence her sympathetic relationship to the Water Element, the womb, and fertility. During the full Moon, she rests opposite the Sun so that she directly reflects its light. In these times, it's common for emotions to express outwardly. Conversely, the new Moon is when she and the Sun are conjunct, or on top of each other, so that she disappears from the sky and leaves us in darkness. This signifies the unconscious part of our being, the internalizing of our emotions and feelings, when what lies within the inner world remains hidden from the light of consciousness.

Silver is the corresponding metal for the Moon, with its gentle, soothing color reminiscent of the silvery Moon. The Moon rules the sign of Cancer and the fourth house, relating to the home, the family, and the relationship to the inner self. Cancer represents the cosmic mother, giving birth to new life as the cardinal-Water sign of summer. Yet the fourth house represents the nadir, the lowest point of the chart, the deepest, darkest recesses of our being isolated from the external world. These seeming paradoxes relate to the waxing and waning cycles of the Moon as she becomes fully illuminated and disappears into the darkness. The Moon is commonly related to the *svadhisthana* or *ajna chakras*.

The Moon's orbital period is approximately twenty-eight days, so she moves rapidly through the birth chart. Her movement represents the development of the emotional body and our interiority, or how we experience ourselves. The Moon provides the evolutionary function of cultivating emotional maturity and buoyancy.

♂ Mars

Mars, being a distinctly yang and dynamic Planet, bears similarities to the Sun, although with its own distinct qualities. Whereas the Sun is the King, Mars is the Warrior, who rides out from the castle to defend and protect the kingdom. He is classically associated with war and "martial" arts, blood, intensity, violence, and anger in its less evolved expressions. Mars is desire in action, representing instinctual impulses to hunt, obtain, seize, and hold territory, food, or mates. Whereas the Sun represents the spiritual will and central "I am" consciousness, Mars is the physical muscle and energy that carry out the orders of the kingly solar purpose and Earthly desires, both low and high. But without that higher guidance from the Sun, Mars can be disastrous.

The glyph of Mars—the arrow pointing above the circle—shows the upward and outward movement of the vital force. Its metallic element is iron, which is plentiful on the red planet and signifies its correspondence to the blood. Interestingly enough, most implements of war in traditional times were made of iron.

Mars governs Aries and Scorpio, signs associated with the first and eighth houses. The word "Mars" is the root for the month of "March," when the spring equinox occurs. The Aries season initiates growth and upward movement throughout Nature as life expresses the dynamic energy of Mars. Scorpio resides in the middle of autumn, representing the descent into the lower world and the destruction that Mars is often related to, as Nature decomposes and breaks down before winter. It is commonly related to the *manipura chakra,* the center of will, action, and strength.

Mars orbits around the Sun in approximately two years. Any parent knows that the two-year-old child develops a new expression of willpower, often by discovering the word "No!" Its location in the chart denotes an area of life that calls for decisive action and represents the evolutionary function of developing strength and willpower, and aligning them with the higher guidance of the Sun.

♀ Venus

Just as the Sun and Moon exist in polarity, so too do Venus and Mars. Each Planet can be understood more deeply in comparison with its opposite. This relationship is often represented in the glyphs: Mars with the cross above the circle (which was replaced by the arrow above the circle), Venus with the cross below the circle. The Venusian glyph represents the spirit rising above matter through the quality of love and sensing the spirit within life through the perception of beauty. The circle above the cross is a symbol for the hand mirror, as Venus understands that all of life is in relationship, and relationship is a mirror. Venus is a key to seeing the whole within the part, the inner within the outer, through the spiritual heart. This is represented by her planetary metal, copper, which has a distinctive shimmering and reflective quality, as well as being highly flexible and able to be shaped into a myriad of forms.

As Mars is like a concentrated version of the Sun, Venus is like an image of the Moon, though with different qualities. She is the Princess as compared to the Queen, as Mars is the Warrior guided by the solar King. She is the third-brightest light we perceive in the sky from Earth, reflecting the light of the Sun more strongly than any other Planet. Venus represents the higher emotional and spiritual aspects of the sensitive heart that opens through attunement of our sensory perceptions and the feeling of love.

Venus is the law of gravitation and attraction, taking two and bringing them together as one through entrainment. Mars destroys;

Venus unites. The process of self-organization in Nature is an innately Venusian function, as she is the harmonizing principle that synchronizes parts into cohesive wholes. She is associated with love, beauty, sensuality, pleasure, affection, aesthetic perception, and creative expression. Her magnetic quality represents what we magnetize to ourselves, which is based upon our desires. It is our inner Venus that says, "I like this and I don't like that," or "this feels good and this doesn't." Based on these declarations, Mars acts. She is commonly related to either the *svadhisthana* or *anahata chakras*.

Venus rules two signs of the zodiac, Taurus and Libra. In Taurus, Venus manifests as Fixed-Earth, the most *kapha* and earthly of the Signs. This sign is simple, concerned with peace, pleasures of the flesh, and building a life of stability and simplicity. In Libra, Venus manifests as Cardinal-Air, giving her a more active and intellectual nature. Libra, the sign of the scales, is all about perceiving balance and harmony, placing a high importance on relationships.

Venus has an orbital period of approximately 225 days around the Sun and roughly a year around the Earth, representing the full development of the sensory faculties and deep bonding with another. Her primary evolutionary function is the formation of harmonious relationships, reception and expression of love, and the establishment of internal equilibrium with the external world.

♃ Jupiter

Jupiter is the largest Planet in our solar system, a "gas giant" primarily composed of hydrogen and helium. Jupiter represents expansion. Like the Sun, he is a "kingly" Planet, but where the Sun represents our essential nature, Jupiter radiates it beyond ourselves and into the world where it has an actual impact, giving us a vision, dream, or aspiration to work toward.

The ancients considered Jupiter to be the "Great Benefic," meaning that he brings all things good, joyous, and uplifting. Kingly

Jupiter bestows gifts and blessings upon our lives, making us feel genuinely happy. We get the word "jovial" from Jove, another form of Jupiter's original Latin name as rendered in modern English. In the natal birth chart, Jupiter's placement is an area where we are blessed and gifted, where our talents flow naturally and with ease. Jupiter relates to work and abundance; as we focus on our gifts and talents, our path and purpose naturally unfold. He also relates to the faith and belief we must cultivate in ourselves to see our purpose through.

Jupiter can be likened to a bird soaring through the sky overlooking the Earth. From this perspective he sees the bigger picture of our lives and can make wiser decisions than we can. Hence he is often related to the archetype of the teacher, and in India his name is *guru*. The radiant quality of Jupiter is represented in his glyph: the crescent rising above the cross, showing the vital force rising above physical matter and expanding beyond boundaries. Jupiter carries us beyond what we know, bringing new perspectives, beliefs, and understanding. The one downside of Jupiter is that he is often so busy looking at the big picture that he can overlook the details.

Jupiter's higher perspective is also represented by his rulership of Sagittarius, the archer, whose glyph is the arrow that soars through the sky. This Mutable-Fire sign contains the radiant, expansive quality of the gaseous Planet, who likes to explore new territory both externally and internally through travel and philosophy. Traditionally Jupiter was also the ruler of Pisces, though today it's associated with Neptune. The Pisces correlation is rooted in our spiritual connection, and believing in something higher than ourselves. Sagittarius is philosophy; Pisces is wisdom. The alchemical metal associated with Jupiter is tin, which is a lightweight metal, much like the semimaterial gaseous Planet. It is common associated with the *ajna* or *sahasrara chakras,* where we receive our vision and expand into the beyond.

Jupiter moves in an approximately twelve-year cycle, bringing about new opportunities, visions, and life dreams that dawn in our awareness. When Jupiter touches our lives, he expands us into new territories beyond our current circumstances and limitations. Thus, he represents the evolutionary function of developing faith and belief in ourselves, having a higher vision and aspiration for our life. The three yang Planets of Jupiter, Sun, and Mars represent the harmony of our inner dynamic nature, three reflections of Celestial Niter within our being. Through their harmonious integration, these Planets bridge our essential nature (Sun) with our aspirations, goals, and visions (Jupiter), and instill the strength to act upon them (Mars).

♄ Saturn

To contrast with the expansion of kingly Jupiter, Saturn rules the opposing force of contraction. The ringed Planet is the most distant one we can see, and it is considered the receptacle for the cosmic forces of the outer Planets, which are organized and distributed throughout the physical world. Saturn is the boundary between the visible and invisible Planets and is thus the gatekeeper between the physical and spiritual worlds—the ruler of tangible reality. Saturn governs the materializing aspect of creation, of fixing spirit down into matter; and yet, according to the Hermetic tradition, Saturn is also the liberator of form, stripping spirit from matter, and in this way is related to death. He is the final Planet we visit in the soul's journey through the seven spheres as it is liberated from the body. This is represented by its glyph, the cross above the crescent (note that it mirrors Jupiter's glyph), showing the spirit contained in matter or the scythe carried by death, which liberates it from form.

As the ruler of the material world, Saturn usually doesn't leave you scratching your head wondering whether it's influencing you; Saturn's touch is always experienced *physically*. Whether through a car accident, a life-threatening illness, your home burning to the ground, or losing your job, Saturn typically shakes things up in your life, restructuring your reality as you know it. Although these life lessons are often harsh, they are ultimately our most profound teachers. Called the "Great Malefic" by the old astrologers, Saturn always got a bad rap because of the deep challenges it presents, often represented mythologically by the tyrannical father. However, these challenges are the experiences that shape our character and restructure it in accordance with who we truly are. But that process often requires us to remove what is false.

Saturn represents our personal boundaries and limits, signified by the icy rings that surround it. As Saturn's opposite, Jupiter's role is to expand us beyond these boundaries just enough so we can see beyond them. If we do not get this expansion through Jupiter, Saturn comes in and simply destroys them. With Saturn, *something has to die.* This is what occurs during the often-feared Saturn return, when it comes back to where it was in your chart at your birth. We reap what we sow, either from this life or from past lives (or from epigenetics, karma, or ancestral patterns, if you don't subscribe to reincarnation).

The signs attributed to Saturn are Aquarius (also co-ruled by Uranus), ruler of the eleventh house, and Capricorn, who rules the tenth house. In Aquarius, Saturn is in Fixed-Air, symbolizing the materialization of spiritual principles to affect the greater good. In Capricorn, Saturn is in Cardinal-Earth and the striving for dominion over our physical world. Its metal is lead, the heaviest and densest of the seven alchemical metals, representing the base level of the self to be transmuted into the gold of soul. It is commonly related to the *muladhara chakra.*

Saturn's orbital period takes approximately twenty-nine years and represents the development of new levels of maturity, self-respect, discipline, and boundaries that enable us to anchor the life vision of Jupiter in the material world. The primary evolutionary function of Saturn is the ability to see life itself as a school, as long as we see our experiences as the teachers.

☿ Mercury

The previous six Planets exist in polar dualities with each other: Sun and Moon, Mars and Venus, Jupiter and Saturn, creating a threefold polarity. With Mercury, we have the seventh Planet, which from a philosophical perspective represents the balance point, the androgynous being, neither masculine nor feminine.**

Mercury's nature is always threefold, represented by his glyph: the crescent above the circle above the cross—the only inner Planet to contain all three symbols. This relates to Mercury's relationship to Thrice-Great Hermes, messenger of the Gods, the only archetype who could travel between the upper, middle, and lower worlds. For this reason he is considered the weaver of the worlds, translating the above and below, the inner and outer. Mercury also goes retrograde three times a year for approximately three weeks at a time. It is interesting to note that both the Principle Mercury and the Planet Mercury represent the balance point and bridge between Heaven and Earth.

This concept of mediation and the messenger is central to understanding Mercury. He acts as the medium between the visible (outer) and invisible (inner) worlds, which we express physically through our breath; hence he rules the respiratory system as well as communication, which ties him to the rational mind. Mercury's function is to connect various parts of our being to each other. Each archetype therefore has a "voice" inside our Mercury (our mind). Because of this rulership over communication and Mercury's association with travel, our fast-paced modern world is constructed with Mercurial technologies such as cell phones, the internet, social

---

** Although Mercury is generally considered androgynous from a cosmological perspective, archetypally and mythologically this Planet is generally considered to be male; thus, masculine pronouns are often used to describe the winged messenger.

media, email, cars, and planes. The dynamics of communication correlate Mercury to the *vishuddha chakra* or the throat center.

The signs under Mercury's rulership are Gemini and Virgo. In Gemini, we see a *vata* quality of Mercury as it manifests through Mutable-Air and the qualities of communication represented by the third house. Virgo is a more grounded representation of Mercury as Mutable-Earth, shown as a highly organized and practical mind.

Being the closest Planet to the Sun, Mercury completes his revolutions in only eighty-eight days, the fastest of the Planets—hence his relationship to the metal mercury, or quicksilver, which moves seamlessly between solid, liquid, and gas. This is also a signature for his ability to move between the worlds and the mutable quality of our minds. The primary evolutionary function of Mercury is the development of an intelligent, rational intellect, effective communication, and reception of information.

The Seven Planets encompass a wide range of correspondences with different cultural sevenfold patterns, their archetypal representations woven into the fabric of the ancient stories and mythologies of the world. At their core, they represent seven fundamental layers of our psychological and spiritual being, each one having both positive and negative influences. The goal of alchemical medicine is to develop and transform each inner Planet, refining it to its purest embodiments and highest virtues.[††] This is achieved by understanding planetary characteristics within people and plants on a deeper level of detail, which we will further explore in part III, "Universal Herbalism." We will discuss how this overarching pattern of energetic architecture is the substratum of many herbal traditions and healing models around the world.

[††] This is quite similar to how Ayurveda aims to transform each *dosha* into its refined attribute as *tejas, prana,* and *ojas.*

	SUN	MOON	MERCURY	MARS	VENUS	SATURN	JUPITER
Day	Sunday	Monday	Wednesday	Tuesday	Friday	Saturday	Thursday
Constitution	Pitta	Kapha or Vata (full or new)	Vata	Pitta	Kapha or Vata	Vata	Kapha
Organs	Heart, Blood	Brain, Stomach	Lungs, Mind	Blood, Adrenal	Kidney, Bladder	Spleen, Bones	Liver, Artery
System	Circulatory Vital Force	Nervous, Digestive	Respiratory	Immune	Genito-urinary	Skeletal/Structural	Metabolic
Tissue	Plasma	Mucus	Nerve	Muscle	Reproductive	Bone,	Fat
Plants	Hawthorn St. John's Wort Rosemary	Milky Oats Marshmallow	Fennel Peppermint Osha	Nettle Echinacea Cayenne	Lady's Mantle Motherwort	Red Root Horsetail Oak	Burdock Dandelion Lemon Balm
Metal	Gold	Silver	Mercury	Iron	Copper	Lead	Tin
Energetics	Hot	Moist	Dry/Tense	Hot	Moist, Relaxed	Cold, Dry, Tense	Moist, Warm
Tissue State	Heat/Excitation	Damp/Stagnation	Wind/Tension, Dry/Atrophy	Heat/Excitation	Damp/Relaxation	Cold/Depression, Wind/Tension, Dry/Atrophy	Damp/Stagnation
Actions	Heart Tonic	Demulcent	Expectorant	Stimulant	Diuretic	Astringent	Alterative
Taste	Pungent, Sour	Sweet	Acrid	Pungent	Sweet, Salty	Astringent Salty	Oily, Bitter
Greek	Apollo	Artemis	Hermes	Ares	Aphrodite	Kronos	Zeus

Figure 8. Table of planetary correspondences

PART III

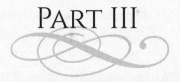

Universal Herbalism

Planetary Herbalism is a term that denotes the integration of the world's most developed systems of traditional herbal medicine. It integrates the traditional differential classification of diseases with the energetic classification of herbal medicines, and includes all useful contributions, past or present, including scientific knowledge.

—MICHAEL TIERRA[1]

For thousands of years herbal traditions have mostly been contained to their particular geographical and cultural regions—until now. The modern-day herbalist has access to vast amounts of information, perspectives, and traditions that have never before been so widely available. We have the capacity to see outside our own models and learn how other traditions came to similar conclusions about people and plants while developing their systems of herbalism. We can synthesize and integrate these seemingly different traditions into a cohesive, comprehensive system of plant medicine, one that unites the core principles and practices of true holistic herbalism in a perennial philosophy. We now have the ability to create a system of universal herbalism.

This concept of integrating different traditions into a universal system first came to me while I was studying Michael Tierra's groundbreaking modern classic, *Planetary Herbology*.[2] In it Tierra reveals the underlying patterns within Ayurveda, traditional Chinese medicine, and Western herbalism, applying Eastern systems of energetics to Western herbs. I was further influenced by the work of Dr. Vasant Lad and Dr. David Frawley in their synergistic approach to Ayurveda and Western herbalism. Through their work I realized that these traditions are not limited to their geographical regions or specific materia medica; rather, they constitute *universal truths* of medicine and plants.

I was further inspired and influenced by the work of Paul Bergner[‡‡] and Matthew Wood,[3] both of whom have done extensive research on Western vitalism as expressed in North American traditions, most notably Thomsonianism, Physiomedicalism, Eclecticism, and homeopathy. Their groundbreaking work has translated the older language of these traditions into modern concepts, enabling the new era of herbalists to integrate the perspectives, practices, and models of these skilled physicians. My goal in this section is to further elaborate on this idea of synergy among herbal traditions by integrating the Western esoteric traditions of medical astrology and alchemy with both Eastern and Western herbalism, and to elucidate their connections to the energetic architecture model.

Traditional Western herbalism is incredibly refined in its understanding of the vital force and the clinical application of plants, but it often lacks a metaphysical background. Western herbal systems were, for the most part, strictly physiological and often didn't integrate a greater cosmology or a spiritual understanding. This was one element of medicine that Paracelsus sought to revolutionize in

---

‡‡ Recommended works of Bergner's include three audio courses: *Vitalist Treatment of Acute Symptoms, Materia Medica Intensive,* and *Advanced Herbal Actions and Formulations.*

the seventeenth century. Interestingly, alchemy and medical astrology are quite similar to Eastern traditions that also maintained a connection between their medicine and metaphysics. It's not that Western herbalism lacks a cosmology; it has just been hidden or outright suppressed.

The foundations of alchemy are rooted in the same patterns upon which these herbalist systems are built, both Eastern and Western. Alchemy, like Chinese medicine and Ayurveda, seeks to understand the deeper meaning behind form, tracing the relationships of people and plants to the macrocosm. Alchemy gives us a physiological model that corresponds to a metaphysical or spiritual model of plant medicine. This correspondence enables us to see the relationship between the body, energy, and soul forces of people and plants, giving our practice of plant medicine a metaphysical backbone.

My goal in the coming chapters is to outline a holistic model for understanding people and plants in a way that integrates their physical, energetic, and spiritual properties while corresponding them to the pattern of energetic architecture. I will draw upon various traditional models, such as Ayurveda, Chinese medicine, Western herbalism, medical astrology, and alchemy, showing their correspondences and relationships with one another.

It's important to understand that each of these systems is complete, whole, and intact unto itself. We don't have to synergize traditions to have an effective practice of herbalism. One can solely understand Chinese medicine, Ayurveda, or Western herbalism on its own and practice with precision and efficacy. It's not my intention to dilute these traditions in any way, nor to remove them from their cultural context, but rather to show that beneath these systems are universal principles revealed to those who astutely follow the Light of Nature. I believe that by studying these universal principles and patterns, we can achieve a holistic, well-rounded understanding of the human and botanical kingdoms that will allow us to bring about transformational levels of healing.

The Principles of Vitalism

*Vitalism is not just a philosophy, but a strategy.... Hippocrates
called this "the healing power of Nature." Nature is much more
multidimensional than just a force. Nature is a force with intelligence. A force with transcendent wisdom. A force with a pattern
and a design beyond our comprehension.*

—PAUL BERGNER[1]

The main approach to the practice of traditional medicine, including herbalism, has always been vitalism, which evolved from the
original "spiritism" approaches common in indigenous medicine,
whereby spirits are seen as the causes and cures of disease. The vitalist approach is found in folk practices as well as the great organized
systems: Ayurveda, Chinese medicine, Greek, Unani-Tibb, and North
American medical traditions such as Thomsonianism, Physiomedicalism, and Eclecticism. It is also the basis of homeopathy. While there
are distinctions among these traditions, upon closer observation we
find more similarities than differences.

Vitalism is founded upon the idea that the living body is intrinsi-
cally different from the cadaver, most notably in the presence of a life
force that animates it. This vital force imbues the body with life and
possesses an innate intelligence that maintains the organism's proper
functioning and self-organization. According to vitalist traditions, if

the body is sick, we can rely upon it, in some measure, to heal itself; accordingly, we work with this life force to restore the organism to health. A universal principle among vitalist traditions is that *medicines are used to support the body's innate, self-regulating healing power*. This is in contrast to the mechanistic model of medicine, which treats the body as a machine: if a part isn't functioning correctly, we can either fix it or take it out and replace it.

Vitalism is more than a model of medicine; it is a perceptual and strategic approach to the practice of medicine and to the world. This way of seeing life is rooted in acknowledging the intelligence of Nature, commonly referred to in the West as the *vital force*. This life force directs the life within a medicinal plant, the organ systems and tissues of the body, and even the patterns of disease—for disease is a part of Nature as well. Everything living contains the intelligence of the vital force, and the healer's duty is to work in accordance with it. The vital force is truly the root of natural medicine, for we are just following Nature. Paracelsus says, "Nature causes and cures disease, and it is therefore necessary that the physician should know the processes of Nature, the invisible as well as the visible man."[2]

This is the opposite approach of modern allopathic medicine, which suppresses the vital force by chemically overriding its innate intelligence. And many herbalists don't realize that *the same suppression can also be achieved with plants*. The practice of allopathy is not dependent upon *what* type of medicine we use but rather upon *how* we use the medicine.

Unfortunately, the practice of allopathic herbalism is quite common in the modern world of phytopharmaceutical products, standardized herbal extracts, and information pervading the internet, all of which emphasize treating superficial symptoms rather than underlying root causes. While herbs are obviously beneficial for certain diseases, when they are only used in this way, we understand less about their holistic nature and about the holistic nature of the patient. We see only the name of a condition and not the whole person; we see only the superficial property of the plant as opposed to its essential pattern that shows us how and why it heals the way it does. We see the curcumin and not the wholeness of Turmeric. We see the inflammation and not the dryness at its root. It is important to understand the parts, but not at the expense of losing sight of the whole.

In order for us to develop a new paradigm of plant medicine, we must integrate the wisdom of the vitalist herbalists so that we work in accordance with the natural intelligence of plants and of people. Medicine was practiced successfully for thousands of years before we knew anything about pharmacological mechanisms of action or biochemical constituents. We must take what we gather from following *natura sophia* and apply it practically in our understanding of the holistic person and plant so we don't get stuck in allopathic herbalism.

Principles of the Vital Force

The vital force has been known by a wide variety of names throughout cultures; in China it is referred to as *qi* or *chi;* in India it is called *prana;* many indigenous people call it *spirit;* in the West, we often simply call it *life force.* It is a universal energy that flows through all things, from the celestial to the molecular, and as such is mercurial or spiritual in nature. It's the animating factor that gives all forms their unique expression of life. It is invisible, but it can be seen through its effects upon a physical organism.

We assess the vital force of things all the time. Imagine taking a stroll through the produce aisle at the grocery store. If you pick up a bunch of Kale and it's brown around the edges, limp and floppy, you can immediately tell that it's not as vital as a bunch that is dark green, crisp, and erect. When you see a friend who's enthusiastic and full of energy, they are clearly more vital than someone who is tired and unmotivated. These are simple indications of the general expression of the vital force, or the *quality of life* that is moving through the vegetable or the person. Yet there are more specific ways the vital force expresses itself throughout living beings that determine the nature of the life flowing through them.

Because the vital force is, in its essence, life, a good way to see how it influences an organism is to observe the difference between a live being and a cadaver. In people, this is commonly observed based on the three vital signs, which directly relate to the Three Philosophical Principles of alchemy. The first vital sign is **circulation**, or the beating heart, governing the movement of the life-giving blood, and its fullness in the tissues, primarily expressed through our complexion and pulse. All things have circulation, from cells to plants and animals, and even minerals and metals, although on a much slower time frame than we are able to perceive. Circulation corresponds to the Sulfur Principle.

The second vital sign is **respiration**, or breathing. All things breathe in their own unique ways; plants, for instance, take in carbon dioxide and release oxygen, and cells engage in cellular respiration. One of the quickest ways we can tell if someone is alive is if they are breathing. Respiration corresponds to the Mercury Principle.

The third vital sign is **motion**, relating to the Salt Principle. Physical movement is another expression of the vital force, and again, all things move in their own ways and at their own speeds, whether it's a human lifting her arm or a deposit of minerals accumulating within the Earth.

The Three Philosophical Principles constitute a fundamental pattern of vital expression correlating to the soul, spirit, and body of any being. This can also be stated as the essence, energy, and substance of a being. These are the three core expressions of the vital force organized within the pattern of Nature, because everything has identity (Sulfur), intelligence (Mercury), and a physical form (Salt).

The vital force also correlates with the Seven Planets, each of which relate to archetypal forces present within every expression of life, creating functional focuses of energy that constitute an organism. Every living thing has a degree of self-awareness and the ability to differentiate self from nonself. In this way, everything maintains a sense of identity, corresponding to the Sun. Everything communicates (Mercury), reproduces (Venus), occupies a physical body

(Earth), assimilates nutrients (the Moon), moves (Mars), eliminates and metabolizes waste products (Jupiter), and maintains boundaries (Saturn). These seven layers of the self are present within people, plants, animals, and even individual cells.

Another functional pattern of the vital force includes the "four qualities," which date back to ancient Greek medicine and were the foundation of Western medicine for more than two thousand years. The four qualities are based on temperature (hot and cold) and moisture (damp and dry). These qualities were used to assess the medicinal properties of plants, the constitution of a person, and other natural factors such as weather, ecosystems, seasons, and foods. When holistically assessing people and plants we can think of the relative state of temperature and moisture within them as primary expressions of the vital force. These qualities are also used in Chinese medicine, where they were expressed through the polarity of yin (moisture) and yang (heat) in either a state of excess or deficiency. The four qualities are also generally related to the Elements.

These qualities of the vital force and their correspondences to the energetic architecture model are summarized in the table below.

THE PLANETS	THE ELEMENTS	THE PRINCIPLES
Identity (Sun)	Heat (Fire)	Motion (Salt)
Communication (Mercury)	Cold (Earth)	Respiration (Mercury)
Reproduction (Venus)	Moisture (Water)	Circulation (Sulfur)
Physical Form (Earth)	Dry (Air)	
Assimilation (Moon)		
Movement (Mars)		
Metabolism (Jupiter)		
Boundaries (Saturn)		

The energetic architecture of the vital force

The vital force expresses through each pattern of energetic architecture in a way that determines the fundamental principles of life itself. These are the specific forces and factors that reveal to us that life is flowing through an organism. All things have circulation, respiration, and motion, or consciousness, intelligence, and form. Everything contains identity, communication, reproduction, assimilation, action, elimination, and boundaries, and all things express and respond to heat, cold, moisture, and dryness.

It is important to remember that the vital force, while invisible, is not merely an ethereal, spiritual quality; it also has a physical quality. It generates, moves, and eliminates actual substances, and it directly correlates to the function (and malfunction) of the body. The vital force is not separate from the physical tissues but is an integral part of them. Because it relates to form, it follows particular governing laws that are universal in nature. While it is not necessarily physical itself, it is the guiding operative force that influences matter.

The Vital Force Within People

The vitalist sees the body as an incredibly complex, intelligent, self-organized system comprising multiple organizational layers. The largest layer is the constitution, which is a universal principle among vitalist traditions. According to this perspective, each person is imprinted with a particular pattern of energetic qualities that determines the overall form of the body, expressions of organ systems and tissues, psychological dynamics, and predispositions toward health and disease. The constitution instills within us certain strengths and weaknesses that are either accentuated or diminished by how we live our everyday lives: the foods we eat, the thoughts we think, the environments where we spend our time. *Everything* influences our constitution.

The next layer is the vital expression of the organ systems, each of which has its own particular set of physiological *and* psychological attributes. Every part of the body contains a unique type of intelligence, a particular form and function that maintains its innate biological equilibrium as well as that of the whole system. When this equilibrium is disturbed, we get sick, as the vital expression is perturbed to the point where it loses its self-organization with the rest of the body's ecosystem. The part is no longer in synch with the whole. To inform us that something is wrong, the body speaks to us through the language of symptoms, which are its intelligent dialect informing us how to come back to "homeodynamis."§§

Vitalism sees symptoms as a language. They are not enemies to fight; instead, they are intelligent communications to listen to, translate, and follow to their roots in order to enact an appropriate cure. This perspective lays a foundation for effective diagnosis and informs a therapeutic approach that follows the innate wisdom of the body rather than suppressing it. As we come to understand the balanced and imbalanced vital expressions of the organ systems—their excesses, deficiencies, strengths, and weaknesses—we learn to perceive their holistic nature and how to regain their innate homeodynamis. The vitalist achieves this by perceiving the specific energetics of the tissues, expressed through patterns of temperature, moisture, and tone, which then give rise to certain symptomatic constellations. These vital qualities of the tissues lie beneath the symptoms and constitute a critical distinction between the allopathic and vitalist herbalist, whether we acknowledge them or not. The symptom, the message, is ultimately the vital force trying to

---

§§ The word "homeostasis" is commonly used to denote physiological balance, but it contains the word "stasis," indicating a static state. The word suggests that once you get there, you've arrived at the top of the mountain—you've achieved balance and will never lose it. But a slight breeze might blow and disturb that short-lived homeostasis. A much better term is "homeodynamis," a term used by herbalist Stephen Harrod Buhner. This term indicates that *balance is a dynamic state*, ever changing with the flux and flow of the natural world, a constant reassessment of the internal state with the outer environment. Homeodynamis is the process all organisms use to maintain their self-organization and internal coherence. I believe it is a better representation of our holistic balance than homeostasis.

get our attention and teach us how to live in balance with our inner constitution and the outer environment.

A great example of this is a fever, which is a brilliant response of the body's vital intelligence. When a pathogen enters the system, the immune system reads its specific nature and signals the hypothalamus, the higher regulatory center in the brain, to respond in two primary ways: first by opening or closing the pores of the skin, and second by increasing the basal set-point body temperature to the precise degree necessary to denature the pathogen. The heat of the fever is supported by increasing the rate of circulation of the blood, which causes heat through friction on the walls of the vessels; thus, it is regulated by our old friend, the sensitive heart.

Unfortunately, modern medicine sees a fever as the enemy, not as an intelligent vital response. Thus, modern physicians give febrifuge drugs to lower the fever and suppress the vital force, or an herbalist gives something like Willow bark. You may feel better in the short term, but the period of suppression allows the pathogen to reproduce, prolonging the symptoms in ways that wouldn't occur were the vital force simply allowed to do its job. Luckily for us, we have the category of herbs called diaphoretics, which support the vital response of the fever by increasing baseline temperature, dilating peripheral vasculature, and stimulating circulation.

In addition to using plants for healing, vitalist traditions also emphasize appropriate diet and nutrition. The vital force is directly integrated into the tissues, and the state of the tissues is related to the proper digestion and assimilation of food. Most of the vitality we generate internally is dependent upon both the foods we eat and our ability to properly digest and assimilate their nutrients and eliminate their wastes. Thus, the vital force is, in a general sense, related to metabolism. Vitalist traditions see that food is our first medicine, and proper digestion is critical to optimal health. The true vitalist herbalist is also a nutritionist—and not in the sense of counting calories.

We also inherit a certain degree of vital force from our family. This can be referred to as the "vital reserve," a term I learned from herbalist Paul Bergner.[3] Vital reserve can be likened to our inner savings account of vitality. Much of this reserve is instilled into our constitution at birth and is influenced by our parents' level of vitality at the moment of conception, throughout pregnancy, and at the time of birth. Astrologers look to the specific day, time, and place of birth to get a snapshot of the overall vitality of their constitution through the birth chart. We can either preserve or deplete our vital reserve through the particular lifestyle we choose to live. Activation of the vital reserve is seen especially in periods of stress, enabling us to exert a significantly greater amount of energy than in a normal state, such as a soldier carrying a wounded comrade in combat. Certain rejuvenative therapies can be used to replenish a depleted vital reserve, as is the case with the adaptogens, *chi* tonics of Chinese medicine, or the *rasayanas* of Ayurveda.

This vital reserve is similar to the concept of *yuan qi* in Chinese medicine, which is referred to as "primordial *qi*" and considered the "vital foundation of life."[4] In Ayurveda the vital force can be likened to the transformed expressions of the three *doshas: prana (vata), tejas (pitta),* and *ojas (kapha).* David Frawley notes that *"Prana, Tejas,* and *Ojas* are the rejuvenative forms of *Vata, Pitta* and *Kapha dosha,* which in turn are the disease-causing aspects of *Prana, Tejas,* and *Ojas."*[5] The vital reserve specifically relates to *ojas,* which is considered the most refined vital fluid essence of the body that confers longevity, endurance, health, and vitality. Further elaborating on *ojas,* Vasant Lad states: *"Ojas* is the vital energy that controls the life-functions with the help of *prana. Ojas* contains all of the five basic elements and all the vital substances of the bodily tissues."[6]

Paracelsus referred to the vital force as the *archeus,* which he defines as "an essence that is equally distributed in all parts of the human body, if the latter is in a healthy condition; it is the invisible nutriment from which the visible body draws it strength, and the qualities of each of its parts correspond to the nature of the physical parts that contain it."[7] According to his philosophy, the *archeus* manifests through the *mumia,* or the inner balsam, the life power inherent within flesh, which is more like the substance or vehicle for the vital force.

The vital force of a person has multiple points of contact with both the inner and outer worlds. When exposed to external factors discordant with the baseline homeodynamis of the body, the vital force responds to maintain equilibrium. For example, when we feel too cold, shivering mechanisms are triggered, or when we get too hot we start sweating. When a pathogen invades, the vital force responds with a fever. When we are around an unsafe person, we get an instinctual bad feeling in the pit of our stomach (the instinctual gut brain). These perturbations include environmental and weather changes, social situations, thoughts and feelings we experience, and literally anything we put into our bodies or are exposed to. The vital force is aware of everything.

That's why, from an herbalist's perspective, we must consider the role played by the vital force when we administer a remedy. It's popular to think that when we ingest an herbal medicine, the medicine works in a biochemical fashion through molecular compounds binding to receptors in a way that alters the body's functioning. This would be seen as the primary response. But from the vitalist's perspective, it is not only the plant acting upon the body, but the body's vital force responding to the vital force of the remedy by influencing the temperature, moisture, and tonal qualities of the tissues. These are the secondary responses of the body to the remedy.

The holistic herbalist always works in accordance with the vital intelligence of the body, preserving and protecting it, building and strengthening it. We want to do more than ameliorate symptoms; we also aim to increase the person's innate vitality so they can reach vibrant states of health throughout their whole being.

The Vital Force Within Plants

There's an innate intelligence within plants that determines their overall qualities, including their preferred habitats, growth patterns, morphology, and medicinal properties. From the vitalist's perspective, there is an underlying identity, consciousness, or archetype of the plant, along with its own particular intelligence, which is flowing through and actually generating its physical structure and form. In this way, everything about a plant is a communication, an expression of its consciousness and intelligence imprinted and signed in its form. This fact enables us to see patterns of connection among its natural habitat, morphological characteristics, medicinal actions, organ system appropriations, energetic virtues, and even spiritual qualities. The vital force is the golden thread that allows us to weave seemingly separate elements of a plant together into a cohesive, comprehensive understanding of its essential pattern of wholeness.

A vitalist sees that a plant heals a person not just through its biochemical mechanisms of action that lead to predictable effects, but also through the overarching intelligence expressing through those chemicals. There is a dynamic communication between the vital force of the plant and the vital force of the person. Based on the constitutional variances amongst individuals, plants interact with different people in different ways. What is remedial for one may not be remedial for another, even if they have the same symptom. To study a medicinal plant entails developing a relationship with its vital force and its unique patterns of influence upon the vital force of the person, allowing the practitioner to see the communication that is occurring and to know when that particular conversation is appropriate for healing a specific person.

Communication between plant and person also occurs through the energetics of the plant and its impact upon the ecological status of the tissues. This is universally recognized as the plant's temperature (warming or cooling), moisture (moistening or drying), and tonal (relaxing or tightening) qualities. Although the energetic properties of a medicinal plant are related to its chemistry, they are often overlooked in favor of the modern biochemical model. Through these energetic properties we know how a plant will influence tissue state patterns and the patient's constitution. Vitalism is an ecological model of physiology and medicinal virtues, seeing both plants and people as reflections of Nature.

We can also understand the vitality within a plant by observing how it moves the vital force of the body, which I like to think of as its "directional flow." This flow can move up, down, inward, or outward. Some remedies tend to sink our energy down and in, a quality common with intensely bitter plants, indicated by a shiver down the spine. Others will send our vital force up and outward, commonly seen in pungent, aromatic plants that make you flushed or sweaty. Some plants contract and tighten the vital force inward, as with astringents, and others will relax it outward, as with antispasmodics. An important therapeutic approach for the vitalist is to see the directional movement of someone's vitality, where it is excessive and deficient, and know how to administer plants to move it back into a balanced directional flow.

Because the vital force is infused into all aspects of people and plants, this principle influences not only the body but also the spirit and soul. Many vitalist traditions recognize that by enacting changes in physiology we also generate changes in the psychological sphere. For example, in Chinese medicine the liver is a hot organ commonly related to the emotional state of anger. If people have problems with the liver and start using herbs to move stagnations there, it can manifest as a flare-up of irritability or frustration. Similarly, the lungs are said to store grief. Each organ system has specific psychological and emotional qualities attributed to it, which are a part of the organ's archetypal form. In Western esoteric medicine, this is understood through the astrological relationships to the various parts of the body.

What occurs in the physical body can directly affect our psychological and emotional states, and the reverse is also true. As plants shift our perception and psychological/emotional orientation, the effects trickle down and manifest within the body. Understanding the holistic nature of a medicinal plant involves seeing how its vital intelligence influences the wholeness of the person, which necessitates sensitizing ourselves to their impact upon our hearts and minds. These patterns of influence can be determined by seeing into the energetic architecture of the plant—its unique embodiment of the Planetary, Elemental, and Principle forces.

Practicing Vitalist Herbalism

Central themes throughout systems of vitalism point toward an effective approach to healing. Most important is that the vital force is *never* to be suppressed in any way whatsoever, unless it is necessary for the survival of the person, such as in the case of a dangerously high fever. The subtle art of therapeutics rests in the ability to perceive and follow the body's vital intelligence and to work with it in a way that supports the innate wisdom of the organism to autoregulate and self-heal. This ultimately translates into the Hippocratic maxim: "**First do no harm.**" When treating a person, it is essential to use the mildest medicines instead of the strongest medicines, to focus all of our work on the preservation of the person's vitality, and to never use medicines that will damage or disrupt the life force.

Beyond the therapeutic context, we must also focus on strengthening and revitalizing the life force. Most traditions of healing have specific principles related to the the promotion of health, vitality, and longevity. These medicines are often called "tonics," though the word is overused and diluted in Western herbalism. Chinese medicine has highly refined *chi* tonification protocols that replenish and revitalize a depleted system. In Ayurveda, rejuvenative therapy is referred to as *rasayana*. As Lad and Frawley note, "*Rasayana* is what enters *(ayana),* in the essence *(rasa)*. It is what penetrates and revitalizes the essence of our psycho-physiological being."[8] This therapeutic approach aims to rejuvenate the body, spirit and soul of the person, achieving an optimal state of radiant health on all levels of being. The process involves educating each individual about their own unique physical and psychological disposition, what types of foods are best suited for them, what parts of the self are in need of development, and how to cultivate a lifestyle that maintains their internal and external balance. This approach to herbalism helps people reach their most optimal physical and spiritual health, expressed through vitality and energy, psychological clarity, emotional balance, and a connection to a greater life purpose.

To develop this model of plant medicine, we must understand the holistic nature of people and plants on a deeper level. We need a system of classification that describes how plants function through their vital force. This helps us understand how and why herbs are therapeutically active for certain symptoms and diseases through their operations upon the whole person. We also need to know how to perceive a person holistically, to get beyond the context of symptoms and develop an integrative model of physiology, psychology and spirituality. This enables us to effectively apply herbs in a therapeutic and transformative context. In our goal of universal herbalism, we can consider these subjects through the lens of various traditional models of plant medicine and consider their relationships within a cohesive and comprehensive system. In this light, the next chapters will focus on the holistic person and the holistic plant and how to understand both within the context of energetic architecture.

The Holistic Person

*A physician who knows nothing more about his patient than what
the latter will tell him knows very little indeed. He must be able to
judge from the external appearance of the latter about his internal condition. He must be able to see the internal in the external
man.... He must have the normal constitution of man present
before his mind and know its abnormal conditions, he must know
the relations existing between the microcosm of man and the macrocosm of nature, and know the little by the power of his knowledge
of the great.*

—PARACELSUS[1]

When people begin studying herbalism, they commonly focus on the
plants, but we must not forget the other half of the herbal medicine
equation: *the people we heal.* In order to understand the holistic nature
of plants, we must first understand the holistic nature of people and
the various layers of being that plants influence. Through knowing
the whole human we can learn the whole plant. This entails seeing the
relationships between the human body, psychological structures, and
the evolutionary potentials of the soul (if we can), so we can fit them
together into a whole pattern.

Just as plants are often pigeonholed into isolated categories, it's easy to become overly linear and reductionist in assessing and understanding a person. Too often this attitude manifests as a narrow focus on symptomatic expressions of the body. If the herbalist sees only the symptom, they lose sight of the whole person, including how their state of mind, emotions, relationships, daily life, diet, and spiritual outlook are affecting their health.

On the opposite end of the spectrum, there is currently a slew of herbalists focusing solely on the psychological, emotional, and spiritual spheres, using subtle forms of herbal medicines such as flower essences or plant-spirit healing to support these more "volatile" layers of the self. While this approach can be powerfully healing and supportive, it's important to understand that the psyche cannot be seen—or treated—as separate from the body. Our goal is an integrative model that sees both psyche and body as essential aspects of our whole being. Approaching a person with this holistic lens may enable us to decipher the core underlying patterns, guiding us to select the most appropriate plants that will lead to transformational healing.

The Three Functional Layers of the Human Organism

In general, we can consider the most basic underlying structure of the human organism through the Three Principles: Salt, Mercury, and Sulfur, or body, spirit, and soul. The spirit in this context refers to the psychological and emotional layers of the self, which translates the qualities of the soul into the physical body. The soul is the essential self, the consciousness seeking growth, transformation, and a deeper connection to the divine principles of life. The body refers to the various layers of our physiological organization, from the large-scale patterns of the constitution down to the cellular level. Evaluation of the whole person involves assessing the Salt,

Mercury, and Sulfur levels, searching for the central patterns that are most influential in their life and particularly in their current circumstances. The ultimate goal is to seek each level's unique pattern of energetic architecture.

Sulfur: The soul's evolutionary potential, karma, ancestral patterns, epigenetics

Mercury: Psychological temperament, emotional disposition

Salt: Constitution, organ systems, tissue states

From the perspective of many medical traditions, the roots of imbalance can grow from any of these three functional layers, and each directly influences the others. Many people think that all health issues arise directly from the soul and gradually manifest down into the body, but while the vital force does move from spirit down into the body, it also rises from matter up into the spirit. In this way, health conditions with a primary root in the physical body can move up and affect the emotions, mind, and soul. A good example of this is food intolerance, wherein consuming a food that is unacceptable and pathogenic to the body can lead to an entire constellation of psychological symptoms such as anxiety and depression.

If we choose to work with a person on only one of these functional layers, then we are likely to overlook the other two-thirds of the person, which greatly reduces our chances of finding the root cause and thus a therapeutic approach that leads to transformational healing. Yet at the same time, through the doctrine of correspondence ("as above, so below"), treatment of one layer may be able to reach all three levels.

Herbal traditions are all looking at the same thing, but based on their unique perspectives they end up with a different picture, a different system or model of practice that seems different from the others on the surface, even though it's describing the same thing. Universal herbalism is based on cultivating a 360-degree view of herbal medicine so we can integrate the various perspectives and

practices of the larger and better-known traditions of plant medicine into a cohesive and comprehensive system that ultimately
facilitates the healing of the body and the evolution of the soul.

Salt: Integrative Physiology

We can understand the physiological level of the human organism
based on three primary organizational layers: the constitution, the
organ systems, and the ecological state of the tissues. These provide
a precise and holistic understanding of the wholeness of the body
and how its various forms and functions interact with one another.
As we will see, this ability to observe patterns of relationship within
the body is not based on a strictly linear understanding of anatomy;
instead it relates the different elements of the body to the patterns
of energetic architecture. We can think of this as a more esoteric
model of physiology in which organs, systems, and tissues are not
only physical in nature but are also carriers for subtle forces that
directly influence the mind and soul.

CONSTITUTIONAL ASSESSMENT: THE FOUNDATIONAL PATTERN

The term "constitution" describes a set of governing foundational
principles, deriving from the same root as "constituent." Thus, a
person's constitution represents the foundational constituent parts
and governing principles that determine the state of the whole
organism. We can think of the constitution as a particular pattern of
physiological tendencies, including the overall shape and structure
of the body, predispositions towards health and disease, and organ
system weaknesses and strengths. Constitutions generally also have
psychological tendencies.

The importance of constitutional assessment rests in the ability
to perceive patterns of wholeness within the person, preventing us
from focusing too narrowly on superficial symptoms. We want to
be able to see what's *behind* the symptom, what's underneath the
surface. This critical practice must be deeply integrated into our

perception when we are working with people. Constitutional systems enable the herbalist to see how a person expresses particular symptoms or disease patterns in ways that are unique to them. This is important because different constitutional types can express the same symptoms but with differing underlying causes that would be treated differently.

There is a wide variety of constitutional systems throughout medical traditions, each one focusing on a different layer of energetic architecture. For the most part, we see a primary orientation around the Three Principles as the fundamental constitutional pattern. Quite popular in modern herbalism is the tri-*dosha* system of Ayurveda—*vata, pitta,* and *kapha*—which correlate to Western physiognomy's endomorph, ectomorph, and mesomorph types developed by William Sheldon. Dr. D. H. Jacques developed three temperamental types based on primary expressions of the nervous system: the nervous/mental, motive, and vital/visceral constitutions. These constitutional models have been used by both alternative and conventional physicians in the West since the 1800s. Interestingly enough, these practitioners had no concept of the tri-*dosha* system but arrived at the same conclusions. As Matthew Wood points out in *The Practice of Traditional Western Herbalism,* the threefold pattern is a natural approach for health because thin, medium, and thick people tend to manifest the same general problems: thin (nervous, atrophic), medium (overactive, hot), and thick (overeating, lack of exercise).

Greek medicine had a constitutional system composed of the Four Humors, which were related to four primal fluids of the body: choleric, phlegmatic, sanguine, and melancholic, corresponding to red bile, white bile, yellow bile, and black bile, respectively. Until the seventeenth century this was the primary model used in European medicine, which, after some time, was ultimately uprooted and replaced with a simpler threefold model. The Chinese use the Five Elements of Earth, Water, Fire, Metal, and Wood.

The general correlations between these constitution systems are outlined below, as per the work of Matthew Wood.

DOSHA	WESTERN	AYURVEDIC ELEMENTS	TCM ELEMENTS
Vata	Ectomorph	Air (dry) Ether (nervous)	Metal
Pitta	Mesomorph	Fire (hot) Water (oil)	Fire Wood
Kapha	Endomorph	Water (water) Earth (cold)	Water Earth

Figure 9. Constitutional systems

Innate and Acquired Constitution

An important concept from Ayurvedic constitutional theory is the idea that we have an innate constitution we are born with, called *prakruti,* and an acquired constitution that we develop over time, called *vikruti*. *Prakruti* is the set of patterns infused into us at the moment of birth. *Vikruti,* on the other hand, is the set of patterns we acquire over time as we experience environmental perturbations, eat certain foods, and engage in specific activities. The *prakruti* is our unique and individualized embodiment of balance, whereas the *vikruti* is the imbalanced dynamic that develops as we live incongruously with our core constitution. The ultimate goal of natural therapeutics is to restore the *vikruti* and *prakruti* to harmony with one another so we can express the highest virtues of our constitution. Astrologically, we can say that *prakruti* relates to the natal birth chart, and *vikruti* relates to the dynamics of transits and progressions that affect and influence that core pattern.

The process of determining one's primary constitution involves assessing every minute detail of the body, the person's overall disposition, and characteristic patterns that express themselves consistently throughout the life of the individual. This involves looking at the structure, shape, and form of the body as a whole; the specifics of the hair, skin, and nails; the arms and legs; the temperature (hot/cold), moisture (wet/dry), and tonal (tense/relaxed) dynamics; the quality of digestion; appetite and thirst; psychological and emotional patterns; and disease tendencies. The goal of this in-depth analysis is to look for the core pattern that is most consistently expressed through the individual's life *(prakruti)*, as well as the pattern that is currently manifesting *(vikruti)*.

Generally speaking, we have one primary constitutional mode of expression. However, the doctrine of correspondence tells us that we have *all* of the Elemental, Principle, and Planetary patterns within us. Thus, it is common for people to have a primary and a secondary "ruler" for their constitution. In Ayurveda, this is summed up by various combinations of the *doshas,* which lead to seven expressions: *pitta, vata, kapha, pitta-vata, pitta-kapha, vata-kapha,* and *vata-pitta-kapha* (i.e., tri-*doshic)*. It is interesting to note that there are seven possible combinations of the *doshas,* which I relate to the seven Planets of astrology as follows:

Pitta	Sun
Kapha	Moon
Vata	Saturn
Pitta-kapha	Jupiter
Pitta-vata	Mars
Vata-kapha	Venus
Vata-pitta-kapha	Mercury

ORGAN SYSTEMS: STRUCTURAL ORGANIZATION

From the constitutional level we move down into the primary structural organization of the body. Whereas the constitution tells us *why* someone expresses certain dynamics and qualities, the organ-system level points to *where* in the body those patterns will manifest.

The study of anatomy and physiology is an important task for the budding clinical herbalist. Knowing the physiological functions of the organ systems, as well as their anatomical locations, is vitally important in aiding our understanding of pathological expression and deepening our awareness of how herbal medicines work. However, as our knowledge of the body's forms and functions has developed throughout history, there has been a gradual replacement of an ecological model of anatomy and physiology with a mechanistic one. Today, this approach has reached an extreme level, wherein we focus primarily on biochemical imbalances, or what Wood refers to as "molecular lesions," rather than overarching disease patterns. As Wood explains, "Modern biomedicine left behind the idea of general patterns of disease located in the general functions, organs, or systems of the body. That was the break that alienated biomedicine, not only from its roots in earlier Western medicine, but from all other systems of natural therapy."[2]

To effectively treat these pathological patterns as opposed to specific diseases, we need to understand the basic physiological functions of the body in a state of health so we can recognize when they are imbalanced. This involves seeing the organizational layers of the body, starting with the basic cellular units, which self-organize to form particular types of tissues. These different types of tissues generate different organs with specific functional purposes, which then couple together to form organ systems. The organ systems connect and communicate with one another to maintain the dynamic equilibrium of our entire organism, constantly interacting with the external and internal ecosystems, responding to perturbations, and crafting intelligent responses. When communication between the systems fails—when the perturbations become so intense that the tissue, organ, or system cannot maintain its homeodynamis—disease occurs. For our purposes as herbalists, these latter three organizational structures—systems, organs, and tissues—provide the most useful patterns for understanding the body in a holistic manner.

Tissues

Tissues are the primary functional units that come together to form the organs of the body. They are formed by various types of cells— such as hepatocytes, chondrocytes, and lymphocytes—that perform specific physiological functions. Western anatomy and physiology define tissues rather differently from traditional systems of medicine. In Ayurveda, tissue types are called *dhatus,* meaning "constructing element," and they constitute one of the primary foundations of Ayurvedic anatomy and physiology. These primary tissues are plasma, blood, muscle, fat, bone, nerve, and reproductive. The *dhatus* are formed in a progressive manner from gross tissues (plasma) to the most subtle (reproductive) and finally into the refined essence of the body *(ojas).* Blood is formed from the by-products of plasma, muscle from the by-products of blood, and so on. In this way, improper nourishment of one *dhatu* will adversely affect the subsequent tissues derived from it.

The formation of these *dhatus* is dependent upon proper digestion and assimilation of foods. From the perspective of Ayurveda, the principle of *agni,* or digestive fire, facilitates the nourishment and sustainment of these seven tissues, which in turn nourish the organs of the body. Thus any deficiency of digestive fire can lead to a loss of strength and vitality within the tissues, ultimately leading to imbalance and disease.

In *Ayurveda: The Science of Self-Healing,* Lad notes:

> *The seven dhatus are understood in a natural, biological, serial order of manifestation. The post-digestion of food, called "nutrient plasma," ahara rasa, contains the nutrition for all the dhatus. This "nutrient plasma" is transformed and nourished with the help of heat, called dhatu agni, of each respective dhatu.... Rasa is transformed into rakta, which is further manifested into mamsa, meda, etc. This transformation results from three basic actions: irrigation (nutrients are carried to the seven dhatus through the blood vessels); selectivity (each dhatu extracts the nutrients it requires in order to perform its physiological functions); and direct transformation (as the nutritional substances pass through each dhatu, the food for the formation of each*

subsequent dhatu is produced). These three processes—irrigation, selectivity, and transformation—operate simultaneously in the formation of the seven dhatus. The dhatus are nourished and transformed in order to maintain the normal physiological functions of the different tissues, organs and systems.[3]

This process of serial transformation from one *dhatu* to the next is quite similar to alchemical processes and transformational healing principles. In esoteric astrology and alchemical medicine, the Planets within the astral body must be gradually purified, nourished, and transformed in order to lead to physiological and psychological health—a principle reflected in the seven *dhatus* of Ayurveda. Below is a list of the seven *dhatus,* their correlation to Western tissues, and the Planets. It's worth noting here that the right column is the traditional correspondences of the Planets to the *dhatus* in the Jyotish astrology tradition, whereas the other columns are correspondences based on the Western medical astrology rulership of body tissues.

DHATU	SUBSTANCE	PLANET	VEDIC CORRESPONDENCES
Rasa	Plasma	Moon	Mercury
Rakta	Blood	Sun	Moon
Mamsa	Muscle	Mars	Saturn
Meda	Fat	Jupiter	Jupiter
Asthi	Bone	Saturn	Sun
Majja	Nerve, Marrow	Mercury	Mars
Shukra	Reproductive	Venus	Venus

Note: In Western medical astrology, Mars rules both the muscles and the blood. As the Sun rules the heart, it is correlated here to the blood, with muscles correlating to Mars, which gives us strength. Further clinical experience will verify these correlations.

The Ayurvedic scheme closely corresponds to some of the primary tissues and fluids recognized in the West, such as blood, lymph, mucosa, muscle, fat, nerve, bone/connective tissue, and skin. To observe a person holistically, it's important to keep tissue types in mind when assessing the primary area of the body that is afflicted; sometimes the imbalance is not rooted in a particular organ or system, but in a type of tissue. Of course, everything in the body is interconnected, and tissue types are deeply integrated into specific organ systems, such as the mucosa relating to the digestive, respiratory, urinary, and reproductive systems; the nerve tissue relating to the nervous system; and lymph fluids relating to the spleen, lymphatic system, and immunity. As we will see, this is also important because some plant medicines have affinities for specific tissue types rather than for specific organs or systems.

Organs

Organs are divided into different categories in traditional models. In the West, there's a general division based on their relative depth within the body, radiating from the core to the periphery. These are the regulatory (nervous, endocrine), functional/vital (heart, lungs, kidneys, etc.), and defensive (skin, mucosa, immunity) organs. The regulatory organs are really best defined as systems, which we will explore momentarily. The functional or vital organs are those we will focus on here. Defensive organs, such as the skin, mucosa, and immunity, can be also likened to either a particular tissue type or a system.

In the West, we can delineate the following functional organs and their primary physiological functions, along with their correspondences to the Western Elements, the three *doshas,* and the Seven Planets, as shown in figure 10.

ORGAN	PRIMARY FUNCTION	ELEMENT	DOSHA	PLANET
Lungs	Respiration	Air	Vata	Mercury
Heart	Circulation	Fire	Pitta	Sun
Stomach	Digestion	Water	Kapha	Moon
Small Intestine	Assimilation	Fire	Pitta	Virgo
Large Intestine	Elimination	Air	Vata	Scorpio
Liver	Metabolism	Earth	Pitta	Jupiter

ORGAN	PRIMARY FUNCTION	ELEMENT	DOSHA	PLANET
Gallbladder	Bile Secretion	Earth/Fire	Pitta	Saturn/Mars
Kidneys	Fluid/Solid Regulation	Water	Kapha	Venus
Bladder	Fluid Elimination	Water	Kapha	Venus
Pancreas	Digestion/ Metabolism	Water	Kapha	Virgo
Brain	Neural Regulation	Ether	Vata	Moon/ Mercury
Spleen	Filtration	Earth	Kapha	Saturn

Note: Not all organs are attributed to a particular Planet in medical astrology, but rather have specific sign correspondences. This is true for the small and large intestines as well as the pancreas.

Figure 10. The energetic architecture of organs and functions

In Chinese medicine, we see an organ system classification dividing them into yin or yang organs. The solid yin organs are located deeper in the body and are associated with processes of transformation, whereas the hollow yang organs are superficially located and are associated with processes of transportation. The Chinese model of anatomy connects yin and yang organs together through the Five Elements, forming the functional systems of the body.

YIN ORGANS	YANG ORGANS	ELEMENT
Lungs	Large Intestine	Metal
Kidneys	Bladder	Water
Liver	Gallbladder	Wood
Heart	Small Intestine	Fire
Spleen	Stomach	Earth

Figure 11. The yin and yang organs of Chinese medicine

The Chinese organ system, or "five-phase" theory, is a highly refined and complex system that sees patterns of interconnectivity within the physiological organism, as well as its relationship to the psychological self. The Chinese terms for these organs do not necessarily refer to the Western physiological equivalent. For example, the Chinese Spleen refers to the digestive process as a whole, not necessarily the Western anatomical spleen, an aspect of the lymphatic and immune systems. The Chinese physiological model is far too complex to present in significant detail here, but two excellent introductory books to Chinese medical philosophy are *The Web That Has No Weaver* by Ted J. Kaptchuk and *Between Heaven and Earth* by Harriet Beinfield and Efrem Korngold.

In Ayurveda, each *dosha* has five particular modes of expression, which govern particular anatomical regions and physiological processes in the body, as outlined in figure 12.[4]

KAPHA (5 WATERS)	PITTA (5 FIRES)	VATA (5 AIRS)
Kledaka- Water of Stomach, digestion	*Pachaka-* Fire of Gallbladder, digestion	*Prana* -Air of Lungs, inhalation
Avalambak- Water of Chest, stabilize heart	*Ranjaka-* Fire of Liver, blood formation	*Udana-* Air of Throat, exhalation
Bodhaka- Water of Tongue, taste	*Sadhaka-* Fire of Heart, mind	*Samana-* Air of Stomach, assimilation
Tarpaka- Water of Head, brain	*Alochaka-* Fire of Eyes, vision	*Apana-* Air of Colon, excretion
Slesaka- Water of Joints, mobility & lubrication	*Bhrajaka-* Fire of Skin, peripheral venting	*Vyana-* Air of Circulation, blood flow

Figure 12. The five anatomical elements of the doshas

Although they don't encompass the specific physical organs we often consider in the West, these manifestations of the three *doshas* provide insight into the Elemental composition of central organs of the body. For example, we can observe that the stomach has all three *doshas* present within it: Fire through hydrochloric acid, Water as the protective mucosal membrane, and Air through neural innervation and churning movements. When assessing an imbalance within the stomach, we need to see into the deeper order and structure of the organ so we can see which Element is imbalanced and select the appropriate herbal remedies. This is ultimately what the tissue-state model does for us, which we will explore after organ systems.

Systems

In the context of the West, we can consider a few different layers of organ systems: first are the regulatory systems, dispersed throughout the whole body, as opposed to centrally located systems. Regulatory systems include the nervous, endocrine, musculoskeletal, and immune systems, which are connected by the universal medium of the body: blood. These four regulatory systems can be seen as the primary overseers of the body because they influence the functional or vital systems. They relate to the four Elements: immunity/Fire, musculoskeletal/Earth, nervous/Air, and endocrine/Water. From these overarching regulatory systems, we have the systems formed by connecting vital organs, such as the genitourinary system (kidneys, bladder) and the digestive system (stomach, small and large intestines).

Chinese medicine divides the organ systems in correspondence with their associated twelve meridians, which relate to the Western astrological signs of the zodiac. Western medical astrology correlates the signs to general areas of the body and the organs they contain. These correspondences are outlined in figure 13.

SIGN OF THE ZODIAC	AREA OF THE BODY	ORGANS/ SYSTEMS	TCM
Aries	Head	Exterior Thermoregulation	Heart Protector
Taurus	Lower Jaw, Throat	Interior Thermoregulation, Thyroid	Triple Burner

SIGN OF THE ZODIAC	AREA OF THE BODY	ORGANS/ SYSTEMS	TCM
Gemini	Arms, Shoulders	Respiratory	Lungs
Cancer	Upper Abdominal Cavity	Stomach, Upper GI	Stomach
Leo	Chest, Upper Back	Heart, Spine	Heart
Virgo	Central Abdominal Cavity	Small Intestine	Small Intestine
Libra	Lower Back	Kidneys, Pancreas	Kidneys
Scorpio	Lower Abdominal Cavity	Bladder, Reproductive, Large Intestine	Large Intestine
Sagittarius	Hips, Upper legs	Liver, Arterial Circulation	Liver
Capricorn	Knees	Musculoskeletal, Gallbladder	Gallbladder
Aquarius	Lower Legs, Ankles	Nervous System, Peripheral Circulation	Bladder
Pisces	Feet	Lymphatics, Immunity, Spleen	Spleen

Figure 13. The twelve signs, body areas, organ systems, and meridians

Medical astrology provides interesting insights into the coupling of organ systems by observing opposing signs of the zodiac, which represent a spectrum of influence that governs a particular physiological process. For example, Taurus represents the throat and the act of swallowing. Scorpio, its opposite, represents the elimination and detoxification faculties, with its rulership of the large intestine and bladder. Taurus brings things in, and Scorpio lets things out, the anabolic and catabolic sides of metabolism. Scorpio also rules the reproductive system, which develops into full maturity during puberty, along with the structure of the vocal cords and the voice (Taurus).

Another example is how Cancer represents absorption and nourishment, as well as the fluids that deliver nutrients, whereas Capricorn
represents the bones and the formation of structural elements of the
body. Cancer is the mucosal membranes and the gums; Capricorn is
the teeth. Cancer is the synovial fluids; Capricorn is the connective tissues and bones of the joints. The opposites within the zodiac come
together to form functional physiological processes, which correspond
to archetypal forces that represent evolutionary pathways we walk in
this life, effectively connecting soul, spirit, and body. Figure 14 outlines
these sign polarities and some of their organ-system representations, as
per the excellent work of Judith Hill, with a few additions of my own.[5]

SIGN POLARITY	FUNCTIONAL PROCESS
Aries-Libra	PH balance of tissues, Fire and Water balance, Head-Kidneys, hormonal axis (HPA)
Taurus-Scorpio	Ingestion and elimination of food, reproductive-voice development, anabolic-catabolic phases of metabolism
Gemini-Sagittarius	Respiration and distribution of oxygen throughout tissues. Lungs-arteries. The nervous system.
Cancer-Capricorn	Assimilation and nourishing physical structure. Stomach-Gallbladder
Leo-Aquarius	Heart and peripheral circulation. Neuro-muscular junctions
Virgo-Pisces	Neural-gut, Gut Associated Lymphatic Tissue (GALT), Systemic immunity rooted in intestines

Figure 14. Sign polarities and functional physiological processes

The three primary organizational levels of the body—tissues,
organs, and systems—provide a holistic framework for observing
physical structures when assessing a person. But knowing *where* an
imbalance is located in the body isn't enough; we must know specifically *how* and *why* the imbalance is expressing in the organs, which
requires us to look at the state of the tissues that constitute the
organs. This is where we shift into an ecological model of physiology, relating the state of the organs to the natural world.

TISSUE STATES: ECOLOGICAL PHYSIOLOGY AND PATHOLOGY

Whereas both traditional and modern medicine have some sort of organizational understanding of how the body functions, what differentiates them is that traditional cultures saw the human organism as a microcosmic embodiment of the macrocosm of Nature. Rather than seeing the body as a machine made of millions of biochemical gears, they saw the body as an ecosystem or a garden: rivers flowing through our lymphatics and veins, mountains constructing our bones, lakes pooling in our joints and kidneys, winds blowing through our lungs and minds, fires burning in our hearts and stomachs. In this way, they related pathological states to ecological patterns.

This level of specificity gets us beyond seeing superficial symptoms and into understanding a person's unique expression of that symptom, because different people can have the same symptom for different reasons. This understanding ultimately rests in the ecological status of the tissues, or the tissue state, which can be thought of as the constitution of the tissue itself. For example, someone can be constipated for a wide variety of reasons: excess tension preventing proper evacuation, lack of moisture in the mucosal membrane, or having too much cold and lack of digestive secretions. Each of these unique tissue states would be treated quite differently, even though they all cause constipation. There is a wide variety of herbs that relieve constipation, but holistic treatment consists of selecting remedies that balance the excessive tissue-state pattern, based on differences of herbal energetics. This is what makes herbal protocols work due to their specificity—or fail due to their generality.

According to the Western tradition of the Physiomedicalists, there's a general division of six primary tissue-state pathologies, representing ecological patterns of organ, system, and tissue imbalances. Wood outlines this model in significant depth in *The Practice of Traditional Western Herbalism*. It's based on three central tissue dynamics—moisture, temperature, and tone—each of which is divided into two qualities: hot and cold, wet and dry, tense and relaxed. As we will see later, these patterns also form the foundation for herbal energetics. Some of the general qualities and characteristics of these tissue states are summarized in figure 15 and will be explored in depth in subsequent chapters.

TISSUE STATE	GENERAL QUALITIES	PULSE AND TONGUE	COMMON SYMPTOMS
Heat/Excitation	Hypermetabolic, excessive tissue breakdown, oxidation, hypersensitive, reactive, overstimulated	Rapid, superficial. Red coloration, yellow coating, sharp, pointed, "flame shaped"	Fever, hypersensitivities, hyperthyroid, burning pain, ulcers
Cold/Depression	Lowered functioning, slow and sluggish	Slow, low, hidden. Pale with white coating	Cancer, diabetes, constipation, poor digestion, depression
Damp/ Stagnation	Toxic and hyper-accumulating	Sluggish and thick. Damp, thick, wide, swollen	Skin conditions, toxicity, infection, "bad blood"
Dry/Atrophy	Weak, emaciated, malnourished	Dry and cracked	Arthritis, muscular weakness, dry skin, nervousness
Wind/Tension	Overly constricted, changeable symptoms, move throughout the body	Quivering and tense	Stress, anxiety, nervousness, spasm, cramping,
Damp/ Relaxation	Weakness of structural tissues, fluid leakage	Scalloped edges, damp, streamers down the edge	Prolapse, varicose veins, hemorrhoids, runny nose

Figure 15. Physical patterns of the six tissue states

The six tissue states can be related to Elemental, Planetary, and *dosha* imbalances, as well as patterns of excess and deficiency of yin and yang, as shown in figure 16.

PRIMARY QUALITY	TISSUE STATE	EXCESS ELEMENT	EXCESS DOSHA	EXCESS PLANET	CHINESE
Temperature (Pitta)	Heat/Excitation	Fire	Pitta	Mars, Sun	Excess Yang
	Cold/Depression	Earth	Kapha	Saturn	Deficient Yang
Moisture (Kapha)	Damp/Stagnation	Water	Kapha	Jupiter, Moon	Excess Yin
	Dry/Atrophy	Air	Vata	Mercury, Saturn	Deficient Yin
Tone (Vata)	Wind/Tension	Ether	Vata	Mercury, Saturn, Uranus	Excess Chi
	Damp/Relaxation	Water	Kapha	Venus	Deficient Chi

*Chinese practitioners don't often refer to this as "excess yin," but rather simply, dampness.

Figure 16. Energetic architecture of the six tissue states

To get a holistic picture of what's going on within someone's body, assessing tissue-state patterns within the afflicted organs and systems is of paramount importance. Such assessments enable us to see what's occurring behind the symptom and in the constitution of the organs themselves. This knowledge, coupled with a knowledge of herbal energetics, provides a holistic framework that allows you to match the corresponding patterns between the herbs and the person in a way that's suited to their unique situation.

Mercury: Natural Psychology

Modern herbal practitioners are becoming more sensitive to the psychological and emotional climates of the people they work with, because it has become increasingly apparent that our minds and bodies are inextricably tied together. The use of homeopathics, flower essences, and plant-spirit healing to tend to the psychological sphere has become more popular. If done properly, such practices will always attempt to see the connection with the Salt level of being.

Many practitioners who incorporate this approach lack a system for understanding psychological patterns that allows them to find an appropriate remedy. Some resort to computer programs to find the correct homeopathic remedy; others rely solely on their intuitive faculty to diagnose and prescribe. This is indeed a valid approach, but strictly intuitive prescribing may lack a rational basis for using a particular plant, which can lead to potential conflicts with the plant's physical level of action. Many times herbalists have told me about times when they gave a tincture of an herb to support someone psychologically or spiritually, only to find out later that the herb was completely contraindicated for that person's physical constitution and was indeed aggravating their physical imbalances. *We must never neglect the body in the treatment of the mind and emotions.*

Having a framework for understanding psychology can be incredibly helpful. To remain holistic, we must ensure that any framework we use is in accordance with the patterns of Nature. There are as many flower essences as there are flowers, and often there is no organizational pattern for how those medicines line up with specific constitutional and temperamental patterns, making the process of remedy selection convoluted and occasionally overwhelming. The energetic architecture model provides an organizational pattern for understanding primary psychological temperaments that we can use to find remedies sympathetic to those forces, making them a closer match with the specific needs of the person.

Just as we work toward determining the constitutional characteristics of a person's body, we want to do the same for their minds and hearts, and there are quite a few models for doing so. As we will see, the pattern of the three *doshas* provides a valuable model for very generalized psychological characteristics, as do the Five Elements. The Seven Planets also have psychological reflections that are even more specific in their delineations. The beauty of these models is that they are holistic systems of psychology that relate the structure of the mind and emotions to Nature, linking the macrocosm and microcosm. Figure 17 provides some of the general psychological characteristics of the *doshas* and the Elements, with significantly more detail in the next three chapters.

DOSHA & ELEMENTS	PSYCHOLOGICAL & EMOTIONAL PATTERNS
Vata, Air & Ether	Ungrounded, flighty, spacey, experiences fear, uncertainty, lack of psychological and emotional boundaries, nervous, anxious, difficulty in self-expression
Pitta, Fire	Anger, frustration, irritability, patterns of control and domination over others
Kapha, Water & Earth	Greed, possessiveness, stubbornness and rigidity, envy, jealousy, control issues, overall difficulty making changes, resistance

Figure 17. Elemental and dosha psychological patterns

Sulfur: Evolutionary Pathways

The Sulfur layer of the self represents the essential soul, the unique and individualized expression of consciousness. It is the place where we are most deeply wounded and represents the core healing work we have incarnated on this Earth to achieve. According to the soul, we come into this life to grow in self-awareness, seeing life as a hospital, a school, and a church—a place where we come to heal, learn, and worship. This is the part of the self that perceives the specific lessons life presents us to facilitate the development and evolution of our consciousness. In the assessment of the whole person, observing the Sulfur peers into the particular archetypal forces that most strongly influence someone's life.

Just as Sulfur represents the most volatile element of the self, it also represents the most volatile layer of the energetic architecture, which in this context would be the planetary level of organization. The Planets represent seven primary evolutionary pathways of the human organism, seven aspects of the self that we are required to develop to their highest virtue. Each of us embodies and expresses particular planetary forces in a variety of ways—some healthy and coherent, and others more challenging. The forces that give us a hard time are those that aren't well integrated, the aspects of ourselves we don't understand or know how to work with. They are our blind spots. They show us where we need to stretch beyond our comfort zone and develop untended aspects of our lives.

Sulfur on its own is too volatile for physical manifestation; it requires the bridging quality of Mercury to influence the physical world. The patterns of Sulfur as represented by the Planets trickle down and affect our unique perspectives of the world and thus the ways we think and feel. It can sometimes be difficult to differentiate the Sulfur and Mercury levels based on how our soul needs to evolve and what is present in our hearts and minds. But it is through the vehicle of Mercury that Sulfur reveals itself, and in this way, the quality of our psychology directly reflects the quality of the soul, pointing us toward our most relevant evolutionary pathways.

Yet the soul of a person is different from their psychology in certain ways. If we look at psychology only from the perspective of Mercury, all we see is how we want to think and feel differently. But the wisdom of the soul takes us further, asking what life is trying to teach us, what we are being shown that opens us into developing lost, forgotten, or untended aspects of our lives. Sulfur shows us how we can take an unhealthy psychological pattern and transform it into a more balanced expression. It's only through the healthy expression of each of the seven Planetary forces—which ultimately prepare us to integrate the more spiritual virtues of the three outer Planets—that we can come into a place of inner and outer harmony, to become truly whole unto ourselves.

Figure 18 presents a brief outline of the evolutionary pathways of the Seven Planets, with significantly more detail in chapter 12.

PLANET	EVOLUTIONARY PATHWAY AND DEVELOPMENTAL STAGES
Sun	Unique path and purpose in life; knowing one's true essential nature
Moon	Emotional expression, intuition, inner relationship, self-reflection, feeling intelligence
Mars	Will, courage, personal power, taking action in the world, strength
Venus	Formation of healthy and harmonious relationships, creative expression, love
Jupiter	Visions, dreams, aspirations, goals, ability to learn life's lessons
Saturn	Self-discipline, formation of structures, healing karma and ancestral patterns
Mercury	Development of intellect, communication, rationality and intelligence

Figure 18. Evolutionary pathways of the Seven Planets

Although we can divide the human organism into various layers of tissues, organ systems, constitutions, psychology, and soul, it is critically important to remember that each of us is a *whole being*. For this reason, the levels of organization described previously are inseparable from one another. Esoteric traditions see the body as the most condensed form of the soul, and the soul as the most volatile part of the body. While we divide them for the sake of study, they are, in essence, inseparable. We are whole unto ourselves. And on another level, we are exquisitely connected to the wholeness of creation itself. This is what constitutes a truly holistic understanding of the human organism.

The Elemental Human

Just as a man can see himself reflected exactly in a mirror, so the physician must have exact knowledge of man and recognize him in the mirror of the four elements, in which the whole microcosm reveals itself.

—PARACELSUS[1]

We will begin our exploration of the energetic architecture of the holistic person through the lens of the Elements, observing the Elemental forces and how they manifest within people's constitutions, organ systems, and tissue states in the body, as well as how they imprint upon our psychology and serve in the evolution of the soul. The correspondences in this chapter are based on the Ayurvedic and Western Elements—Earth, Water, Air, Fire, and Ether—as opposed to the Chinese Elements. Correspondences between the Elements and plants will be explored in chapter 14.

Earth

On the most basic level, the Earth Element represents the physical body. In the constitution, it manifests in people with a larger frame, heavier build, thicker bones and muscles, greater physical strength and resilience, and broader shoulders and hips. They often have thick hair, lustrous eyes, oily skin, and thicker fingers and toes, and they tend to feel cold and damp. When the Earth Element becomes excessive, it accumulates as adipose tissue leading to obesity, stagnations within the body, sluggish organ system function, and an accumulation of toxins and metabolic waste products. Many common chronic health issues in the Western world, such as diabetes and heart disease, are related to excess accumulation of Earth. Its deficiency generally shows as weak constitutions lacking in vigor and vitality, and a smaller build.

The primary organ-system attribution is the skeletal system, comprising the bones, teeth, tendons, ligaments, cartilage, and other connective tissues. These are the densest tissues of the body, and they form its structural integrity. Without the skeletal system, we would simply be a puddle of tissues and fluids. This connection also relates Earth to mineral nutrition, especially minerals concerned with structural development, such as calcium and silica.

The digestive system relates to Earth because its sole responsibility is absorption and assimilation of vital nutrients that nourish and strengthen the body. Nevertheless, the digestive system is quite complex and has each of the Elemental forces present within it, such as the fires breaking down foods into primal constituents, the waters of digestive juices, and the airs that move the digestate through the canal. The pancreas also has some relationship to the Earth Element, specifically in its regulation of sugar metabolism through the hormones insulin and glucagon, which directly nourish and build up the body. This generally correlates to the Chinese understanding of the Stomach and Spleen, which are related to the Earth Element and processes of digestion, absorption, and assimilation.

With regard to the tissue states, an excess of Earth generates cold/depression, wherein the tissues exhibit depressed activity, functioning, movement, or stimulation, affecting their ability to properly perform their physiological duty. The term "cold" doesn't simply refer to degrees on a thermometer, but rather a qualitative state marked by a lack of stimulation. There is often a reduction of blood flow, difficulty expelling waste products, diminishment of cellular activity, and ultimately deterioration of the tissues from lack of hydration, nutrients, and oxygenation. This results in pale skin, cold extremities, poor digestion, and an overall lack of vitality within the organism. The tongue is pale and the pulse slow and low. Just as the psychological state of depression is characterized by heaviness, sluggishness, and lack of inspiration, a depressed liver, kidney, or other organ exhibits similar qualities. If you can take the psychological state of depression—how it *feels*—and imagine that quality expressing in an organ system, you have a clear picture of the cold/depression tissue state. Common symptoms of cold/depression include lowered metabolism, hypothyroidism, constipation, poor digestion, fatigue, and cold hands and feet through lack of blood circulation.

Psychologically, an excess of Earth manifests as stubbornness, rigidity, greed, inflexibility, melancholy, and depression. Earth is solidity that sinks down and in, so when it excessively influences the mind and heart, there's a sense of being weighed down, of being stuck or rigid in a certain way of thinking. We all know people who are completely inflexible and unyielding in their set-in-stone ways, unable to open to something new. There can be a certain coldness to their emotional nature, a bluntness and directness in speech, and a potential for being immobile in their routines.

On the brighter side, a balanced expression of the Earth Element conveys an incredible capacity to be highly organized, structured, and logical in thought. There's a grounded, practical stability to the mind. When a person with balanced Earth performs a task, it's done in an orderly fashion and seen through to completion with little to no distraction. Earthen minds have an impeccable memory because they deeply integrate information not only by mental organization but also through sensory understanding. Individuals with

Earth Element psyches tend to plan ahead, create lists, and stick to them, while still maintaining a degree of flexibility and spontaneity when the Element is in balance.

Spiritually speaking, the Earth Element is the teacher of this physical world, showing us how to care for our physical bodies and for the Earth itself. In our modern world, with its emphasis on the intellect, most people are disconnected from the vital intelligence of the body and don't trust it. This means we're disconnected from the body of the Earth as well and lack trust in the intelligence of Nature. The Earth Element teaches us to be embodied beings, reminding us that this physical form is our temple, the natural world is filled with meaning and communication, and we are a part of it. From Earth we learn to respect our bodies again. It teaches us to attune to the ecological system we are a part of and how the external ecosystem directly influences the internal ecosystem of our body.

It also shows us the importance of our homes, our families, our food, and of tending to the practical aspects of life that keep us alive—the foundations of our lives that we may overlook or take for granted. The Earth Element ultimately teaches us to see the living, vital spirit within all physical forms. It shows us that heaven is not a far-away place, and enlightenment isn't achieved on the mountain-top—it's right here and now. Through Earth our spirituality and practicality become deeply integrated.

Water

Whereas Earth is the physical body, Water is the flowing spectrum of emotion. Without Water, we would be bodies and thoughts, intuition and consciousness, but life would be monotonous and shallow, for it's the emotional dimension that gives our lives a deeper sense of purpose, meaning, and connection. Imagine a life without happiness, sadness, excitement, joy, fear, or frustration. It would be unbearably drab.

The Water constitutional type is typically phlegmatic, according to the Greeks, or what Ayurveda would refer to as *kapha*. Water types commonly have soft, smooth, and moist skin, and a tendency to accumulate fluids in their tissues; thus they often have rounded, teardrop-shaped bodies. The face and cheeks are full and round, with thick earlobes, round eyes, and thick hair. The tissues lack tone, definition, and structural integrity, with a certain lackadaisical or flabby appearance. The voice is often soft, sweet, and infused with palpable caring and compassion. It's common for Water constitutions to be cold, heavy, and excessively damp. Central to Water constitutions is that their primary response to life is based on feeling and emotion rather than sensation or thought.

Because of the changeable nature of Water, it can manifest in different ways on the physical level. On the one hand, it can produce the thick, round body shape common to *kapha* types, but it can also generate thin, sensitive individuals with highly responsive and active emotional natures; this is commonly seen in the water signs Cancer or Pisces, respectively.

The primary organs governed by Water are the kidneys and bladder. The urinary system is responsible for excretion of water-soluble toxins and the regulation of fluids and solids. The mucosal membranes also come under its domain, like a protective moat surrounding the organs that are open to the exterior world: the respiratory, urinary, digestive, and reproductive systems. The fluids secreted by these tissues act as a protective mechanism; the high levels of immunity present within them trap potential pathogens and prevent them from entering deeper parts of the body.

The lymphatic system, considered the "internal ocean," is responsible for cleansing and filtering the bloodstream and transporting immunity throughout the body. The lymph nodes are like lakes, and the ducts like rivers. The cleansing action of the lymphatics reflects the archetypal purifying nature of Water. The stomach also has an important relationship to Water as the seat of initial chemical digestion of food through fluid secretions, along with its sensitivity to phlegm accumulation, which reflexes into the respiratory system. Anyone who is intolerant to dairy knows that after drinking a glass of milk, they will soon develop a mucusy cough as the Water Element becomes disturbed.

The reproductive system, in particular the uterus, is also associated with Water. This is partly because of the fluids generated by the reproductive glands, the presence of mucosa, and the watery fluids of the womb that encase the developing child during pregnancy. In Ayurveda there are five primary locations of the Water Element: *kledaka* (stomach), *alambaka* (chest), *bodhaka* (tongue), *tarpaka* (brain), and *shlesaka* (joints).[2]

Water manifests in two primary tissue states—damp/stagnation and damp/relaxation—which point to its changeable dynamics and how it can exist in multiple states. Damp/stagnation occurs when fluids become thickened and congealed, congesting the channels and circulation, and accumulating metabolic waste products. Another name for this state is torpor, or toxic; it almost always involves the generation of an inflammatory or immunological response. Indeed, this tissue state is the perfect environment for the breeding of bacteria, viruses, and other microbial pathogens. We can see damp/stagnation in overly wet, mucus-laden coughs; edema; lymphatic swellings; headaches; pus accumulation; lowered immunity; greater susceptibility to infection; puffy, arthritic joints; all manner of swellings; and weepy skin conditions like eczema. Other terms for this tissue state include catarrh, excessive humors, or what Ayurveda refers to as *ama*.

Where damp/stagnation results from the slowing and putrefying of Water, damp/relaxation is Water overflowing, either out of the body or into areas where it doesn't belong. This is caused by an impairment in the structural integrity of the tissues, resulting in their inability to hold fluids, as if the banks of a river were eroding.

A prime example of damp/relaxation is a runny nose: the upper respiratory mucosal membranes become lax; thin, watery secretions are unable to be contained; and they leak out of your nose like a stream. The fluids of damp/relaxation are typically thin, clear, and prolific, whereas the fluids of damp/stagnation are thick, congealed, and yellowish-green or white in color, and they do not flow easily. Varicose veins are another great example of damp/relaxation, as venous integrity is insufficient to move the blood back to the heart. Thus, blood pools and settles in the overly relaxed vein, causing it to swell and bulge. This tissue state is best thought of as a deficiency of Earth, leading to an inability to properly hold in Water. Interestingly enough, when relaxation occurs over a prolonged period of time, it can lead to the dry/atrophied tissue state as too many fluids leave the body. This occurs with relaxation of the skin pores leading to excessive sweating, kidneys leading to excessive urination, or bowels leading to diarrhea.

In the psychological and emotional sphere, Water people have strong emotions. This leads to a high degree of sensitivity: they experience life through their feelings as opposed to their intellect. These individuals are commonly regarded as "irrational," and while this is often true, it's unfortunate that this reaction is regarded as an inferior response to life. Rationality has its place, but so does feeling. The emotional life of Water types is rich, deep, and sometimes turbulent like the ocean, but it can also be calm, peaceful, and serene like a still pond.

These are people with deep levels of empathy and compassion for others because they feel the heart of another and thus can sympathize in ways that the mind cannot grasp. While this empathetic nature is their gift, it can also sometimes be their challenge because they can exhibit poor energetic boundaries, picking up on everyone else's feelings without differentiating what's theirs and what's not. The trick for Water types is to know their own baseline emotional and feeling tone, to know themselves so well that they can differentiate between the feelings of others and their own. Their capacities give them an incredible ability to gather information from people, as well as plants and Nature, through the feeling heart rather than through logic.

The spiritual aspects of the Water Element run deep, teaching us to be in harmony within ourselves and with our external relations. Water teaches us to accept life as it is, to move and flow with life as it occurs moment to moment, to respond to these moments directly instead of reacting out of our past conditioning. It teaches us emotional integrity—the idea that feelings are internally generated, and we shouldn't splash our emotional Waters onto others in the form of blame, judgment, and criticism. Through Water, we learn to honor what we feel, take responsibility for those feelings, and express them in healthy ways that maintain harmonious relationships within our own bodies, hearts, and minds, as well as with our families and communities. Water teaches us not to stagnate through the suppression of our feelings, and not to flood our ecosystem by leaking them out onto others unawares.

The Water Element calls us to become open and intimate with the world around us, to break down the walls we unconsciously build around our hearts so we can feel the touch of the Earth upon us. This requires us to become vulnerable again, to open our hearts— even just a crack, even if it hurts—to let something enter the feeling dimension of our lives. Water teaches us to wash ourselves clean and live in a pure way, letting go of our attachments and our blind clinging to the way we think things should be, and accepting things as they are. This living in a pure way radiates into the sphere of our sexuality, for this Element governs the creation of life itself, as all things are formed within and born of Water. This Element teaches us to venerate sexuality as sacred, to honor the sacred Waters of our own bodies and of others, and to revere and respect the power held within the cycles of reproduction.

Air

The Air Element brings thought to consciousness. Just as the air around us is invisible, just as the wind blows, so too are our thoughts invisible and constantly moving. In the same way wind can ripple the waters of a lake and bend trees back and forth, so too can our thoughts influence our emotional and physical bodies. But unlike the feelings of Water and the body of Earth, the thoughts of Air are intangible, a primary distinction between the volatile and fixed Elements.

Because Air is formless, a strong Air Element constitution generates a physical form significantly smaller than Earth and Water types. They tend toward thin, small frames, with long, slender arms, legs, fingers, and toes; prominent joints, connective tissues, and veins due to thin skin; a thin face, lips, and earlobes; dry, rough skin; and coarse hair. Because they don't have much insulation in the form of muscle or adipose tissue, they are commonly cold and have paler skin. Generally speaking they are often cold, dry, light, mobile, changeable, and tense within their bodies. Air Element types are synonymous with the *vata dosha*.

Air governs the lungs and respiratory system, the seat of gaseous exchange in the body. The lungs are filled with tiny alveoli, small sacs surrounded by capillary beds, where the heart delivers oxygen-depleted blood laden with carbon dioxide to be exchanged with fresh oxygen. Upon inhalation our blood is reoxygenated, and upon exhalation we eliminate carbon dioxide, which in turn becomes the inhalation of the plant kingdom and completes the cycle of the Air Element. Just as Air mediates between Fire and Water and thus between above and below, so too does it mediate the interior and exterior worlds as embodied by the respiratory system. With each breath we take, the inner and the outer blend together in a communicative relationship that is the essence of this Elemental force.

The large intestine is another primary organ under its ruler-ship. Just as Air is predominantly drying in its influence, the large intestine is responsible for the absorption of water into the body and thus the dehydration of the stool. This organ is particularly susceptible to an accumulation of air and wind, as anyone who has experienced gas and bloating unfortunately knows all too well.

In a Four-Element system of energetics, the Air Element relates to the brain and nervous system.*** As the lungs mediate the inner and outer worlds through respiration, so too does the nervous system function as an intermediary. The nerves are one of our body's primary methods of internal communication, achieved through chemical and electrical signaling as sensory inputs gener-ate internal responses, and these internal responses in turn affect the outer world through our conscious and unconscious reactions. According to Ayurveda, there are five primary seats of the Air Ele-ment: *prana* (inhalation), *udana* (exhalation), *samana* (assimilation), *vyana* (circulation), and *apana* (excretion).[3]

An energetic understanding of physiology, such as that achieved through an Elemental perspective, reveals patterns of relationship to organ systems that seem otherwise disconnected. The Air Ele-ment demonstrates this principle quite clearly, for when the ner-vous system is overstimulated from stress, anxiety, or nervousness, it directly influences our pattern of breathing. Conversely, what's one of the first things everyone does (or at least should do) when trying to calm down? *Take a few deep breaths.* Consciously attun-ing to the breath is one of the quickest ways to still the mind and settle an overstimulated nervous system. People who experience chronic constipation often experience a degree of mental confusion, brain fog, and difficulty concentrating. Anyone who has smoked Tobacco knows that one of the first physiological responses (after

---

*** In a Five-Element system, the brain and nervous system are related to Ether/ Quintessence.

the coughing) is to run to the bathroom. This is because these organ systems are connected through the archetypal force of Air.

On the tissue-state level, an excess of Air generates two patterns: dry/atrophy and wind/tension. The first is just what it sounds like: dryness in the tissues. Water is the carrier of life, the primary delivery mechanism for oxygen, nutrients, and waste products throughout the body. When tissues are dry, they're less able to receive the vital nourishment they need for optimal functioning, and their capacity to expel waste products is diminished. This leads to overall weakness within organs afflicted by dryness, which can gradually progress into atrophy, or loss of organ function. This worsening health is perpetuated by their inability to effectively detoxify, because they lack the water to cleanse waste products.

This tissue state includes not only dryness of water but also of oils. Dryness of oils affects the skin and the nervous system, which is coated with oils to help conduct the electrical impulses of neurons. Oils also form a delivery mechanism for many fat-soluble compounds in the body, especially hormones. The dry/atrophy tissue state also profoundly influences the mucosal membranes, which by their nature are designed to be moist. Common manifestations of dry/atrophy include dry, itchy skin; dandruff; dry, bloodshot eyes; nervous irritability; insomnia; dry cough; constipation; and overall weakness, fatigue, and emaciation of the constitution.

Wind/tension manifests as both psychological and physiological tension, such as musculoskeletal spasms, cramping, tightness and constriction, nervousness, anxiety, and overall stress. This condition primarily afflicts the nervous and musculoskeletal systems, the latter of which is directly innervated by the nerves through the neuromuscular junctions. This is commonly seen as a state of sympathetic excess, or the fight/flight/freeze reaction in response to stress.

Because the nervous system afflicted by wind/tension is in a heightened state of sensitivity, it overstimulates the smooth and skeletal muscles, leading to contraction and thus muscular tension.

This can be as mild as a stiff neck and shoulders or as severe as the intense cramping of the smooth muscles around the ureters when passing a kidney stone, around the gallbladder and bile ducts when passing a gall stone, or around the uterus during menses. Many organs surrounded by smooth muscles are influenced by this tissue state, and those that are not (such as the kidneys or liver) can still be affected, as smooth muscles surround our vasculature and thus determine the amount of blood flow to the organ. In such a state of tension, vascular constriction reduces blood flow to these organs, impairing their proper functioning.

In the psychological and emotional sphere, the Air Element—being predominantly associated with thought—tends to manifest as a highly analytical and intellectual mode of perception. Somewhat opposite to Water types, Air people are often disconnected or even dissociated from their feelings, preferring a rational orientation toward life based on reason and logic. When in balance, this can manifest as a high degree of intelligence, the ability to learn quickly and retain information, and highly developed communication faculties. In its more evolved expression, these people may also have highly developed imaginations and visionary capabilities, enabling them to leave behind the tangible world and enter invisible realities. They have the crystalline perception of dreamers, creatives, and visionaries.

Yet when imbalanced, they become ungrounded, flighty, nervous, or scattered; have difficulty with self-expression or communication; and become disconnected from the practical world of responsibilities. Air can sweep them off their feet, lifting them up and out of their bodies; thus, they lose track of where they put their car keys, forget to eat, stay up too late at night, never balance their checkbook, neglect to pay their bills, or show up late for work. They get wrapped up in their own intellectual world and lose touch with the practical concerns and realities of daily living. This disconnection makes it harder for them to create the boundaries and the discipline to manifest those visions, ideas, and inspirations in tangible form.

The evolutionary teachings of Air have everything to do with the proper use of our intellect. Air leads us toward a mind in alignment with the emotional and physical self and ultimately in service to a higher good that surpasses our individual will. The rightful place of the mind is to serve the heart. Air teaches us to consciously use our thinking—to treat it like a tool, picking it up when needed and putting it down when we are done using it. Our modern cultural narrative is the story of a highly excessive Air Element: sophisticated in technology, but disconnected from the Earth.

Intellect is fundamentally about communication—how we communicate with ourselves in our inner dialogue, as well as how we communicate with others. Words and language are powerful, and the Air Element shows us that words work like magic; they are spells we cast upon others and ourselves, formed and shaped through Water and Earth until they become reality. The way we think—and thus the way we communicate—directly generates the way we feel, emotionally and physically. We can use our words consciously or unconsciously, for good or for ill. Air is a means of translation between our inner and outer worlds, with language and communication allowing us to transcend our sense of isolation and establish rapport with another.

Unfortunately, many feel inhibited in their communicative faculties because so much of their experience seems to elude expression in words. In order for Air to be truly balanced, for communication to establish connection, it must be fused with the Water Element; it must encapsulate the dynamic feelings that ebb and flow in the tides of our lives, giving it depth and meaning. To communicate effectively, our language cannot just be mind to mind; rather, it must generate feelings within another, so they see and feel what we mean. In this way we can learn to speak from the heart.

Fire

According to Jung, the Fire Element represents the intuitive faculty, our capacity to synthesize information into cohesive patterns of wholeness, an ability beyond that of the rational intellect. In this way, it is connected to our hearts. What many commonly refer to as intuition is actually the empathic sensitivity of the Water Element, rather than the higher faculty of the intuition, which blends feeling and thought.

On the constitutional level, Fire brings in unique qualities and characteristics unlike those associated with the other three Elements. Whereas Earth and Water types are often larger and thicker in their frames, and Air types tend to be thinner and smaller, Fire types land in the middle. They are of medium build, neither excessively thick nor thin, displaying prominent musculature, whereas Earth and Water tend toward fat and fluid accumulation, and Air reveals through thin skin. Fire types can be described as having an athletic build. Their skin is often red, warm, and oily, with brightly colored eyes. Fire types have strong digestion and appetites, and they are generally energetic, outgoing, and somewhat intense.

The primary parts of the body associated with Fire include the heart and cardiovascular system, the blood, the small intestine, the gallbladder, the adrenals, immunity, and the thermoregulation system, or internal temperature mediation, governed by the hypothalamus. As Fire relates to the essence or center of all things, the heart and circulation are of prime importance to the body's health and survival. Just as the Sun in the center of our solar system disseminates heat, light, and the vital force to all life, so too does our heart radiate and circulate life and vitality throughout the organism via the blood. When the Fire Element becomes active, it is common for the heart rate to increase and blood to flow to the surfaces of the body, such as during a fever or exercise.

The small intestine is the seat of Fire within the digestive system, the location of chemical digestion through bile, pancreatic and intestinal enzymes, mucosal secretion, and a host of microflora. Just as Fire breaks down materials during combustion, so does our small intestine break down foods into their principal components. In Ayurveda, this is referred to *agni,* or the core metabolic flame of the body. Although its primary seat is in the small intestine, it is microcosmically embodied within every cell of the body, as each cell performs the same functions as the whole body: ingesting, digesting, absorbing, and expelling wastes. This vital heat in the gut radiates outward and distributes warmth throughout the organism; hence, clients with chronically cold hands and feet are often seen as having a deficiency in *agni*. This principle also relates to the flame of perception in terms of "digesting" information, acuity of awareness, and a certain light behind the eyes and a glow of vitality.

Another component of this digestive fire is found within the gallbladder, responsible for the storage and secretion of bile, the chemical substance that emulsifies and digests fats and oils. Many traditions view the gallbladder as being the seat of willpower, such as when we refer to someone who has a lot of "gall." Bile is produced in the liver, the physiological seat of metabolism and the hottest organ in the body. The liver has a twofold nature with regard to metabolism: on one hand it prepares the digestate absorbed from the intestines to be shipped out to the rest of the organism (anabolic), and on the other it metabolizes waste products for detoxification (catabolic). When the metabolic fire of the liver is reduced, a common result is the accumulation of waste products and stagnations within the body, likened to an excessive buildup of the Earth Element due to a deficiency of Fire.

Immunity and the thermoregulatory system function as the body's protection mechanism by identifying foreign pathogens and differentiating between self and nonself. (On the spiritual level, the Fire Element represents the core self in a Four-Element model.)

When immunity is acutely triggered, the classic signs and symptoms of excessive Fire manifest, primarily inflammation, which is characterized by heat, redness, pain, and swelling, as well as fever. The latter is governed by the hypothalamus, which controls our internal temperature. When the immune system detects a pathogen, it signals the hypothalamus to close the pores of the skin, which act like peripheral vents, and increases the internal temperature set point to produce a fever. Observing someone in an acute febrile state is one of the best ways to immediately see the activation of the internal fires.

The adrenal glands also relate to the Fire Element and are a prominent topic in the modern alternative health world. The adrenals sit atop the kidneys and are where the nervous system and endocrine system "plug in" to one another. They secrete hormones that stimulate the fight/flight/freeze response of the sympathetic nervous system. This instinctual process is evolutionarily encoded as a mechanism to protect us from predation and threats to our survival by enabling us to fight off potential enemies, run away, or play dead. Once triggered, this stress response initiates a systemic cascade of physiological events, including an increase in heart rate, dilation of the pupils, stimulation of the central nervous system, and a shunting of blood flow away from the digestive system and into the periphery, which has highly detrimental effects upon digestion when chronic. A key term for understanding the adrenals and their relationship to Fire is *stimulation*.

According to Ayurveda, there are five primary fires within the body: *pachaka* (gallbladder and digestion), *ranjaka* (liver and blood formation), *sadhaka* (the heart), *alochaka* (the eyes), and *bhrajaka* (pores of the skin).[4]

With regard to tissue states, Fire generates heat/excitation or irritation. The term "excitation" yields insights into this pattern, which is essentially overstimulation of a particular tissue. If we think of how it feels to be excited and imagine that feeling in a tissue, we get a sense of what this tissue state does. It leads to aggravation, degradation, and physiological hypersensitivity. As the opposite of cold/depression, it is marked by hyperactivity, increased circulation, and overstimulation. It's important not to simply equate this tissue state with inflammation, which can manifest due to a variety of underlying tissue states, such as dry/atrophy or damp/stagnation. As with cold, heat is not just a degree on a thermometer, but a *quality*.

Characteristic patterns include red coloration of the skin and mucosa, sharp pains, burning sensations, increased body temperature (as in hyperthyroidism); fever and immunological hypersensitivities (allergies, systemic inflammation from food intolerance); oily, inflamed skin conditions; nervous excitability (rapid heart rate, sweating, insomnia); and an overall sensitivity to warm weather and spicy foods. The tongue is often red, especially at the tip, and flame shaped, and the pulse is rapid and superficial.

In the psychological and emotional arena, Fire expresses in individuals with a strong drive, willpower, and energy exerted upon the world. As the fire in your fireplace radiates heat and light outward, so do Fire people expand outward and impose their will upon the exterior. They are purposeful and motivated to achieve their goals, with a highly energetic character. Their minds are quick, sharp, and intelligent, able to digest experience and turn it into wisdom and understanding. They often display qualities of leadership.

On the other hand, the internal flame can burn out of control and lead to less desirable traits such as anger, frustration, irritability, and a heightened egoic identity that's primarily concerned with itself and doesn't take others into consideration. It's common for Fire individuals to burn with intensity, leading to rushed actions (sometimes acting before thinking), talking quickly, and living a fast-paced lifestyle. When in balance, they embody a warm and caring disposition, with all the qualities necessary for good leadership and innovation; but when out of balance, the self often trumps the needs, feelings, and thoughts of others, and there is a tendency toward arrogance, superiority, and pomposity. When in deficiency, there is little willpower, low self-esteem, weakness, fatigue, a poor sense of self, and feeble desire to aspire toward higher achievements in life.

From an evolutionary perspective, Fire bestows an acuity of perception that can burn through the false and see the truth. It activates a higher mode of cognition that is planted in the heart and flowers through the intuitive faculties. Fire is the primary force of transformation and lives at the center of every living thing. This is why it opens our capacity to penetrate into the living essence of any being, see the patterns of wholeness within it, and understand how the whole is greater than the sum of the parts. Fire teaches us to know beyond reason, to understand beyond logic. Only when we activate the internal flame by accessing the heart as an organ of perception can the logical mind be put in its rightful place, its artificially constructed language replaced by the living syntax of the natural world.

Many cultures say that Fire is the spark of life and that at the heart of Creation a fire has been burning since the beginning of time—a fire that witnesses *everything*. This fire holds the secrets of life itself, can see into the core of any living thing, and holds Truth. Fire relentlessly burns through the illusions that prevent us from clearly seeing the world around us. This purification calls us to live in accordance with our truth, from the core of our heart, and in alignment with our essential nature.

Ether

The Ether Element corresponds to pure consciousness, which pervades every aspect of the self. Every cell, organ, tissue, thought, and feeling is a different expression of consciousness. Whereas the other Elements relate to our intuitive, thinking, feeling, and sensation faculties, Ether is the container that holds them, the consciousness that mirrors these layers of the self. Jung related Ether to the imagination, the dreaming awareness that enters the archetypal landscape.

In a Five-Element model, Ether takes up some of the correspondences related to the Air Element in a quaternary model. Its organ correspondences include the brain and nervous system, and it governs movement within the body, relating to Wind. It generally forms a similar constitution as the Air Element: thin, cold, dry, light, and mobile, with a smaller form and stature. It generally produces the wind/tension tissue state, leading to patterns of nervousness, tension, spasm, and overall constriction within the body. It may also produce the damp/relaxation tissue state, as relaxation and tension form the polarity of tissue tone, which ultimately relates to space. Too much space leads to relaxation, and insufficient space leads to tension.

Each Element can only be perceived externally by orienting ourselves with the corresponding force within. Fire perceives Fire. Water perceives Water. Yet as we connect to our inner Quintessence, we perceive the Quintessence in the outer world—the essential consciousness that contains all Elemental forces. When we come into direct contact with the Ether within, we are able to perceive in a way that unlocks the innate power and wisdom of each Elemental force. We see the Elemental pattern within what we perceive. This is achieved through synesthetic perception, which is directly correlated to our inner resonance with Ether because it blends intuition, thinking, feeling, and sensation, opening a multifaceted state of consciousness that perceives the underlying pattern of anything we come into contact with. Through Ether we merge our essence with the essences of what we perceive.

When assessing the Elements within a person, an essential parameter to consider is their relative states of excess and deficiency, both in the whole constitution and in afflicted organ systems or tissues.

As one Elemental quality becomes excessive, it draws energy away from the opposing Element, and the body responds to maintain its dynamic equilibrium. For example, when the vital force becomes depleted from lowered metabolism, it results in an accumulation of waste products, dampness, and stagnation within the tissues. This could be seen as a deficiency of Fire leading to an excess of Earth and Water. The body may respond by creating an inflammatory process in the local area or may initiate a fever systemically. This is a vital Elemental response to increase Fire and regain balance between it and the fixed Elements. Most traditional systems of medicine rely on antipathetic principles, using opposing Elemental qualities in their remedies to reestablish balance.

We can also use elemental synergy to relate organ systems with tissue states. When observing the correspondence of an organ system—e.g., the lungs and the Air Element—we can look at the specific state of the tissue and its Elemental patterns, such as excess accumulation of fluids and stagnation of mucus. This is an excess of Water within Air. We could then apply a plant that is both sympathetic and antipathetic to these Elemental forces, using a remedy with an affinity for the lungs (Air) that is also warming, stimulating, and drives off the Water (Fire), such as Osha *(Ligusticum porteri)*. In reverse, an excess of Air within the Water Element manifests as musculoskeletal cramping (excess Air) in the ureters of the urinary tract (Water). A remedy such as Kava Kava *(Piper methysticum)*, with its strong spasmolytic action (Air) and affinity for the urinary tract (Water), would be a choice remedy. These Elemental dynamics can be translated into the psychological and emotional spheres as well. With this model, we can cultivate an Elemental mode of assessing the human organism, which guides our remedy selection when we classify and understand our materia medica based on this same pattern (see chapter 14).

This raises an important point in the study of the energetic architecture: it functions as a *translation mechanism*. Because the energetic architecture directly influences the state of our soul, spirit, and body, it shows how they relate to one another. The state of our body is the most fixed expression of the soul, and the state of the soul is the most volatile expression of the body. *They are not separate;* they are just opposite ends of one spectrum that is our holistic being. The ultimate goal is to assist the person in finding their own unique Elemental balance, which is achieved by creating customized herbal strategies and holistic health protocols. The Elements form an indispensable framework for doing this.

The Triune Human

*An understanding of tridosha greatly contributes to recognition of
a person's constitutional predisposition, assisting the practitioner in
creating a therapeutic program that integrates all aspects of that
individual's life.*

—MICHAEL TIERRA[1]

While the Elemental pattern has been used throughout both Eastern
and Western traditions of medicine to understand the person holistically, the threefold division is widely used as a simpler constitutional
system. The triune pattern forms the foundation of Ayurvedic medicine in the three *doshas* and was also adopted in traditional Western
medicine, as we saw in chapter 9. According to energetic architecture, threefold energetic patterns are seen as being born of specific
combinations of Elemental forces, as revealed in both Ayurveda and
alchemy. While Western physiognomy may not directly correlate its
constitutional systems to the Elements or other esoteric forces, its
descriptions and understandings of these patterns are a perfect match
with what the ancients said. Here we will explore some of these constitutional patterns as outlined by both Ayurveda and the Western
understanding. The following material has been strongly influenced
by the work of Dr. Vasant Lad, Dr. David Frawley, Michael Tierra,

Matthew Wood, and Todd Caldecott (whose training is rooted in traditional Nepalese Ayurveda by the teachings of Vaidya Madhu Bajra Bajracharya).

Vata

Vata is formed through the combination of the Air and Ether Elements and is best understood as the mobilizing force of the body. All movements are governed by *vata*. It is characterized by a thin body frame, with long, slender arms, fingers, and toes, with prominently protruding joints, an oval-shaped face and head, a prominent forehead, and thin ears and lips. They tend to have an overall wiry appearance and often have difficulties gaining and maintaining body weight. The skin is often thin, with visible veins and connective tissues and protruding joints. These qualities are all due to *vata*'s composition of the most ethereal Elements.

Their primary energetic qualities are coldness, dryness, and lightness, which can influence the joints, skin, nervous system, and mucosal membranes. This constitutional type has a highly nervous and anxious disposition, with a proneness to mental confusion, nervousness, or being ungrounded and spacey; but they also have potential for creative genius and intellectual prowess.

Vata correlates to the respiratory system and large intestine, both governed by the Air Element. The bowel is the main site of accumulation for vata within the body. When it is "overfilled" with this dosha, it "spills over" into the body proper and lodges in other parts of the body ruled by vata, such as the joints and hips. Hence this constitution is prone to stiffness and dry, popping, clicking joints. When imbalanced, there's dryness of the skin, hair, and mucosa, and an overall lack of secretions. The nervous system is also important, as this is the most anxious and nervous of the three doshas. Vata conditions commonly disperse randomly throughout the body, come and go, or have an overall changeable quality to them, due to an excess of wind.

This constitution tends toward the dry/atrophy and wind/ tension tissue states. It corresponds to the Air and Ether Elements and the mutable mode of astrology, and it has a connection to the Mercury Principle of alchemy. The Planetary forces that often generate an excess of vata include Saturn (dry, cold), Mercury (tension), Uranus (tension), and Neptune (weakness).

In Western constitutional systems, it relates to Sheldon's ectomorph type. It's interesting to note that in fetal development, the ectoderm forms the sensory aspect of the nervous system, which vatas generally have an excess of due to their sensitivity. They tend toward emaciation, weakness, difficult digestion, an excess of coldness and dryness, and an overall upward and outward movement of the vital force that can sweep their feet out from under them. Other terms used for this constitution are the visionary/seer, sensitive types, or nervous types. Its highest expression or transformed state is *prana*.

Kapha

Our second constitutional type is composed of Earth and Water, being somewhat opposite to *vata*. This *dosha* is characterized by the "nutrient source of bodily energy"[2] and is best translated physically as mucus. *Kapha* expresses through heaviness, sluggishness, and dampness, though it is similar to *vata* in its coldness. This constitutional pattern is the "thick" type, with a larger physical frame, big bones, broad shoulders and hips, round faces, and thicker arms, legs, fingers, toes, earlobes, and nose. Whereas *vata* often has a prominent forehead, *kapha* is more prominent in the lower jaw and chin. The skin is often pale and moist, the hair thick, oily, and lustrous. *Vata* tends to display highly visible veins and connective tissues, whereas *kapha* is predominantly adipose tissue or fat. People commonly equate *kapha* with obesity, but we must realize that obesity was not likely a major issue for people in ancient India. Thus, *kapha* more precisely equates to a well-developed and strong body.

With its predominance of Earth and Water, *kapha* is prone to water accumulation, fluid imbalances, stagnation, buildup of toxins, and an overall heaviness and slowness. Its general characteristics are heavy, cold, soft, stable, viscous, and greasy. It's interesting to note that in the *doshas*, Water exists in both *kapha* and *pitta*. This is because Water, in its magic, has the ability to exist in all three states of matter: solid, liquid, and gas. It's unique in that its dual nature has an ability to dissolve substances but also to join them together, stabilize them, and create cohesion. Within the body, the Water Element also manifests in two primary fluidic forms: water itself and oils. Thus, the *kapha* aspect of Water manifests as water accumulation and its cohesion property, whereas the *pitta* aspect of Water manifests as oil accumulation and its dissolving property. *Pitta* causes Water to boil, rise up, and disperse, as it is Water combined with Fire, whereas *kapha* causes Water to freeze, slow down, coagulate, stagnate, and bind, as it is Water combined with Earth.

Earth and Water patterns are reflected in the mind as well, leading to stubbornness, greed, and inflexibility on the negative side, or dependability, reliability, calmness, tolerance, sweetness, and kindness on the positive side. These positive psychological characteristics related to *kaphas* have a stronger predisposition towards parasympathetic excess. This *dosha* accumulates in the stomach, which is the moist component of the digestive system, where it can then overflow into other parts of the body, most notably the lungs, liver, lymphatics, spleen, and interstitial fluids.

Kapha tends towards the damp/stagnation, damp/relaxation, and cold/depression tissue states, which we explored in the previous chapter. It generally relates to the Salt Principle of alchemy, the fixed mode of astrology, and the Earth and Water Elements. The dynamics of the Moon (damp), Saturn (cold, heavy), Jupiter (stagnation), and Venus (relaxation) can all lead to accumulation of *kapha* in their own unique ways.

The "vital" or visceral type in the West was associated strongly with the digestive organs and nutrition, which produced a larger, well-nourished individual. This correlates to Sheldon's endomorph type, as the endoderm layer generates the digestive organs and intestinal tract. A key point to note with this type is that everything tends to operate significantly slower than for the other two constitutions (ectomorph and mesomorph), which is both its strength and its weakness. The highest expression of *kapha* within the human is referred to as *ojas*, or physiological essence.

Pitta

Pitta is the "medium" constitutional type, neither too large and thick nor too small and thin, but poised in the middle. *Pitta* is best summarized as the physiological property of heat, or "biological energy,"[3] which is achieved through bile. *Pitta* constitutions have a medium-structured body, with prominent muscular development and an athletic build. Because they are formed through the synergy of Fire and Water, they tend toward heat patterns: hot, rapid digestion, active immunity, proneness to sweating, redness of the skin, and an overall hypermetabolic pattern that leads to inflammatory issues and excessive tissue breakdown. The face can be flushed or coppery, the skin warm with moles and freckles, the hair red, and they have an accentuated middle part of the face—eyes, nose, cheekbones—whereas *kapha* has predominance in the lower part of the face and *vata* is shown in the forehead. The general characteristics of *pitta* are hot, oily, spreading, mobile, and light.

As the only *dosha* with the Fire Element, *pittas* tend to be hot. While both *kapha* and *pitta* are formed from the Water Element, *kapha* typically expresses moisture through a surplus of water, whereas *pitta* expresses moisture through excess oils. This is commonly seen in oily skin conditions, like acne, or issues with the gallbladder and liver. In the digestive system, *pitta* governs the Fire dwelling within the small intestine, where it accumulates and enters the entire system, burning its way through other organs and tissues, especially the heart, blood, and cardiovascular system. Because of this Fire in the intestines, *pittas* often have strong digestion and excessive hunger. As we also saw with Fire, the cardiovascular system, heart, and blood are all strongly affected by an excess of *pitta,* as is the immune system.

The psychological disposition of *pitta* tends toward intensity, anger, irritability, and frustration when in excess. On the positive side we see leadership, ambition, motivation, drive, and heightened energy—the classic type A personality. The highest virtue of *pitta* is referred to as *tejas,* the refined flame of perception.

This *dosha* generates the heat/excitation tissue state and relates to the Fire and Water Elements, the cardinal mode in astrology, and the Sulfur Principle of Alchemy. The Planets most prone to generate an excess of *pitta* are the Sun (warm), Mars (hot, stimulating), and Jupiter (oily).

In the West, *pitta* closely correlates to Sheldon's mesomorph type. Interestingly, the mesoderm layer of the embryo forms the muscles, heart, vasculature, and kidneys, the first three being traditionally related to *pitta*. This type is also referred to as the "motive" constitution. It's fascinating that Sheldon's three constitutional types, based on the layers of the embryo, describe the same basic types of people as traditional Ayurveda—even down to the functional organ systems generated from the particular embryonic layer that relates to each *dosha*. Such insights reveal that universal patterns of Nature are not limited to certain cultures or traditions; they are overarching truths of the natural world.

12

The Celestial Human

*Astrology is a highly refined and comprehensive symbolic language,
based on a set of archetypes. It can be applied to reach a profound
understanding not only of the human psyche and its transformations, but also of physiology, pathology, healing and various phenomena in nature.*

—SAMUEL SAGAN[1]

According to esoteric traditions around the world, the human being
contains the entire pattern of Nature, including that of the cosmos.
It has long been understood that the structure of our solar system
reflects human nature. While modern astrology has focused on personality characteristics and our spiritual path, traditional astrology
had a strong foundation in the physiological reflections of the Planets
and Signs, constituting the tradition of medical astrology. It was standard training for physicians throughout the Renaissance era to be well
versed in astrological language, which formed a central axis in their
diagnostic and therapeutic models. While some argue that astrology
is not scientifically valid or "proven" to work, the fact that it has been
successfully practiced for thousands of years to help people speaks to
its validity, whether it can be explained by reductionist means or not.

Some astrological texts focus on its spiritual applications and others on its medical uses, but there are few that bring both approaches together into a cohesive understanding. From the alchemical perspective, the Planets represent archetypal forces imprinted upon the body, spirit, and soul. We can observe how a planetary energy manifests in the organs of the body and generates health or pathology, along with specific psychological and emotional states, and then observe a pattern of relationship between these events and the lessons the soul needs to learn to advance its evolution. Our goals are to understand the core patterns, signatures, and correspondences of the Planets, understand how they affect the wholeness of our being, and draw correlations with other energetic systems such as the *doshas* and Elements.

This chapter will introduce a comprehensive constitutional system based upon the Seven Planets (Sun, Moon, Mars, Venus, Jupiter, Saturn, and Mercury) and the Three Alchemical Principles. This is not to negate the significance of the three outer Planets (Uranus, Neptune, and Pluto) but rather to focus on the forces demarcated in the Western alchemical tradition. This material has been strongly influenced by the groundbreaking work of my personal mentor in medical astrology, Judith Hill, whose understanding of astrophysiognomy is stellar. Other sources of inspiration include Steven Forrest, Jane Ridder-Patrick, H. P. Cornell, Matthew Wood, Robert and Karen Bartlett, Tyler Penor, and Steve Dahmus.

What follows is a breakdown of each Planet into its three constituent parts: Salt, Mercury, and Sulfur. Salt corresponds to the body (constitutions, anatomy and physiology, and tissue states), Mercury to the psychology and emotions, and Sulfur to spiritual development. Although there are multiple layers of correspondence in astrology, with certain patterns being related to Planets, signs, and houses, for the sake of simplicity I will only address correspondences with the Planets. Further detail on sign correspondences will be outlined in a future work.

The Sun

Salt

Solar constitutions tend to be of medium height, with a strong, athletic, graceful physique. They have well-developed musculature and are generally *pitta*. They usually have a broad, full chest, wide shoulders, bright eyes, light-colored hair, and a chiseled appearance. Solar types are well proportioned and warm due to strong circulation. The primary associated organ is the heart, the root of the inner Sun. It also rules the thymus, where our immune system gets trained and our baseline level of vitality is set, as well as the eyes, responsible for perception of visible light.

The Sun represents our deepest level of vitality, governing the overall energy that relates to our core immunity. As our vitality is lowered through depleting activities, improper digestion, lack of sleep, and overexertion, there's a corresponding lowering of immunity and overall energy levels. This is an important aspect of the Sun, for it is associated with our core vital force, our *chi* reserve. When this reserve is full we have peak immunity. This vitality is what disseminates life throughout the body, achieved through the circulation of blood by the heart.

The solar force has many traditional centers in the body, one of which is the "solar" plexus, or the general region between the diaphragm and the navel. This is similar to the vital heat referred to as *agni* in Ayurveda, the *manipura chakra,* or the alchemical furnace of Paracelsus. This vital heat radiates from the core out to the periphery, circulating blood, nutrients, and oxygen throughout the body, as well as removing metabolic wastes. While the heart is physically central to circulation, it depends upon this vital fire that resides in the abdomen. When the vital force circulates throughout the subtle channels with ease, there's a sense of strength, energy, and vitality.

The heart is the central organ governed by the Sun. Just as it sits at the center of the solar system, distributing life throughout the cosmos, so too does our heart rest at the center of our being, emanating life throughout the organism. As the perceivers of light, the eyes also have an intimate relationship with the life force, and their relative health is highly dependent upon proper circulation of blood through the small capillary beds that nourish them. The eyes and heart are thus bridged through the Sun, and as we embody the deeper soul qualities of the Sun, we learn to see with the eyes of the heart.

Diseases of the Sun are rooted in the heat/excitation tissue state, which commonly afflicts the heart and circulatory system. This manifests as high amounts of inflammation, which oxidizes the bloodstream and makes it acidic, damaging the blood vessels. Many heart and circulatory conditions often involve the Sun, or his ruling sign, Leo. Excess solar influence can overheat the system, leading to agitation and aggravation, adversely affecting the nervous system and leading to high blood pressure. Imbalances may cause a rapid metabolism, with the need to eat more frequent meals as a result of a high digestive Fire that burns too quickly and impedes absorption. In general, Sun excesses are similar to an excess of the Fire Element.

Solar deficiencies manifest as decreased vitality and weakness. Metabolism is lowered, resulting in accumulation of waste materials, especially in the cardiovascular system, as if the Fire has dimmed, allowing Water and Earth to accumulate. This leads to coldness and depression, directly affecting the heart and circulation, digestion, vision, libido, and overall energy and vitality. Everything starts to slow down. Whereas an excess of Sun overly excites and agitates through too much heat and activity, a deficiency of Sun causes symptoms of cold and depressed functioning.

Mercury

The Sun relates to our willpower, individuality, and soul. It is our essential self, the light we shine into the world. This is why modern pop astrology focuses on the Sun sign, because it generally reflects the core personality, although we often don't truly step into it until later in life as we learn to live in accordance with our inner truth. It's all too common that the light of our inner Sun becomes dimmed by the clouds of cultural conditioning, as we internalize externally imposed truths that mask our true nature. The purpose of an evolutionary model of healing is to peel back these layers of conditioning so the inner Sun can radiate its glory from the soul.

In the Sun's positive expression, we see individuals who are vitally confident in themselves, cheerful, positive, and warm-hearted, exemplifying good leadership both within themselves and of others. They have strong willpower and express it without fear of judgment, but they do so in a way that isn't egocentric or arrogant. The testing point of the Sun is to have confidence with humility and to live in alignment with our truth while honoring the truth of others. A person with a well-integrated inner Sun knows who they are and why they are here, and they have the courage to express that in the world.

In its negative expressions, an excess of the Sun is overpowering, domineering, bossy, egocentric, and self-centered—a psychological orientation in which the world revolves around them. They want to be the center of attention and for all the wrong reasons. Deficiency will display as shyness, lack of confidence, chronic avoidance, or downright fear of one's strength and power. Depression is a very common symptom of a deficient Sun on the Mercury level, which anyone living in the Pacific Northwest can attest to. There is a disconnect with our inner spiritual source, our portal to the divine, which causes us to wonder where we are going, what we are doing, why we are here, and the biggest solar question of all: who am I?

Sulfur

The Sun reveals the inner light of our essential self that dwells within the spiritual heart. The truth that shimmers within the heart instills a vision that shows us who we are at the core. Trusting and following the center of our inner solar system bring us into alignment with the highest virtues of our true self. We develop our true identity from within.

As we enter the territory of the heart and build a bridge to our essence, we begin to see ways in which we're not living in accordance with that essence. We see the conditioned patterns imprinted onto our minds and the ancestral patterns we carry that shroud our inner light. The healing journey is thus initiated, as the inner Sun shines outward from our hearts and vaporizes the falsities piled up around our true self.

This healing process is the essence of our life journey. As we grow and evolve, our actions and willpower come into alignment with our essence, which is connected to the essence of all things. Our will thus transcends our individual ego and becomes a vessel for something beyond ourselves. We act in service to the greater good, not just our own. We embody our purpose and live it with strength and humility. Through the Sun we become who we really are.

The deeper we go into our hearts and connect to the inner light, we open our eyes and see that this same light is infused within all of Creation. Through our hearts we are connected to everything, and each part contains a mirror image of the whole. Nature comes to life as we perceive the Light of Nature and its living language. We see that everything has its own unique kind of heart, and through it we enter into communion with life, participating in existence and transcending our isolated perceptions. In this way, heart awareness connects us to all of life and thus generates compassion. For how can we blame, criticize, or judge another and destroy the Earth when we realize we are a part of everyone and everything around us? Through the heart, we directly feed the good, true, and beautiful in all things, as the light of our inner Sun is connected to the same light within everything.

The Moon

Salt

There are two primary constitutional reflections of the Moon: the full Moon and the new Moon. The full Moon is *kapha:* round and full in shape, prone to fluid retention, fullness in the abdomen and hips, and a tendency toward pale, soft skin and a sweet, mothering nature. The new Moon type is more *vata,* with tendencies of frailty, thinness, and a slender body shape. New Moon people can be psychologically distant, imaginative, poetic, and sensitive to their environment. These varied reflections of the Moon are dependent not only on the phase of the Moon present at birth but also its placement within the chart.

The organs ruled by the Moon are the female reproductive system as a whole (along with Venus), but more specifically the breasts, uterus, and menstrual cycle, along with the hormone progesterone, which governs growth and development of the uterine lining. The rhythmic ebb and flow of the female reproductive cycle correlate to the phases of the Moon in that both of their cycles take approximately twenty-eight days. During pregnancy, the developing fetus is surrounded by amniotic fluid, a distinctly lunar quality in the Moon's relationship to the Water Element. Imbalances within the female reproductive system, such as amenorrhea, dysmenorrhea, hormonal imbalances, premenstrual syndrome, uterine fibroids, polycystic ovary syndrome, or endometriosis may have their root in lunar pathologies, or in Venus, who also governs the female reproductive system.

The Moon also relates to the stomach and esophagus, for they are the receptacles of food. Food, diet, and digestion have a powerful relationship to the Moon, as she is the principle of receptivity and nourishment. The digestive system is a relatively complex system, with many organs and therefore different astral rulers. The absorption of nourishment is essential to the pattern of the Moon.

Digestive issues such as vomiting, constipation, and nausea can arise, especially from an excess of cold/damp foods that suppress the digestive Fire, or from excessive dryness (deficient Moon). The bladder also comes under lunar correspondence as the passive storage container for urine, as opposed to the active function of the kidneys, ruled by Venus.

Bodily fluids including tears, urine, reproductive fluids, and mucosa all relate to the Moon. The mucosal membranes lining the respiratory, urinary, digestive, and reproductive systems also bear correspondence based on their moisture. Similar to how the Moon orbits the Earth and mediates its relationship to the other Planets, so do our mucous membranes reside in close proximity to the outer world and protect the body. The underlying structure of the solar system is precisely the same underlying structure of our physiological and psychological organism.

The Moon in excess generates dampness and fluid accumulation, or the damp/stagnation tissue state. This leads to a buildup of metabolic wastes, poor excretion of toxins, sluggish digestion and circulation, and mucus accumulation. In Ayurveda, these accumulations are referred to as *ama,* a thick, sticky, moist substance that congests the body. Interestingly enough, *agni* is the counterpoint to *ama,* which could be seen as the polarity between the Sun and Moon. This can lead to headaches characterized by dull, full, and swelling pain, as opposed to sharp, intense, stinging pain. These patterns are more common in full Moon types, who are more watery and stagnant. When the Moon is deficient, it gives rise to dryness/ atrophy, referred to as yin deficiency in Chinese medicine.

The last traditional rulership for the Moon is the brain. This gets a little confusing, as the brain is part of the central nervous system, which is ruled by Mercury. The lunar aspect of the nervous system is the receptive function of the nerves, the ways we respond and react, and specifically the gray matter and meninges, whereas the Mercury component has to do with the mind and speech centers.

Memory is deeply associated with the Moon; when we engage in a process of self-reflection, we are activating the lunar component of our astral body. The limbic system is also important, as it is the central processing center for emotions.

Lunar pathologies can affect the nerves and consciousness, such as epilepsy, hysteria, nervousness, anxiety, psychosis, and schizophrenia. In the Physiomedicalist understanding, these patterns would most closely relate to the wind/tension tissue state. Indeed, many of these psychological disturbances have been recorded as following the cycles of the Moon. Insomnia, severe fatigue, and disrupted sleep patterns also relate to the Moon.

Mercury

The Moon is the psychological function of feeling and emotion, the receptive faculty of consciousness. Just as the Moon reflects the light of the Sun, so does our inner Moon reflect what we receive from the outer world, generating the emotional tone of our lives. As the Moon goes dark in the new phase, our emotional reality is internalized and associated with our unconscious programming. As the Moon cycles to full, our emotional states are expressed outwardly. Through her waxing and waning, the changing shape of the Moon powerfully influences the shifting inner tides of feeling.

A well-integrated lunar force can be seen in a person who makes you feel really good, welcomed, accepted, and cherished; they know how to acknowledge and attend to the emotional reality of another. This type maintains emotional buoyancy in an overwhelming sea of stimulation. These people are sensitive, yet stable in their sense of self. There is a gentle serenity to lunar types, an emanation of patience and peace; yet on the inside there's a depth of feeling limitless in its sensitivity. This spectrum of feeling is allowed to ebb and flow, to rise and fall with the undulations of life experience, neither suppressed in the closets of the soul nor expressed in unhealthy ways. They have developed emotional maturity.

In its less developed adaptations, lunar people have such high degrees of sensitivity that their lives are governed by reactive patterns based on past conditioning; their memories and encoded reactions determine their courses of action. They have a tendency to perpetuate unconscious patterns and belief systems throughout their lives, reach brinks of emotional meltdown, and have unclear boundaries and hypersensitivities. They are easily overwhelmed in social situations, choosing to timidly isolate themselves from the world so they can retreat into the fluidity of dreams and imagination. They can be highly moody and indecisive, submissive to others' opinions and ideas, and irrational in their actions, choosing to operate from feelings instead. While this sensitivity is the gift of the lunar type, it must be balanced with other Planetary archetypes.

Sulfur

The passage of the Moon through the sky reflects our inner journey between the polarities of darkness and light. The Moon guides us to the depths of our soul if we can become hollow enough to receive it. Through the Moon we learn to let go and flow with the vast currents of the inner ocean. In that surrender, we develop emotional buoyancy, allowing ourselves to consciously feel.

Through the Sun we connect to our purpose and soul essence. Paradoxically, however, we can only connect to the Sun by becoming utterly feminine like the Moon and looking within. In order to be full, we must integrate our lunar magnetic and solar dynamic natures, allowing them to coexist in harmony. The evolutionary function of the Moon is the cultivation of emotional maturity. We learn to be sensitive, allowing the outer world to touch our innermost core—allowing ourselves to feel—yet with healthy emotional boundaries. This sensitivity ultimately turns into compassion and empathy. Through the Moon we learn the grand archetype of the Mother, who teaches us how to nurture and care for life. She helps us realize that everyone has deep inner waters just as we do. The highest state of this awareness is, simply put, happiness. We must consciously feed our inner Moon with things that generate true happiness from the inside out, for happiness cannot be externally dependent; it must be consciously created within.

Mars

Salt

The Martian constitution has medium height and stature, with prominent muscular tone; a square, sharp, or angular appearance; and an athletic build, similar to solar types. They are notably *pitta* constitutions, prone to patterns of heat. They emanate warmth and often have red, oily skin, red hair, freckles, and an intense look in their eyes, with a sometimes furrowed brow. Judith Hill says a widow's peak is a classic Mars characteristic. As they embody a high degree of Elemental Fire, their voice is commonly sharp, loud, and intense. The differentiation between Mars and the Sun is that Mars is more intense in its characteristics, especially with regard to heat.

Physiologically Mars corresponds with the formation, preservation, and circulation of blood. This is a beautiful signature, for Mars is red and full of iron, just like our blood. Mars people are often described as "hot blooded." Just as the King sends the Warrior out into the kingdom to preserve and protect, so too does the heart send the blood out to the system, providing immunity (protection) and delivering nutrients (preservation) to the entire organism. Diseases of the blood, toxicity, sepsis, anemia, the classic "bad blood syndrome," and overall circulatory issues can all be related to Mars.

Mars governs the adrenal glands, which are responsible for the "fight or flight" response, stimulating our vital force for protection. Blood is diverted from the central organs and into the periphery—the arms and legs—so that we can either fight or run away. The face flushes red, pupils contract to pinpoints, heart rate increases, immunity is decreased, and digestion is shunted. This powerful cascade of effects occurs through the neuroendocrine, circulatory, digestive, and nervous systems, which is beneficial in dangerous situations; but when it becomes chronic, it ultimately taxes the body. The modern dynamic of adrenal fatigue directly relates to Mars, specifically in the way it "burns out" the Sun's core vitality. As Mars is essentially energy, it draws upon the Sun's resources.

The immune system is our internal defense mechanism, or the inner warrior. Upon activation, it's often accompanied by the Martian responses of fever and inflammation. This febrile mechanism closes the pores of the skin and increases the basal temperature, trapping internal heat to "cook out" pathogens. Hypersensitivities, systemic inflammation, chronic low immunity (also a Sun deficiency if related to overall vitality), and autoimmune conditions all have their direct relationship to Mars pathologies.

Mars also rules muscle tissue and thus governs our physical strength and stamina (also associated with Saturn), along with the male reproductive system, especially the prostate gland. Benign prostatic hyperplasia is alarmingly common in men older than fifty. Muscular degeneration, weakness, and fatigue are pathological patterns that may relate to Mars, along with low libido, low sperm count, and other male reproductive issues.

The heat/excitation tissue state, with its relationship to the Fire Element, is generated when Mars is in excess, manifesting as excessive sweating, fever, irritation in the tissues, and stress, as excess heat dries out the oils of the nervous system and leads to nervous exhaustion (i.e., burnout). This can occur through hyperadrenalism. Because Mars is energy, its excess can lead to restlessness and insomnia, as well as overstimulation or excitation of the organ systems, leading to hyperactive sensitivity of the organ. The heat/excitation tissue state in the pulse is rapid, bounding, and close to the surface, a sign the blood is pushing towards the periphery. The tongue will be red, perhaps with a yellow coating, and often pointed, or as Matthew Wood commonly says, "flame-shaped." The excess of heat generated by Mars can easily lead to dryness and atrophy as well, as heat cooks off fluids and breaks down tissues. Injuries, accidents, flesh wounds, and traumas—any occasion when blood is spilled—involve Mars as well.

A deficient Mars is cold. There is insufficient circulation to the periphery of the body, manifesting as cold hands and feet, anemia, or blood deficiency expressed as pale skin, fatigue, and lack of oxygenation to the tissues. The demeanor will be slow and sluggish, with a general lack of energy and drive from adrenal fatigue, along with lowered immunity. The pulse will reflect this energy, and the tongue is often pale with a white coating. Often an excess of Mars will tip the scales in the opposite direction and eventually turn into a deficiency, and is thus "burned out."

Mercury

The psychological function of Mars is the ability to use our willpower in action. It represents the dynamic force that drives and fuels our entire being. Without Mars, we would simply be lackadaisical and unable to do anything. In its balanced expression, Mars people have courage, having the self-determination to move through the world and take action. They have the capacity to assert their will in the world, shaping their reality and sculpting their destiny in whatever way they see fit, and they can destroy whatever gets in the way of that. In short, they aren't passive observers of their lives.

However, if the Warrior operates without the guidance of the King, it only serves the ego. Thus Mars in its rightful place is guided by the Sun, aligning our actions with the higher functioning of the heart, which takes into consideration the whole. The highest expression of the Warrior archetype is the willingness to fight for what is good and true in this world. That same energy turned inward gives us the courage to face our inner demons, to conquer the lower parts of the self and rise above our inner conflicts.

The red planet is classically associated with war, and when Mars becomes imbalanced it can wreak havoc on ourselves and those around us. Waging an inner war against the self leads to festering irritations, volatile anger, and explosions of rage. Mars people become highly reactive, the nerves always on the precipice of irritation, lashing out at their families, friends and communities, only considering their own egos—what *they* want to do for *themselves*. They often forget to realize that true power is not domination and control over others through intimidation, but rather power generated from within that is guided by a higher power beyond the self.

On the flip side, people with deficient Mars lack courage and strength, trudging through life in a state of helplessness and fear of the unknown, often blaming others for the problems they don't have the courage to face themselves. With a flaccid will and feeble strength, deficient Mars people can't get out of bed in the morning because they're afraid to take action and haven't found a higher purpose worth fighting for.

Sulfur

Mars teaches us how to properly express ourselves in the world. It's the hard journey of cultivating a warrior spirit that overcomes our internal demons and shadow so we can find the light of the Sun within. Mars gives us the energy and determination to find something worth fighting for. And if we don't find it, we'll create fights within ourselves or in our relationships. Mars in its most evolved state has the courage to face *anything,* to generate the energy to climb mountains and find the truth that resides at its peak—and to overcome the fear of what might be dwelling in the valley on the other side. Mars teaches us to stand strong in who we are, to walk directly on our path of purpose, and to not buckle under pressure or cower in the face of challenge. He teaches us that courage is not the absence of fear but the strength to face it. It is the spiritual strength to cut out our bad habits.

The soul healing that occurs through Mars is not necessarily the reclamation of our power (power is part of the Sun) but reconnecting our will to the vital source of power that exists beyond us. Mars brings that strength back so our actions are guided by the higher self that dwells in the heart. In this way, through courage and strength we harness the innate power of our traumas and abuses, transmuting them into our unique gift to share with the world.

Venus

Salt

The physical constitution of Venus-type people will vary depending on her unique placement within the chart, which is true for all the Planets. But in general, Venus people can be medium to tall, with slender, graceful, and smooth appearances (a Libra expression, more airy), or they can be full and thick with accentuated curvature (a Taurus expression, more earthy). There is often a symmetry and beauty to Venus types, a pleasantness to the eye that exists beyond our skewed cultural definitions of beauty.

As the Planet associated with love and sensuality, it's no wonder that Venus rules the female reproductive system (along with the Moon), whereas the male system is governed by Mars. More specifically, she relates to the ovaries and estrogen, whereas the Moon corresponds to the uterus and progesterone, although in general Venus rules the entire reproductive system. Indeed, the term "venereal disease" comes to us from medical astrology. Imbalances in the female reproductive system are commonly Venusian at their root.

She also rules the kidneys, which relate to Libra, the sign of the scales, and the principle of balance. The kidneys are responsible for maintaining the balance of fluids and solids within the body, especially minerals, as well as pH balance. They constantly survey the quality of the blood, sense its dynamic fluctuations, and adjust as necessary to maintain physiological harmony. This shows the relationship between Mars (blood) and Venus (kidneys). While the kidneys are one of the primary organs, Venus also governs the urinary tract as a whole (whereas the Moon and Scorpio rule the bladder specifically). Kidney infections, excessive urination, urinary tract infections, incontinence, and other kidney imbalances all relate to Venus.

She also rules the venous side of the cardiovascular system, the passive aspect of circulation that returns blood to the heart. The term "vein" also derives from Venus. We can see the relationship between the Sun, Mars, and Venus in the circulatory system, with the Sun being the heart, Mars the blood, and Venus the veins. Jupiter, discussed later, is the arteries. Venous issues, most notably varicosities and hemorrhoids, are a common imbalance of Venus.

She also rules the skin (along with Saturn), and especially the face. The skin is the carrier of our inner beauty, reflecting how we care for ourselves and the internal state of the body. The premise of facial diagnostics holds that the entire inner body is reflected on the face through coloration, hydration, and specific lines. Chronic skin conditions such as eczema or acne can have their root in a poorly aspected Venus in the birth chart.

A common word used to define Venus psychologically is "sweetness," which also relates physiologically to a tendency to crave sweet foods. Anything with a sweet taste triggers the pancreas to secrete the hormone insulin, which opens the cells to receive the excess sugars in the blood. While traditionally the pancreas is placed under Jupiter, I propose that it may also be attributed to Venus. A dysfunction in cellular sensitivity to insulin is called insulin resistance, which leads to these cellular channels not opening properly, elevating blood sugar levels and ultimately resulting in type II diabetes. While Venus rules sugars in general, most sources attribute insulin to Jupiter, which builds the body, and the pancreas to Virgo, ruler of digestion as a whole. Because Venus relates to desire and magnetism, it can lead to patterns of overindulgence, whether of food, sex, shopping, or any other habitual pattern.

Whereas Mars is the intense Warrior with a highly charged, dynamic quality, Venus is the opposite: relaxed and receptive. As such, she manifests as the damp/relaxation state, wherein tissues become structurally weak, lose their tone, and become leaky, saggy, and apathetic. This particularly affects the veins; as they lose their tone, fluids leak into the surrounding tissues and pool there, congesting the area and leading to engorgement of the tissues. This tissue state is clearly expressed in varicose veins and hemorrhoids. The relaxed tissue state also causes fluids to leak out of the body, as with a runny nose, diarrhea, or excessive urination. There is a lack of boundary, a weakness in the structural integrity of the tissues that cannot hold fluids in. When the relaxed tissue state affects the connective tissues, we see organ prolapse, hyperextension of the joints, and overall structural weakness. These all point towards the boundaryless quality of Venus.

Mercury

Psychologically, Venus is the principle of relationship and harmony. When in balance Venus conveys social graces, deep and heartfelt connections, and being a genuinely loving, good person. Venus types commonly have a relaxed, easygoing, sweet, and friendly disposition that thrives in social situations. Venus maintains harmony between our inner and outer worlds and thus creates health within our relationships. Just as the health of an ecosystem is based on its biodiversity and capacity for self-organization and harmony, so too is the health of our lives strongly influenced by our relationships. This is rooted in our heart's ability to harmonize with other hearts, to transcend our sense of isolation in the world by being open and vulnerable. Venus brings a deep intimacy with the world, moving beyond superficial relations that tiptoe through the shallows of the self and diving into the true depths of connection that reveal our true nature to the other. She is the essential psychological faculty of being in relationship with life and maintaining that harmony. Her highest attribute is love and the healing journey toward loving ourselves so we can learn to love another.

This deep intimacy with the world often leads to creative self-expression, in which the essential heart of something is touched and encapsulated in a particular creative form; where the words reach off the page, the colors lift off the canvas, or the harmony moves through the notes to touch the heart of the observer.

In its negative reflections, Venus becomes disharmonious with the other, and as such can become judgmental, jealous, envious, and resentful. She can become cold and inconsiderate, selfish and vain, as well as perfectionist, self-critical, and obsessed with appearances. There is a certain wall that can be felt in someone with an underdeveloped Venusian function, as they pull back and isolate themselves. There can be a misuse of sexual energy as a way of manipulation and power control, as well as unhealthy patterns around intimacy that can be excessive or deficient. There can be fear of intimacy and relationship, a coldness around the heart that prevents connection and can be turned inward on the self. Sexual promiscuity can be an element of an excessive Venus, focused on the mere physical pleasure of the act rather than on the deeper sense of connection and love present in sexual union. Venus in her darker moments can tend towards laziness, shallowness, self-absorption, greed, and indecisiveness.

Sulfur

The evolutionary process governed by Venus has its access point in the center of our hearts, although not the physical heart like the Sun; we are speaking here of the relational and spiritual heart. Through Venus we are initiated into the ways of the heart, a process that touches our deepest wounds, as we all carry scars from experiences of rejection or lack of love. As we enter into the territory of relationship, we enter the heart of our healing, with deep roots in our childhood, families, ancestry, and the patterns that form the hearts of our future generations, because it's up to us what we pass down to our children.

Through Venus we heal our relationships. The deepest relationships we carry are those with our families. This is the truest testing ground of our spiritual development, where we integrate our spiritual ideals into how we relate to others, especially our families. We embody compassion, seeing our families outside the stories of our wounding, blame, or trauma. We shed suppressed tears so our hearts can reopen and we can trust in love again. We learn to forgive our mothers and fathers. We learn to forgive our partners. We learn to forgive those who created our deepest pains. Ultimately, we learn to forgive ourselves.

By connecting us to beauty, Venus teaches us that all of Nature is not only alive and filled with meaning, but beautiful. Life touches us when we perceive beauty, stirring something inside where we understand that the external beauty of Nature is a mirror for what we carry within. As the mirror, she shows us how everything reflects a part of who we are.

The evolutionary function of Venus involves the healing of our sexual nature, corresponding to qualities of *svadhisthana chakra*. We learn to accept our sexual identity, heal any shame or guilt we carry, and ultimately come to a place of respect for the power of Creation held within our internal sacred Waters. As we harmonize with this Planetary power, we magnetize relationships into our lives that are in accordance with our true heart.

Jupiter

Salt

Jupiter, being the Planet of growth, manifests as a large frame and stout build, with a tendency toward obesity and weight gain. Judith Hill once noted to me that "Jupiter types are usually either very fat or very tall."[2] Generally associated with the *kapha dosha,* Jupiter types display broad shoulders, chests, and hips, with thick legs, although slightly different manifestations are expressed through Sagittarius and Pisces, the two signs ruled by Jupiter. Pisceans tend to be thinner and more sensitive if they display its mutable aspect, or short, round, and prone to fluid accumulation if they display the Water aspect. Sagittarius has a strong and lean athletic build (mutable-Fire), with prominent hips and thighs and longer legs. Sagittarius, along with Jupiter, rules arterial circulation. They tend to be warm blooded, as they are often well insulated with adipose tissue, which is a primary tissue ruled by Jupiter. In this warm aspect, they can sometimes display *pitta* qualities, though this is rarer. They commonly have thick, oily, ample hair, both on the head and elsewhere on the body, although some male Jupiter types tend to be bald. They have a big personality, and they fill a room with their radiant energy, loud voices, and booming laughter.

Jupiter specifically rules the anabolic side of metabolism, along with the liver. The overall process of distributing and utilizing nutrients comes under his dominion. The liver is a central part of this process, as it receives nutrients from the gut and distributes them throughout the organism, primarily through arterial circulation. If the digestive Fire is low or food intake is excessive, the liver receives poor-quality materials and has to do all the work itself, leading to poor digestion, gas, bloating, and abdominal distention, as well as liver stagnation and lowered bile production, which affects fat absorption. The liver is thus less able to provide nutrients required for anabolism and to detoxify the body of wastes for catabolism.

This leads to the damp/stagnation tissue state, also called toxic or torpor. This tissue state is characterized by an accumulation of metabolic wastes that congest the channels of elimination, leading to what the old doctors called bad blood. This state also affects the lymphatics, which the Piscean aspect of Jupiter relates to. Many of today's chronic diseases, such as cancer, hypothyroidism, type II

diabetes, heart disease, and strokes can all be traced back to underlying damp/stagnation, with the liver and lymphatics playing a significant part. Damp/stagnation is often the result of imbalanced
metabolism, with an excess of the anabolic side and a deficiency
of the catabolic side, the latter of which is governed by the heat of
Mars. Anabolism supports growth, a key signature for Jupiter.

Arterial circulation is also of prime importance, as the arteries
are the "long-distance roads" by which the blood travels, which
relates to the archetype of Sagittarius. As the anabolic function,
it's through the arteries that oxygen and nutrients are delivered to
the cells so they can be optimally nourished. This is a signature of
the supportive and generous quality of Jupiter, as well as the fact
that the arteries expand and fill with blood with the rhythms of the
heart to further propel blood through the vasculature.

Jupiter types tend to seek escape from reality, preferring their
palace in the clouds to the practicalities of the mundane world,
which can lead to patterns of escapism and addiction. They can
escape through food, drugs, and alcohol, but also through shopping,
pornography, gambling, or any type of addictive behavior. This relationship to excess is an important aspect of Jupiter, because doing
whatever feels good isn't always what's best for us. Excesses of rich,
fatty foods, alcohol, and drugs are particularly stressful for the liver
and can lead to accumulation of fat, which Jupiter also rules.

A deficiency of Jupiter can lead to undereating and poor digestion of fats and oils, which affects every cell in the body, as the phos-
pholipid bilayer of the cell membrane is composed of fats. This can
also adversely affect the nervous system, as the myelin sheathing
of the nerves is coated with oils to properly conduct the electrical
signals of neurons. Whereas excess Jupiter will tend toward obesity,
weight gain, and excess damp/heat, and often requires strengthening the catabolic side of metabolism, people with deficient Jupiter have difficulty gaining weight, are malnourished, and need to
strengthen the anabolic element of metabolism.

Mercury

Jupiter in the psychological sphere manifests as joy, hope, and faith—not necessarily faith in a patriarchal God in a sky palace, but *faith in life itself* and our unique purpose. Jupiter instills aspirations and goals to attain, expanding us beyond our self-imposed boundaries with a curiosity to explore life's mysteries. There is an optimism, enthusiasm, and positivity in the air surrounding a healthy Jupiter person, as well as a philosophical orientation toward pondering the greater meaning of things. As a kingly Planet, Jupiter is the benevolent social impulse that acts for the good of all.

In its negative manifestations, Jupiter's expansion dynamic can afflict the ego, leading to boastfulness, arrogance, overoptimism, overextension, overconfidence, and pride—a person who considers themselves to be above everyone else. Through Jupiter we learn to express our truth tangibly in the world, to share our message, but if we mistake the messenger for the message, we get in our own way and arrogantly think it's all about us. For those who don't learn this lesson, they often fall as far as they have risen.

As mentioned earlier, excess Jupiter can lead to patterns of addiction and overindulgence because the gas planet has few boundaries. Jupiter says "yes!" to life, but when he overextends himself he ultimately meets his opposite Planet, Saturn, who comes in with discipline and boundaries, providing the harsh lessons bound to occur when addiction rages out of control.

On the other end of the negative spectrum, a deficient Jupiter leads to psychological rigidity, an inability to expand beyond the known. These mental stagnations narrow their perceptions of the world and restrict Jupiter's expansive function to see beyond the self. The job of Jupiter is to carry out the essence of the Sun, and Mars provides the strength and energy to do it. But if we are not connected to our truth (Sun), what we are carrying into the world is just a reflection of the ego and ultimately not in service to the greater good. This greater good is an essential part of Jupiter's evolutionary function.

Sulfur

The initiatic process of Jupiter cultivates inner trust and faith in our life purpose, teaching us to see beyond ourselves and to serve a higher power and the greater good. Jupiter enables us to transcend our ego; hence, the negative attributions of Jupiter are associated with having an overinflated ego. We learn to be happy and joyous, not based on external circumstances of our finances or personal achievements, but by connecting to something with deeper meaning. Jupiter facilitates the initiation into our life's work and what we are meant to do with the precious life we are given. He gives us a *vision* for our lives, something to orient ourselves toward moving into the future.

The evolutionary function of Jupiter is to expand beyond our self-imposed limits and boundaries. He lifts us out of our limited preconceptions so we can see the bigger picture of our lives. We reach into the mystery, expand into uncharted territories of the self, and see beyond what we think is possible. This unknown landscape can be intimidating, yet Jupiter instills the faith, trust, and belief that guide us. If we ignore the evolutionary function of Jupiter, at the end of our lives we may not be happy with the biggest question he asks: "Did I matter?"

Saturn

Salt

Physiologically, Saturn expresses as a solid, rigid, and sturdy physical frame. They tend to be big boned and skeletal in appearance, with distinctly sharp, angular structures that some might describe as bony. Their face can be firm, serious, and even grim. The joints are prominent, with high cheekbones and a chiseled appearance. In some ways Saturn is a *vata*-type constitution: tall, slender, and often cold, dry, and tense. We can think in terms of the vital force moving down and in with Saturn; thus, it is restrictive and contracting. The bodies of Saturn people tend to be cold and stiff, with creaky, cracking joints due to dryness, and sore muscles and bones. Saturn is associated with old age and the end of life, just like *vata*.

As the ruler of form, Saturn governs the hard, dense, structural components of the body: bones, teeth, tendons, ligaments, cartilage, and minerals, and specifically the joints themselves, where many of these tissue types come together. There's a specific influence on the knees in Saturn's relationship to Capricorn, and the ankles, ruled by Aquarius. Because of Saturn's governance of minerals, it has a strong association with the composition of the blood, the formation of stones, and the condensing of physical materials out of fluids. As the ruler of boundary and structure, the skin correlates here, co-ruled with Venus. Traditionally, the spleen and the gallbladder also come under the dominion of Saturn, the latter due to its connection to Capricorn.

As we observe Saturn within the chart, it often indicates a blockage in the flow of the vital force, expressed through its cold, dry, tense energetics. This restriction of vitality makes it a primary indicator of disease predisposition, manifesting in the organ systems ruled by the sign or house Saturn occupies, or in our psychological and emotional patterns. If these patterns remain unbroken, then as we age they will slowly lodge deeper in the body, which is why Saturn rules chronic illnesses.

As the coldest and driest Planet, Saturn generates the tissue states of cold/depression and dry/atrophy. Due to its constrictive nature, it can also produce wind/tension. These are all *vata*-related pathological patterns. The coldness and dryness of Saturn commonly afflict the synovial fluids of the joints, leading to deep-seated pain, stiffness, and rigidity, as well as overall organ depression and

weakness due to a lack of circulation and nutrition. The entire cellular matrix of the body is suspended in fluids, so when dry/atrophy
sets in it affects the body's ability to absorb nutrients, leading to
deficiencies, weakness, and loss of function in extreme cases. This is
the atrophy side of this tissue state. As dryness progresses, Saturn
becomes hardened by materializing minerals out of fluids, causing
mineral deposits such as gout, gallstones, kidney stones, or arthritic
deposits in the joints. Excessive dryness can lead to tension, manifesting as psychological and physical constriction in the form of
cramping, spasm, stress, and nervousness, primarily influencing the
nerves and muscles (although these patterns are also attributed to
Mercury and Uranus).

Mercury

A healthily embodied Saturn yields an individual who possesses a
practical, prudent wisdom that can only be achieved by learning the
lessons life presents to us. They tend to be dignified in their man-
nerisms and, as the vital force turns inward with Saturn, introspec-
tive, conservative, and reserved. In this way they can appear serious,
formal, and perhaps solemn. This is the opposite of Jupiter's expansive, joyous, inspiring qualities.

In its negative attributes, Saturn can be rigid, stubborn, stingy,
and isolated from the outside world. In accordance with its association with the melancholic humor, Saturn can bring depression,
melancholy, and a cold, fearful quality to the mind. Like a constant cloud that hovers over our heads, Saturn can prevent us from
breaking through to the limitless sky where our creativity dwells. As
the opposite of Jupiter, an afflicted Saturn can be faithless, uncar-
ing, unkind, and unsympathetic towards others. It can also lead to
a rigid mind, unwavering in its beliefs and values, whether they are
rational or not.

A deficiency of Saturn can lead to a person having no boundaries or limits, such as sensitive people who aren't grounded in

the practical world—the dreamers and artists who forget to come down from the creative ethers to balance their checkbooks and wash their dishes. There's a lack of discipline, a shunning of responsibility, and an avoidance of seeing life lessons. When Saturn is weak, we lack the discipline necessary to make the changes that improve our lives.

Sulfur

Saturn is one of the fundamental teachers of the soul. Our choice of whether to accept that harsh reality will determine how we navigate the ringed Planet's influences. By carrying us into the architecture behind the bones that shape our form, Saturn unwinds and heals the karmic patterns that bind us to our past and prevent us from embodying our essential spiritual identity. Saturn makes us confront our inner demons, face our ancestral patterning, and peer into the unconscious parts of the self to transform them. Saturn teaches us to turn challenge into triumph, disease into medicine, fear into power, and darkness into light; to approach life with the perspective that everything is our teacher, from the peaks of our joys to the depths of our suffering. To overcome these tests of the soul is to successfully navigate through the territory of Saturn, whose main evolutionary function is to help us *see all of life as a school.*

The tests Saturn offers us repattern our perceptions, thoughts, beliefs, and approach to our daily lives. We often trap ourselves in mental prisons that we believe are made of gold; we become comfortable but unhappy and afraid to change. It's when these illusions come crashing down that we meet our fate with Saturn, who restructures us from the bones outward.

The trick is acceptance—*utter acceptance* of all that is. Saturn shows that everything is absolutely perfect, as long as we do not have any idea of what perfection is. If we carry ideals of how things *should* be, we deny what is and strip life of its perfection. It is only through total acceptance of our life circumstances, within our control and beyond it, easy or hard, fair or unfair, that we begin to transmute them into wisdom. If life was easy, growth would not be possible. Challenge firms us up, gives us strength, and tests our resolve. In Saturn we must always remember: "This too shall pass."

Through Saturn, the soul is shown that all of life is ultimately a great mystery. In the end life is limitless and timeless. But as we exist within physical matter, we are bound by the limits of space and time, by the material world, so in order for our soul to evolve closer to this mystery, we must learn to play by the rules governing this world. Saturn teaches us that our spirituality and our practicality need not be separate; in fact, they are meant to be integrated and embodied as one, so that we walk a spiritual path with practical feet.

Saturn teaches us to take responsibility for our lives. That means making decisions and living with their consequences, for we reap what we sow. A healthy Saturn is always humble and flexible enough to change, to let go of old patterns and beliefs so that newer, more mature ones can be learned. We must be willing to stretch, grow, and evolve with Saturn; otherwise we will be crushed. Yet we also must learn to not go beyond our natural capacities. In this way Jupiter and Saturn work together, helping us see the limits and have the wisdom to know when to move beyond them or stay within them.

Saturn represents the psychological function of the self-discipline necessary to achieve the life purpose received from Jupiter. This is accomplished by creating life habits that help us physically manifest those dreams. Saturn cultivates responsibility, grounding us in the practical elements of life by creating structure and discipline. Without Saturn, through Jupiter we would expand into infinity forever and never actually "land the plane" to do something practical. Whereas Jupiter is philosophy, Saturn is *practice.*

Mercury

Salt

Mercurial constitutions are primarily *vata*, tending toward slenderness, prominent joints, and sharp, angular appearances (nose, face, chin). The face and head are thin, and there is a high forehead, lanky arms and legs, low muscular development, and a highly communicative, dynamic, and active temperament. This communicative nature is often shown in their face, as their emotions and thoughts are revealed through their expressions and constant gesticulations. Mercury is the messenger, so Mercury people often exhibit quick movements and talk a lot, sometimes incessantly, without noticing your yawning and glancing at your watch.

Anatomically, Mercury governs inner parts of the body that are in contact with the outer world. The primary rulership is over the lungs and respiratory system, whose inhalations and exhalations unite the inner and outer environments. The breath holds an important piece in the health of Mercury, for it not only oxygenates the blood but is also the vehicle through which we receive *prana,* or the invisible life force. Just as Mercury is the closest Planet to the Sun, so are our lungs the closest organ to the heart, given that inhalation brings freshly oxygenated blood immediately to the heart. In alignment with the lungs and respiratory system, we have the organs associated with speech: larynx, pharynx, tongue, and vocal cords, the latter of which are co-ruled by Venus and Taurus.

Like the lungs, the nervous system plays an integral role in mediating between the inner and outer worlds. Mercury is classically associated with communication, and the nervous system forms a primary communicative network within the body. As we receive sensory data, it's translated through the nervous system within the heart and brain and then decoded for meaning, leading to an appropriate response to the external stimuli. This process is governed by the afferent and sensory nerves, which are strongly ruled by Mercury. Through our neural networking we construct our perceptions of reality, and our conditioning will determine how well this construction corresponds to reality. The ultimate goal of the Mercurial function is to make our perceptions congruent with reality, which we might describe as psychological clarity. The dual nature of the brain, with its two hemispheres, comes under its rulership, as does the analytical mind itself.††† Indeed, the mind can only operate in the sphere of polarity and comparison, representing the two-sidedness of Mercury. Similarly, Mercury governs other "pairs" of the body: the lungs, the arms, and the hands, which also relate to Gemini, the sign of the twins.

The Virgo aspect of Mercury brings us to the digestive system, as Virgo rules the digestive system as a whole. The gut wall forms another point of contact between the inner and outer worlds, as the digestive tract is technically considered to be outside the body in naturopathic medicine. Mercury provides a link between our nervous system and our digestion, which are very intimately connected, especially through the solar plexus with its high concentration of neural tissue that orchestrates all digestive processes. Researchers are currently establishing many connections between the gut and the brain/mind. What were once considered psychological or brain imbalances, such as schizophrenia, ADHD, depression, and anxiety, are now being directly correlated to the health of the digestive system. This is all linked through Mercury's association with Virgo; its opposite, Pisces; and the connection between the mind and the nervous and digestive systems.

Mercurial pathologies are highly dependent on the sign, house, and aspects of other Planets, as it's highly adaptable and changeable.

---

††† Astrological correspondences can be complex because they are essentially fractal patterns that can be applied on any scale or to any dimension of the body. The nervous system is *generally* under the dominion of Mercury, but in its more specific demarcations we can associate it to the mutable cross: Gemini, Virgo, Sagittarius, and Pisces. Each sign governs different aspects of the nervous system, such as peripheral, afferent, efferent, and sensory nerves, the autonomic and somatic branches, the nerve plexus, and so on.

Mercury is about swiftness and change; therefore, symptoms it produces by transit are typically short lived and acute. This is a property synonymous with "wind." The primary tissue states of Mercury are wind/tension and dry/atrophy, or *vata*. We see tension manifest through the nerves and muscles as cramping and tightness, and through psychological disturbances such as nervousness, attention deficit disorder, a scattered mind, and stress. The dry/atrophy tissue state can arise due to Mercury, as the winds of excessive movement lead to dryness, affecting the nerves, digestion, respiration, and any mucosal membrane that should be moist in quality, along with the joints and skin.

Mercury deficiency can result in lack of movement, shallow respiration, hypothyroidism, poor brain function, and general nervous system disorders. Many language and speech problems are related to an afflicted Mercury, such as dyslexia and stuttering. Excess Mercury manifests as heightened movements, a scattered quality, and random dispersion of the vital force throughout the body. There can be communication difficulties, such as an inability to complete a sentence, veering off subject, or spacing out midsentence. In the body this can manifest as hyperthyroidism, quick digestion, an overactive nervous system (anxiety, insomnia), asthma, tightness in the chest, and respiratory tract infections. This in turn will ultimately affect the heart because excess Mercury overrides the wisdom of the heart with the mind. As my astrologer friend Tyler Penor puts it, "Mercury gets so close to the Sun that he actually thinks he *is* the Sun and that the whole solar system orients around him. When we solely dwell in the mind, our entire being orients itself around the mind as if it is the center—which, of course, it's not."[3]

Mercury

In its positive expression, the mind is clear and able to process information in a logical, timely manner. We're able to take the influx of sensory streams from the outer world, comprehend their underlying meaning, and enact appropriate responses. We have an innate capacity to translate our inner world to the outer world through language, and we feel that we express ourselves in a way that can be understood. A healthy Mercury also listens well.

The mind's essential function is like a computer: it stores data and information with great efficiency. Therefore, a well-integrated Mercury has an innate ability to learn and accumulate information. But therein lies his trickery. As we learn, we can be deceived into thinking that what we know is all we need to know, causing us to ignore other perspectives. We may mistake information for knowledge—or even worse, wisdom. While Mercury is associated with our learning process, the transformation of information into knowledge, understanding, and wisdom is the concern of Jupiter and Saturn.

Mercury is highly mutable and changeable, and when healthy, is able to adapt to changing circumstances, letting go of limited models of how things should be and adopting the one that is most fitting. But this changeability can also become a shadow side of Mercury. In its negative attributes, Mercury can be too mutable, leading to overflexibility where we have no roots to anchor us. The mind scatters in the winds, and repeating thoughts loop in a consciousness unable to grasp or remember them. They become finicky, uncommitted to anything, flaky, and unreliable. They constantly change their minds. People with excessive Mercury can talk too much and forget how to listen. They locate their consciousness strictly within the rational mind, relying on the intellect while neglecting the intuitive and instinctual self. In deficiency, there can be an underdeveloped intellect and difficulty with learning, and in excess they can be too smart for their own good: cunning, crafty, and clever, embodying the archetypal form of the trickster aspect of Mercury.

Sulfur

The evolutionary function of Mercury is the proper development of the intellectual faculty and maintaining its balance. Our culture worships the intellect and trains us well to think logically and rationally, but it ignores other facets of the self that gather information from the world, such as the intuition. In its rightful place, the mind should serve the heart, just as Mercury is the closest Planet to the Sun. Balance cannot be obtained through the mind itself; it requires the synthesizing and unifying force of the heart. Through the heart, the mind connects with our bodies and souls, and with the outer world of Nature. The mind that serves the heart is intricately woven into the inner and outer environments and thus becomes a *natural mind*—one that mirrors the patterns of Nature. That is the most evolved state of Mercury.

As our minds become more natural, Mercury teaches us about our communication faculty, both internally within ourselves and externally in our expression to others. With the mind connected through the heart, we learn to express ourselves truly and clearly, to speak in a relatable manner that generates feeling and transfers our inner world to another. Mercury ultimately helps us use our minds and language to reflect nature (Venus), adequately express our inner world of feelings (Moon), serve the heart (Sun) and our higher purpose (Jupiter), and from that place, take effective action in the world (Mars). In this way, Mercury communicates among the various planetary forces.

Mythologically, Mercury carried the caduceus and was the psychopomp—the guide who conducted the spirits of the dead to the lower world, connecting the visible and invisible realities—and thus corresponds to the *sushumna* circuit of our energetic anatomy. These signatures reveal that as we consciously integrate Mercury into the architecture of our being, we learn to be conduits for the divine to work through. As we hollow ourselves out, we become a receptacle for a vision that guides our life, revealing our sacred purpose on this Earth. This is why Mercury is related to the sixth house, relating to our work in the world. It is only through opening ourselves to the beyond that it may enter and instruct us in the virtues of our soul. The caduceus is also the signature of the archetypal healer, who opens up to the pure medicinal force of the divine so it can move through them and into the client.

As with the other layers of energetic architecture, our goal in the study of planetary forces is not simply memorizing their attributes and signatures, but rather to understand their core essential patterns *by heart* and be able to directly perceive them with our own eyes. This cannot be done by simply reading about them in a book; we must go out into the world and see and experience them for ourselves. Astrology is truly learned when it becomes a lens through which we see the world, where we directly perceive the Heavens within the Earth.

The Holistic Plant

*Each plant has an innate intelligence or core "essence," as the
ancients would have said, binding together the disparate properties and uses into a meaningful and logical or intuitive whole. The
compounds in the plant, its appearance, growth habit, ecological
niche, and medicinal properties are united by this common personality, intelligence, or essence.*

—MATTHEW WOOD[1]

When studying a medicinal plant holistically, it's important to understand its various parts in the context of the greater wholeness of the
plant, seeing how each property and quality come together in its
essence. Instead of limiting ourselves to knowing what conditions or
diseases a plant is good for, a more practical approach is to understand its core physiological and energetic properties first, which work
together to give rise to its benefit for particular conditions. This approach
guides us toward the plant's proper holistic usage for the ecological
terrain of the body, and it helps us find specifically indicated plants
that match the wholeness of the person. This can reduce the feeling
of being overwhelmed that many beginning herbalists face when
attempting to determine which remedies to administer to their clients
and how to craft formulas strategically.

There are five primary aspects of a plant to study in this holistic context, which I refer to as the Five Keys. Each unlocks a particular pattern within the plant that's critical for understanding its wholeness. It's rather common in the study of medicinal plants for only one or two of these keys to employed, which leads to missing puzzle pieces and a less comprehensive understanding of the plant. As we will learn in the next three chapters, to truly understand the whole plant, we must see the relationship between these keys and the pattern of energetic architecture, linking the microcosm of the plant to the macrocosm of Creation.

These Five Keys are 1) taste, 2) affinities, 3) actions, 4) energetics, and 5) special potency. While none of these concepts are new to herbalism, my goal is to review each of these Keys and show how they are dynamically connected to each other to give a picture of the wholeness of plants, as well as their connection to the energetic architecture model. The following has been guided and inspired by the work of Paul Bergner, Matthew Wood, Judith Hill, Michael Tierra, Rosalee de la Forêt, David Frawley, and Vasant Lad.

Taste

The moment a plant touches your tongue is the first point of contact between its vital force and the vital force of the body. When this initial contact occurs, a vast amount of information is exchanged between the plant and the person——the first words spoken in their communication—as their vital intelligences weave together and influence one another. Taste is one of the most important sensory means we have to decipher the medicinal properties of plants and extract meaning from them. Taste is the first Key that opens the doorway of understanding a medicinal plant holistically, which ultimately leads us into the next four. Without using the first, it is indeed quite difficult to use the others so we can step through to the other side.

In the Ayurvedic tradition, taste is an important aspect of understanding a medicine. The term used to denote taste is *rasa,* defined
eloquently by Frawley and Lad in their modern classic, *The Yoga
of Herbs*:

> *The Sanskrit word for taste, rasa, has many meanings. All of them help
> us understand the importance of taste in Ayurveda. Rasa means "essence."
> Taste thus indicates the essence of a plant, and so is perhaps the prime
> factor in understanding its qualities. Rasa means "sap," so that the taste of
> an herb reflects the properties of the sap which invigorates it. Rasa means
> "appreciation," "artistic delight," a "musical note." Thus taste communi-
> cates feeling, which again is the essence of the plant. Through it the beauty
> and power of the plant can be perceived. Rasa means "circulation," "to feel
> lively," "to dance," all of which is reflected in the energizing power of taste.* [2]

In this way, we can see that the taste of a plant has an incredible
level of depth and meaning that goes far beyond what we typically
think of as just flavor. It's a dynamic communication between the
vital essence of the plant and our own, directly transferred via the
nervous system throughout the rest of the organism. Each *rasa*
is a composition of two Elemental forces, but from the energetic
architecture model we can also relate the tastes to the Seven Planets as well.

While Western herbalism and Chinese medicine recognize five
primary tastes—sweet, sour, salty, pungent, and bitter—Ayurveda
includes a sixth: astringent, which technically speaking is not a taste
perceived by the tongue but rather a mouth sensation. This property is often used to describe the sour flavor in Chinese medicine.

Although these are the primary flavors, Chinese and Western
herbalism recognize other flavors, such as acrid, nutty, mucilaginous, earthen or "mineraly," and diffusive. Some Western herbalists
would hesitate to identify tastes with any particular elemental or
metaphysical system too strongly, because a number of tastes can
have different effects. The bitter cyanogens (Wild Cherry, Peach

leaf) are cooling sedatives, whereas the alterative and digestive bitters are mostly also cooling but act on different pharmacological pathways and detoxification mechanisms, and the nervine bitters (Hops, Blue Vervain) sedate the nervous system. Given the exceptions that always occur in Nature, we can outline the overall qualities, major characteristics, and influences over the body associated with the primary tastes.

The **sweet** taste is primarily moistening in quality, leading to the building, nourishing, and strengthening of the body. This is not the sweetness of candy but more like the taste of starch, such as with many grains. It often indicates a remedy that is nutritive, demulcent, or emollient in action, with affinities for the mucosal membranes of the lungs, intestines, stomach, or urinary tract. These plants often contain high levels of sugars, starches, or mucilaginous polysaccharides. In excess, it can overbuild the tissues and lead to stagnation and dampness, or an excess of *kapha*. In Ayurveda it is considered wet, cooling, and heavy. In this regard, we often use the sweet taste to treat an excess of dryness, weakness, and emaciation within the tissues, or an excess of *vata,* Mercury, Mars, or Saturn. Sweetness can generally be related to the Moon and Venus. Ayurveda assigns it to Earth and Water. A few herbs with the sweet taste are Marshmallow *(Althea officinalis),* Licorice *(Glycyrrhiza glabra),* Slippery Elm *(Ulmus rubra),* and Solomon's Seal *(Polygonatum multiflorum).*

Pungent plants are those that are spicy and aromatic. This taste is used to warm up the constitution, disperse stagnation and coldness, strengthen appetite and digestion, and increase circulation of the blood, and it often has antiseptic properties. We use it to treat cold/depressed tissue states and accumulated damp/stagnation, *kapha* or *vata doshas,* and an excess of the Moon, Jupiter, or Saturn. Pungents are considered primarily yang or *pitta*-generating, relating to the Fire Element, Mars, or the Sun. These are often diaphoretic, circulatory stimulant, carminative, or stimulant expectorant remedies. Ayurveda assigns it to Fire and Air. Some classic pungent remedies include Cayenne *(Capsicum annuum),* Ginger *(Zingiber officinale),* Fennel *(Foeniculum vulgare),* and Prickly Ash *(Zanthoxylum clava-herculis).*

Sour plants have some unique influences on the body, and this taste is one where we see some differences among traditions. In Ayurveda, the sour flavor is said to be warming, associated with an acidic quality and relating to the Earth and Fire Elements. Yet in Western herbalism, most of our sour medicines and foods are used to cool down an excess of heat. This difference may be due to vinegar being used a basis for understanding the sour taste in Ayurveda, which is distinctly acidic and warming to the stomach. Another possible explanation for this difference could be in the pre- and postdigestive effects of these plants, because some sour plants are slightly warming to the digestive system yet cooling to heat patterns systemically, such as Lemon Balm *(Melissa officinalis).* Chinese medicine generally relates the sour taste to a cooling property as well.[3] In general, sour plants often act upon the cardiovascular system, reduce heat and inflammation, strengthen vasculature, and slightly tonify flaccid tissues. They are often used for an excess of heat/excitation tissue states, *pitta,* Mars, and Sun, and can be used to treat damp/relaxation for their toning effects, expressed by excess *kapha* or Venus. A few sour plants are Hawthorn berry *(Crataegus monogyna),* Elderberry *(Sambucus cerulea),* Rosehips *(Rosa* spp.), and Lemon Balm *(Melissa officinalis).*

The **bitter** flavor is a highly important taste in Western herbalism, triggering a long chain of physiological processes, most notably in the digestive system. This includes stimulating gastric and intestinal secretions, as well as liver and gallbladder function. Many generally have a cooling and drying effect upon the constitution over the long term. Bitters will also influence immunity, the heart, and the nervous system, as it has been shown that bitter receptors are scattered throughout the entire body. True bitters often have alterative or detoxifying properties and are thus used to treat the damp/stagnation tissue state, excess *kapha,* Jupiter, and the Moon. Ayurveda assigns it to Air and Ether. Examples of bitter plants include Oregon Grape *(Mahonia aquifolium),* Dandelion *(Taraxacum officinale),* Greater Celandine *(Chelidonium majus),* Artichoke *(Cynara scolymus),* and Reishi *(Ganoderma lucidum).*

Salty plants are those that have a "crispiness" to them, a certain heavy mineral-like taste, such as Kale or Celery, or that are just downright salty, such as Kelp. Ayurvedic tradition says this taste is more associated with the mineral kingdom than with plants, and when therapeutically indicated, it is suggested to simply add salt to an herbal formula.[4] Salty plants are generally considered heating in Ayurveda, for salt burns when rubbed in open wounds, but it is considered cooling in Chinese medicine for its yin, moistening, heavy, and downward-bearing motion. This taste tends to influence the kidneys, the heart and circulation, structural tissues, fluid/solid regulation, and the nervous system. Due to the presence of nutrients, it has an overall strengthening and nourishing influence upon the body. It would commonly be used for excess *vata* or *kapha* conditions, the Moon, Saturn, Sun, and Venus. Ayurveda assigns it to Water and Fire. A few salty plants are Nettles *(Urtica dioica),* Bladderwrack *(Fucus vesiculosus),* and Horsetail *(Equisetum arvense).*

The **astringent** "taste" is the mouth sensation resulting from the puckering, tightening, and drying of the mucous membranes. This is due to the presence of tannins, which knit together proteins to increase the structural integrity of tissues, bringing tightness where there is excess laxity. This taste is also an action, primarily used for the damp/relaxation tissue state, excess *kapha,* Venus, and the Moon. Ayurveda assigns it to Earth and Air. Astringents predominantly affect the mucous membranes, as well as connective tissues and the venous side of circulation. It is a distinctly Saturnian quality, yet some Venusian plants also display astringency. Examples of astringent plants include Red Root *(Ceanothus americanus),* Oak

(Quercus alba), Cranesbill *(Geranium maculatum)*, Lady's Mantle *(Alchemilla vulgaris)*, and Horse Chestnut *(Aesculus hippocastanum)*.

	SWEET	SOUR	SALTY	PUNGENT	BITTER	ASTRINGENT
Three Principles-Doshas	Salt Kapha	Sulfur Pitta	Salt Kapha	Sulfur Pitta	Mercury Vata	Mercury Vata
Five Elements	Earth, Water	Earth, Fire	Water, Fire	Fire, Air	Air, Ether	Earth, Air
Seven Planets	Moon, Venus, Jupiter	Sun, Venus	Venus, Saturn, Moon	Sun, Mars	Mercury, Saturn, Jupiter	Saturn

Note: The correspondences between the tastes of herbs and the Planets, Principles, and Elements are based on sympathetic relationships, meaning the tastes are similar to the corresponding facets of energetic architecture. For example, the Three Principles/*doshas* reveal which particular *dosha* will be generally *increased* by an excess of that taste. The Elemental correspondences are the traditional Ayurvedic associations. The Planetary correspondences are taken from my own research. These relationships are not set in stone; rather, they are general patterns. A plant being pungent in taste does not automatically place it under the rulership of the Sun or Mars, though it does help to point us in the right direction. There are always exceptions to any rule. We will further explore the process of determining the energetic architecture of a plant in chapter 17.

Figure 19. The energetic architecture of the six tastes

Affinities

Our second Key is a plant's anatomical affinities within the body, or its primary location of influence—what the ancient Greek doctors referred to as "appropriations." This points toward *where* in the body a plant will exert its predominant medicinal effect. Traditionally, affinities were commonly determined through the doctrine of signatures, according to which the plant resembles the organ to which it is appropriated. For instance, large leaves are for the lungs (Mullein, Comfrey), rhythmic structures are for the heart (Digitalis, Motherwort), and lobed plants are for the liver (Chelidonium, Artichoke, Dandelion). Another approach is to use the taste of the plant, as bitters generally have an affinity for the gastrointestinal tract, pungents for the circulation and blood, and sweets for the mucosa, for example. And of course, experience plays a role in understanding where plants act in the body, as does tradition.

A helpful way to understand affinities is to break down the different layers of organization within the human organism as we did in chapter 9. The most practical of these levels are the tissues, organs, and systems. Some practitioners may consider these delineations to be too specific, preferring to just look at the affected organs; however, some plants may not have particular organ affinities and instead affect a certain tissue type. Some herbs can influence a specific organ, whereas others may influence the entire organ system.

For example, Cascara Sagrada *(Rhamnus purshiana)* has a particularly strong affinity for the large intestine but does not influence the stomach as strongly, whereas Oregon Grape *(Mahonia aquifolium)* addresses the entire digestive system—stomach, small and large intestines, liver, and gallbladder. Marshmallow *(Althea officinalis)* certainly affects the respiratory, urinary, and digestive systems, but it does so because it has a primary tissue affinity in the mucosal membranes. Thus, breaking down a remedy's affinity for tissues, organs, and systems outlines specifically where in the body it will have its primary influence, and it supports the practitioner in selecting the remedy that is most well suited for the person.

While in biomedical physiology we see various tissue types such as mucosa, blood, and nerves, in the Ayurvedic tradition we see seven primary tissues, or *dhatus,* which are the basis for the formation of all the organs of the body. The *dhatus* progress from one to the next, founded upon the proper digestion of food. Thus we see that the digested materials that are absorbed from the gut turn into the *rasa dhatu,* or plasma, which is then transformed into *rakta dhatu,* or blood, moving into *mamsa dhatu* (muscle), *meda dhatu* (fat), *asthi dhatu* (bone), *majja dhatu* (marrow/nerve), and finally *shukra and artava dhatus* (reproductive).[5]

Ayurvedic physiology and therapeutics are strongly rooted in these seven tissue types. Practitioners note where there is inadequate transformation from one tissue to the next, and they use herbal medicines and other therapeutic strategies to clear blockages within these tissues and the channels that connect them to generate a seamless flow of vitality from one tissue to the next. This leads to overall maintenance of the system and ultimately physiological rejuvenation. These seven *dhatus* correspond strongly to the Seven Planets of Western astrology. In fact, the principles of rejuvenative therapy in Ayurveda relate to the initiatic healing process described in the alchemical literature.

Whereas Ayurveda examines tissues affected by a medicinal plant (as well as *doshas*), Chinese medicine focuses on the affected meridians and organs. These are the twelve meridians, which are divided into yin and yang organ categories. (See Chapter 9.)

Most Western herbalists, like biomedical doctors, recognize about a dozen major organ systems: nervous, endocrine, immune/lymphatic, circulatory, respiratory, digestive, metabolic (liver and cells), urinary, reproductive, eliminative, muscular, and skeletal or the connective tissue system. In addition, some tissues are recognized as structures to be treated: mucosa, skin, and blood. One could organize these systems according to the zodiac, and they are so closely analogous to the Chinese system that Western herbalists are increasingly using some Oriental therapeutic concepts. This practice enables us to see connections between organ systems that may, from a strictly physiological perspective, seem disconnected, as well as with their psychological dynamics.

When considering the affinities of a medicinal plant, it is most helpful to note the specific tissues, organs, and systems where it has its orientation. This makes the process of remedy selection significantly more straightforward, as you select remedies that are sympathetic to the imbalanced organ system. For a detailed breakdown of the layers of the body, refer to chapter 9 in the "Salt: Integrative Physiology" section.

Actions

The third Key has to do with what an herbal action is—and what it is not. Through the breakdown of the old traditional medical systems, there came a time when all differentiations in Western herbalism were defined as "actions." Thus, the actions ceased to be anything more than descriptive terms and became a sloppy method of classification. It's quite common these days to look up an herb in a book and under the "herbal actions" section see a massive list of terms, many of which are actually not an herbal action. This list includes terms with origins ranging from ancient Greece to modern pharmacology. This being the case, we need to reestablish some reasonable definitions for herbal actions.

On the positive side, I love that we use the word "action" to define how an herb functions, or directly *acts* upon the body. There is a dynamic quality associated with this term that's essential for understanding what an herbal action is and what it is not, and that dynamism brings a lot of clarity to the question.

A true herbal action is one you can directly feel within the body or perceive with the senses, such as sweating, coughing, fluid secretions, or calming the nervous system. Herbal actions specifically adjust a *physiological process*. I learned this valuable lesson from herbalist Paul Bergner, who denotes three primary categories that are *not* herbal actions that are nevertheless commonly included in the actions section of an herbal monograph.[6]

The first of these "actions" actually refers to affinities, such as hepatic, pectoral, or stomachic. These "actions" don't give us a clear indication of how a plant is acting upon a physiological process; instead they point to the anatomical region they affect.

The second type of nonaction is a disease or symptom the plant treats. Many of these are listed as words beginning with "anti-," which flood the herbal actions listings of most modern monographs: anti-migraine, anti-cancer, anti-inflammatory, etc. This category is best found in a different section of a monograph that focuses on conditions and symptoms treated, or how the plant is used, rather an action listing.

Lastly are terms referring to pharmacological mechanisms of action, which indicate the biochemical properties of a plant, such as COX-2 inhibiting or adrenergic. These terms describe biochemical effects rather than a physiological process perceptible through the senses. In terms of clinical herbalism, these biochemical actions are not always helpful. No one will ever ask you to adjust their cyclooxygenase levels. This is not to devalue the fascinating subject of pharmacognosy and pharmacokinetics, as we are learning more about how plants influence our bodies on the molecular level; it's just that these terms aren't herbal actions and are best located in a section of a monograph that specifically discusses the pharmacological properties of plants.

It's also common for the energetic properties of a plant to be included in the lists of plant actions. The energetic aspects of a plant are really a distinct category. This includes the original Greek concepts such as "warming, cooling, drying, moistening," and their modern reinterpretations: "stimulating, refrigerant, astringent, demulcent." The latter, however, are frequently included.

A true herbal action is one you can sense or feel—a noticeable change in the body. It refers to the specific ways a plant will influence the organs, systems, and tissues it has affinities for and how it will adjust the movement of the vital force in the body. Thus, it is preferable to focus on these "vitalist actions." Matthew Wood offers this description of the original Greek actions:

> [They] were fairly simple "sensory actions": raising, lowering, centripetal, centrifugal, thinning, thickening, opening, closing, etc. These are indeed characterized by physiological effects that we can feel when we are sampling a plant or a client is receiving an herb. Herbalist Karyn Sanders emphasizes "these simple kinds of sensory actions and the longer I practice the more I notice them and the more meaningful they are."[7]

The most important herbal actions today are adaptogen, alterative, astringent, bitter, carminative, cholagogue, choleretic, demulcent, diaphoretic, diuretic, emmenagogue, expectorant, galactagogue, lymphagogue, mucolytic, nervine, spasmolytic (or antispasmodic), and stimulant (circulatory or nervine). In the next three chapters we will delineate the relationships between herbal actions and the Seven Planets, Five Elements, and Three Principles.

Energetics

This fourth Key is unfortunately commonly overlooked in modern allopathic approaches to herbalism. It's common when people hear the term "herbal energetics" to conjure images of a plant spirit, consider an herb's psychospiritual effects, or think of it as a lofty spiritual or esoteric concept. In actuality, herbal energetics is a highly pragmatic and specific approach to understanding the medicinal properties of a plant that we cannot achieve through affinity and actions alone. Energetics gets us to see deeper underlying patterns in both people and plants, and it shows us how to apply medicines with specificity and precision. It is a translation language that describes the link between the physiological expression of the person and the ecological nature of a plant.

According to this perspective, plants are understood in their effects upon the constitution and the ecological state of the tissues. This is commonly achieved through observing three primary plant qualities: temperature, moisture, and tone. An energetic model of plants need not be distinct from a biochemical understanding. Indeed, we can trace distinct relationships between particular chemical constituents in plants and distinct energetic effects, for the chemistry of a plant is merely a vehicle for its vital force to operate through. Examples of this include mucilaginous polysaccharides being moistening; iridoid glycosides being bitter, cooling, and drying; the alkaloid lobeline being relaxant; and tannins being astringent/tonifying.

Energetics is one area where there is universal agreement among traditions. Whether in China, India, the Middle East, Greece, or North America, all vitalist traditions agree that plants do not just enter specific parts of the body and have a physiological action upon them; there is a deeper level of influence upon the overall energetic or ecological aspect of the organism. In North American Physiomedicalism these are the tissue states. The integration of herbal energetics and constitutional theory is at the foundation of the vitalist model: one without the other would be like a plant without roots.

In *The Practice of Traditional Western Herbalism,* Matthew Wood explains the origin of the Western energetic systems.[8] The Greek system was developed by Aristotle, who saw the basic constituents of the world as heat, cold, damp, and dry. According to his perspective, the four Elements were derived from these four qualities, causing them to have less value in traditional Western medicine. Thus, rather than relating a plant to an Elemental force, they were primarily related to the qualities of hot, cold, damp, or dry. Hippocrates adopted the four qualities and derived from them the four humors: choleric, sanguine, phlegmatic, and melancholic. We can see the relationship between the humors, qualities, and Elements below:

HUMORS	QUALITIES	ELEMENTS
Choleric	Hot and dry	Fire
Sanguine	Hot and damp	Air
Phlegmatic	Cold and damp	Water
Melancholic	Cold and dry	Earth

Aristotle's system, on the other hand, is awkward in terms of "reality": Air is damp and hot (which is not true in Norway), and Earth is cold and dry (not true in Louisiana). A certain unreality clings to this model, though it was the norm in Western medicine for two thousand years. I would argue that the shift away from the

Elements to the qualities led to the gradual development of the more mechanical view of medicine that Paracelsus sought to revolutionize in the sixteenth century. From my perspective, the quality of heat is *generated* by Fire, just as moisture is the result of Water, not the other way around. I see the Elements as being the primal manifestations of the cosmos, which then led to the creation of the qualities. When we change our orientation toward energetics so that we see the Elements as the primary cause of the qualities, we perceive deeper layers of meaning within our herbal remedies, as the archetypal forces of the Elements represent so much more than the properties of temperature and moisture.

This results in a slightly different perspective from Aristotle's, which is confirmed by the medical astrologers of the Renaissance era. As astrology is also tied to the Four Elements, the astrological doctors adopted them as equivalent to the qualities, rather than each Element being formed from a combination of two of them. This alignment also relates to the phases of matter as recognized in physics and chemistry, which are also central to the alchemical understanding. Many practitioners find that this system makes more practical sense:

ELEMENT	QUALITY	STATE OF MATTER
Fire	Hot	Combustion
Air	Dry	Gas
Water	Damp	Liquid
Earth	Cold	Solid

The four qualities of Western medicine are the same as the four natures of Chinese medicine and are analogous to the concept of *virya* in Ayurveda.[9] This demonstrates the universal approval of the concept. Virtually every energetic system in the world starts with the duality of temperature and moisture. The table below relates the Greek system (hot, cold, damp, dry) to the Chinese:

CHINESE	AYURVEDIC/GREEK
Excess yang	Heat
Deficient yang	Cold
Excess yin	Damp
Deficient yin	Dry

In the alchemical system, we have Celestial Niter (the yang, volatile principle) and the Celestial Salt (the yin, fixed principle). The duality of Celestial Niter and Celestial Salt generates the Four Elements, which express through the four qualities—hot, cold, moist, and dry. This aligns perfectly with the astrological model, as shown in figure 20.

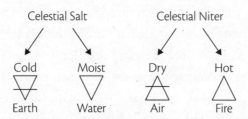

Figure 20. Generation of the four qualities

The Eastern systems also incorporate the fifth Element into their metaphysical models; in the West this Quintessential Element is recognized, but for some reason it is less integrated into their working model. The fifth Element in Chinese medicine is Wood, similar to wind or change; in Ayurveda it is "ether" or "space." This fifth Element acts not through temperature or moisture, as the Four Elements do, but through tissue tone (i.e., tension and relaxation, too little or too much space).

The Ayurvedic system is not binary but rather threefold and fivefold, based on the three *doshas* and the Five Elements. However, there are plenty of analogies:

Vata	Air (dry) and Ether (tension)
Pitta	Fire (heat) and Water (damp/oil‡‡‡)
Kapha	Water (damp/water) and Earth (cold)

It is important to understand that the four qualities were being described long before the advent of the thermometer, so they do not refer to degrees on a thermometer or how much Fire or Water is present within a tissue. They are *effects;* thus, studying the influence of heat or cold, moisture or dryness within Nature lends us further insights into their true properties. Moisture relates not only to hydration but also to flexibility and relaxation; dryness relates not just to desiccation but also the creation of boundaries and a lack of flexibility. Cold is not just the sensation of cold but is contractive, heavy, and "cementing," whereas heat is stimulating, radiant, and volatilizing.

According to the astrological tradition, the Planets also display the properties of hot, cold, wet, and dry. Because there are seven of them, the correspondences are less straightforward than with the Elements, and they become more specific with further subdivisions of their properties. These are the Planets' correspondences, as confirmed by Matthew Wood and Judith Hill:[10]

Sun	Radiant heat (warm)
Moon	Hydrating moisture§§§
Mercury	Neutral, tension
Venus	Relaxing moisture

---

‡‡‡ The Ayurvedic system recognizes two forms of moisture within the body: water and oil. This is one of the few traditions that places a high degree of importance upon oils for proper hydration.

§§§ Water or damp is also considered nutritive, as yin is in Chinese medicine, and this applies to all the moist Planets.

Mars   Stimulating heat (hot)

Jupiter   Volatilizing heat, expansive moisture

Saturn   Dry and cold

Although the terminologies differ among traditional medicine systems, we can see the universality of this principle of energetics based on these primal qualities, which are summarized in figure 21. Note that these relationships are based on sympathy or similarity.

	HOT	COLD	WET	DRY
Chinese Medicine	Increases Yang	Decreases Yang	Increases Yin	Decreases Yin
Ayurveda	Increases Pitta	Increases Kapha, Vata	Increases Kapha, Pitta (oil)	Increases Vata
Elements	Increases Fire	Increases Earth	Increases Water	Increases Air
Planets	Sun and Mars	Saturn, Mercury	Jupiter, Venus, Moon	Mercury, Saturn

Figure 21. The four qualities in Chinese medicine, medical astrology, and Ayurveda

With the historical context in place and the patterns of similarity established between various systems, let's take a look at the energetics of plants.

The **warming** property stimulates organs and tissues into a greater level of activity, increasing their metabolism, cleansing, and dispersing stagnation. They warm the digestive core, thin fluids, radiate heat to the periphery of the body, open the pores of the skin to increase sweating, and in their most extreme form, can burn the skin, as is the case with Garlic *(Allium sativum).* Many of these herbs taste pungent and contain aromatic essential oils and resins. They often influence the heart, circulatory system, and digestion, and they display diaphoretic, circulatory stimulant, carminative, and stimulant expectorant actions. Some examples of warming plants include Fennel *(Foeniculum vulgare)*, Ginger *(Zingiber officinale)*, Black Pepper *(Piper nigrum)*, Angelica *(Angelica archangelica)*, Prickly Ash *(Zanthoxylum clavaherculis)*, and Cayenne *(Capsicum annuum)*.

Cooling plants bring sedation to hypermetabolic, overly agitated, and stimulated organs and tissues, decreasing their innate heat and irritation. They thicken and congeal the fluids, restrain their flow, and anchor the vital force downward and inward when it excessively radiates up and out. This is referred to as "rebellious *qi*" in Chinese medicine. Excessively cold plants, such as Opium Poppy *(Papaver somniferum)*, can lead to intoxication, inebriation, and dulling or numbing of the senses, and it can depress overall organ function. Many cooling plants are bitter or sour in taste. Cooling plants include Hawthorn *(Crataegus monogyna)*, Rosehips *(Rosa* spp.), Lemon Balm *(Melissa officinalis)*, Dandelion *(Taraxacum officinale)*, and Oregon Grape *(Mahonia aquifolium)*.

Moistening plants hold a special place in herbalism, for a majority of herbs have a net drying effect. These increase moisture to hydrate and lubricate excessively dry, contracted, weak, and atrophic tissues. They can also increase transport of nutrients, oxygen, and waste products because fluids are the universal medium through which substances travel. They can increase moisture through either water or oil. Through their hydration they reduce hardness, provide a nutritive effect to the tissues, and promote flexibility, expansion, and relaxation of tissues that are overly constricted and tense from dryness. Primary herbs here are the mucilages and nutritive tonics that often have a sweet flavor and demulcent or emollient action, such as Marshmallow *(Althea officinalis)*, Slippery Elm *(Ulmus rubra)*, Licorice *(Glycyrrhiza glabra)*, Plantain *(Plantago major)*, Milky Oats *(Avena sativa)*, and Solomon's Seal *(Polygonatum multiflorum)*.

Drying plants remove excessive fluids from the body, constrain their outward flow, contract, tighten, and tonify the tissues. They help to "firm up" the body, close the pores of the skin, expel moisture, and protect the body from external pathogenic invasion. These remedies are the astringents, but many herbs dry by promoting diuresis, sweating, and excretion of fluids that leave the body. Many warming plants may lead to dryness as excess heat cooks off fluids. Some mineralizing remedies, like Horsetail *(Equisetum arvense)* and Nettles *(Urtica dioica)*, are astringents, but also dry through diuresis. When used for too long, many astringents, like Oak bark *(Quercus alba)*, are drying and can be damaging. Some examples of astringents are Uva-Ursi *(Arctostaphylos uva-ursi)*, Horse Chestnut *(Aesculus hippocastanum)*, Goldenseal *(Hydrastis canadensis)*, Yarrow *(Achillea millefolium)*, Yellow Dock *(Rumex crispus)*, and Lady's Mantle *(Alchemilla vulgaris)*.

Each of these four qualities can manifest on a spectrum of strength, which in the Greek system was divided into four degrees of intensity. Thus there is warming, cooling, drying, and moistening in the first, second, third, and fourth degrees, with the first degree being a mild influence and the fourth degree being a strong influence. The Chinese adopted a simpler system of degrees, with only two: warm and hot, cool and cold, and so on.

While the fourfold model is a common pattern for herbal energetics, in Western herbalism there's an additional threefold system of energetics from the Physiomedicalist tradition. Here, rather than focusing on the warming, cooling, moistening, or drying properties, an herbal remedy is observed to contain a property of stimulation, relaxation, or contraction. This system is based upon Albert Haller's ECR (excitation, contraction, relaxation) model (see chapter 6 for a discussion of this model of the nervous system). Matthew Wood pointed out this connection to me, which shows that this is not just an energetic system but a *physiological reality*. This model describes the connection between the nervous and musculoskeletal systems, called the neuromuscular junction, whereby motor neurons become stimulated (i.e., excitation) via electrical charges, which triggers muscular contraction through calcium release. When signaling from the motor neuron ends, calcium channels close and the muscles relax.[11] This process occurs in all muscle fibers throughout the body, as they are all innervated by the nervous system. Because the nervous system and muscles are distributed throughout the entire organism, they have systemic effects upon all organs and tissues, either directly or by affecting their circulation.

We can assess a plant based on its influence at this neuromuscular junction level and the resulting effects upon the nerves and muscles—whether they are stimulating, relaxing, or contracting. Because these are systemic actions that directly change the flow of the vital force (via the nerves and blood), I feel they constitute a separate category of herbal energetics that's distinct from the classical qualities of temperature and moisture. This is important because this category brings us to the final polarity in herbal energetics: the tonal quality of the tissues. We can relate this ECR cycle to three primary herbal effects: stimulants, relaxants, and astringents.

I originally learned this threefold model of classification from Paul Bergner, who based it on his in-depth research on the Physiomedicalist tradition of North America.[12] I have associated these three vital actions with the three *doshas* of Ayurveda and the Three Principles of alchemy, based on their overall similarity with one another:****

ECR	HERBAL EFFECT	PRINCIPLE/DOSHA
Excitation	Stimulants	Sulfur/*pitta*
Contraction	Astringents	Mercury/*vata*
Relaxation	Relaxants	Salt/*kapha*

**** Because the *pitta dosha* is warming and intense, it relates to stimulants. *Kapha* is the most relaxed and thus relates to relaxants. *Vata* is by nature nervous and tense, and it relates to tonic-astringents. These three energetic properties of plants will generally increase these *doshas* within the body, although of course there are always exceptions to the rule.

Stimulant remedies are those that increase the vitality within a particular organ or system by stimulating circulation or the nervous system. These two systems directly influence every part of the body and are the conductors of vitality throughout the organism. These are used primarily for depressed tissue states. I used to think that "stimulant" merely indicated something that increased the general activity of an organ. But through the tutelage of Matthew Wood I realized that this would essentially encompass every herbal remedy, as they all stimulate or affect organ systems to some degree. Thus this definition of stimulation is far too general and rests outside the traditional definitions of the word.

Stimulants increase vitality by bringing a greater level of blood flow and circulation to the local area, or by influencing the nervous innervation to that area. As the nerves are stimulated, we feel more alive, as we do when our tissues are full of freshly oxygenated blood, such as after going for a long run. Although most of these remedies are warming, there are some cooling herbs that are also stimulants. A good example of this is Echinacea *(Echinacea angustifolia)*, which stimulates blood circulation, immunity, and the lymphatic system but is also cooling energetically. Yarrow *(Achillea millefolium)* also stimulates circulation and has diaphoretic properties, but it is distinctly bitter and cooling at the same time. Because of this stimulating and often warming quality, I generally associate stimulants to the *pitta dosha* and the Sulfur Principle. The archetypal stimulant in Western herbalism is Cayenne *(Capsicum annuum)*. Other examples include Angelica *(Angelica archangelica)*, Prickly Ash *(Zanthoxylum clava-herculis)*, Ginger *(Zingiber officinale)*, and Black Pepper *(Piper nigrum)*.

The next two vital actions relate to a third qualitative factor distinct from temperature and moisture, which is tissue tone. Here we are looking at the relative tensile property of a plant, that is, whether it helps to relax a tissue that is overly tense, or to contract, astringe, or tonify a tissue that is overly loose. Not all herbs will necessarily have an effect upon tissue tone, but it's an important consideration when selecting herbal remedies. I like to think of the tonal property of a plant as being similar to the tension on a guitar string: a relaxant loosens the string, while an astringent (i.e., a tonic) will tighten it.

Astringents increase tissue contraction and are primarily used for relaxed tissue states. Bergner also uses the word "tonic" here. This requires further definition, as the word *tonic* is a rather nebulous term in Western herbalism. Often it refers to plants rich in minerals or nutrients, to be taken by everyone for overall support of the body. This definition lacks specificity and can lead to people using certain plants that may be incongruous with their constitutional needs. *Tonic* is also used in Chinese medicine, though in quite a different way, more similar to the Western term *adaptogen.*

Tonic derives from the Greek *tonikós,* which relates to the tonicity of muscles or tissue. This is looking at the word from a physiological perspective, as opposed to the more generalized dictionary definition as something that will "restore or improve health or well-being." Thus, a tonic remedy from this perspective is a plant that will increase the tone of the tissue, meaning it will tighten and contract the tissue when it is overly loose and lax. This is typically equated with the astringent property. It's worth noting that many of the nutritive tonics used in Western herbalism, such as Raspberry leaf *(Rubus idaeus),* Nettles *(Urtica dioica),* or Alfalfa *(Medicago sativum)* are also mildly astringent.

Astringents will increase tension within a tissue, like winding a guitar string tighter—and if it gets too tight, it can snap. As the *vata dosha* is primarily related to tension, there is a relationship between the tonic-astringent quality and this *dosha,* which relates to the Mercury Principle. Because these plants are primarily astringent, they are almost universally drying, yet not all drying plants are necessarily astringent. The archetypal astringents in North American herbalism are Bayberry *(Myrica cerifera)* and Goldenseal *(Hydrastis canadensis).* Others include Oak *(Quercus alba),* Red Root

(Ceanothus americanus), Rhodiola *(Rhodiola rosea),* Lady's Mantle *(Alchemilla vulgaris),* and Witch Hazel *(Hamamelis virginiana).*

Relaxants are plants that unwind tension, most notably within the nervous and musculoskeletal systems. These are often nervines and spasmolytics that reduce spasm and excessive nervous tension. Constrictive states restrict the flow of vitality wherever it is located, similar to when the water stops flowing through your garden hose because there is a kink in it. Similarly, blood circulation can be impeded by tension in the neuromuscular junction, contracting the blood vessel and reducing circulation. A relaxant will unkink the hose and allow the blood to flow more smoothly, thus raising the vitality. Because the *kapha dosha* is the most relaxed of the *doshas,* this quality corresponds nicely to its nature. It's common for people to think of a relaxant as having the opposite effect of a stimulant, though the true opposite of a relaxant is an astringent, or the tonic property. Many relaxants are acrid in taste. The archetypal relaxant remedy in North American herbalism is Lobelia *(Lobelia inflata),* although many spasmolytics and nervines fit into this category: Crampbark *(Viburnum opulus),* Black Cohosh *(Cimicifuga racemosa),* Valerian *(Valeriana officinalis,* which is also warming and stimulant), Hops *(Humulus lupulus),* and Blue Vervain *(Verbena hastata).*

Some plants "break the rules" or have seemingly contradictory properties. Wood Betony *(Stachys officinalis)* and Agrimony *(Agrimonia eupatoria)* are both relaxants for the nervous system but are also astringent. Black Haw *(Viburnum prunifolium)* is distinctly antispasmodic but is also a tonic for the uterus. When assessing the energetics of a plant, it is important to consider the three qualities of stimulant, relaxant, and astringent in conjunction with hot, cold, wet, and dry. This alleviates certain contradictions in the herbal literature that can be found when comparing resources on herbal energetics. For example, some sources note that Echinacea is warming, while others say it is cooling. A more accurate representation of its energetics is that it is a cooling stimulant. When we consider these seven energetic qualities together, we gain a well-rounded understanding of a plant's true holistic nature.

Other Energetic Considerations

Chinese medicine and Ayurveda have made a few unique contributions to energetics that are worth consideration. The first is the Ayurvedic concept of *vipaka,* which refers to the postdigestive effect of the plant. Remedies are classified based on their energetic effect upon the digestive system, along with their constitutional effect after the remedy has passed through the gut wall, which can sometimes be different. These properties are divided into three primary categories based on taste: sweet, sour, and pungent *vipaka.* A good example of this is Lemons. Their sour flavor warms the digestive system, but after digestion they cool down and sedate heat in the tissues. This is why lemonade is so refreshing on a hot summer day. *Vipaka* is unique to Ayurveda, and I believe it should be incorporated into our energetic understanding and classification systems in Western herbalism. This is also an important consideration in the long-term usage of an herbal medicine, as the postdigestive effects will become more pronounced over time. In Western herbalism, this differentiation could be equated to the short-term versus long-term effects of a plant.

The four directions of Chinese medicine relate to the directional quality of a medicinal substance, noting whether it will float (expand), sink (contract), ascend, or descend in the body. These properties are related to seasonal qualities as well as the relative density of plant parts; for example, leaves and flowers are more floating and ascending, whereas heavy roots and barks sink and descend. This pattern notes how a plant influences the directional flow of the vital force. Generally, cooling remedies tend to sink and descend, warming remedies tend to float and ascend, relaxants float and expand, and astringents sink and contract.

We can therefore break down the overall energetic properties of medicinal plants into the following categories:

FOUR QUALITIES	THREE PRINCIPLES	DIRECTION	POSTDIGESTIVE*
Warming	Stimulant	Upward (ascending)	Sour (*pitta*)
Cooling	Relaxant	Downward (descending)	Pungent (*vata*)
Moistening	Astringent	Outward (floating)	Sweet (*kapha*)
Drying	N/A	Inward (sinking)	N/A

Note: This energetic property is most important when an herb is taken over a longer period of time. For short-term usage it is best to look to the primary taste and quality of the herb.

Synergizing Herbal Actions and Energetics

The synergy between herbal actions and energetics is a critical element of understanding the holistic nature of a plant. Far too often people will look up herbs to treat a person based only on herbal action, and they'll get an extensive list of remedies that isn't specific enough to effectively treat someone holistically. This leads to a lack of precision in remedy selection, and it increases the potential of choosing plants that may conflict with the person's tissue states and constitutional patterns.

For instance, imagine a client with a harsh, hot, dry, racking cough that's keeping them up at night. You look up how to treat a cough in an herb book, and you note that the main action needed is an expectorant. Under the expectorant category you find an extensive list of herbs. It's far too easy to think, "This person has a cough. Coughs indicate expectorants. Here's the list of expectorants, so I'll just pick a few of them, and they should work." This is far too general an approach. If we are to be successful herbalists, we need specificity in our remedy selection, which can be achieved by coupling the action with the energetics.

That list of herbal expectorants might look like this: Osha *(Ligusticum porteri)*, Lomatium *(Lomatium dissectum)*, Elecampane *(Inula helenium)*, Mullein *(Verbascum thapsus)*, Licorice *(Glycyrrhiza glabra)*, Coltsfoot *(Tussilago farfara)*, Plantain *(Plantago major)*, Skunk Cabbage *(Symplocarpus foetidus)*, Yerba Santa *(Eriodictyon californica)*, Lobelia *(Lobelia inflata)*, Pleurisy root *(Asclepias tuberosa)*, Marshmallow *(Althea officinalis)*, etc. Now if you put together a simple three-part formula consisting of Osha, Lomatium, and Elecampane for this person with the harsh, hot, dry cough, you can almost be certain this formula will *aggravate* their condition, because these three plants are pungent, aromatic, warming, stimulating, and drying. In short, they are *contraindicated* for the respiratory tissue state (in this case, heat/excitation and dry/atrophy).

A more suitable organizational system for differentiating these plants would include linking their energetics with the action so we can get more specific in choosing the right remedy. This further differentiation could look like figure 22:

STIMULANT EXPECTORANTS (WARM AND DRY)	RELAXANT EXPECTORANTS (RELAXANT/ SPASMOLYTIC)	DEMULCENT EXPECTORANTS (MOISTENING AND COOLING)
Osha (*Ligusticum porteri*)	Lobelia (*Lobelia inflata*)	Coltsfoot (*Tussilago farfara*)
Lomatium (*Lomatium dissectum*)	Skunk Cabbage (*Symplocarpus foetidus*)	Marshmallow (*Althea officinalis*)
Elecampane (*Inula helenium*)	Pleurisy root (*Asclepias tuberosa*)	Plantain (*Plantago major*)
Yerba Santa (*Eriodictyon californica*)	Mullein (*Verbascum thapsus*)	Licorice (*Glycyrrhiza glabra*)

Figure 22. Energetic differentials of expectorants

These categories could be expanded upon and some remedies can be in more than one. For example, Mullein is both relaxant and moistening, as are Pleurisy root and Coltsfoot. But as you can see, the integration of herbal energetics with the actions helps to refine our materia medica organization to a greater degree of specificity that will aid in appropriate remedy selection. This results in matching the plants to the constitution of the whole person and the tissue state afflicting the organ system, making it a more refined classification system that's clinically oriented.

So rather than using a triplet of stimulant expectorants for this poor, tired person with the harsh, hot, dry cough, a more beneficial approach would be to use demulcent and relaxant expectorants that will soothe, cool, moisten, and relax the tension in the respiratory system and mucosal membrane. A more suitable triplet might be Coltsfoot *(Tussilago farfara),* Mullein *(Verbascum thapsus),* and Lobelia *(Lobelia inflata).*

Special Potency

The first four Keys we have observed are, in essence, linear, reductionist aspects of the plant. The taste of the herb is the first doorway we step into, which leads us to seeing its anatomical affinities, physiological actions, and unique energetic influence upon the constitution of the tissues. This synergy of tastes, affinities, actions, and energetics gives us a nearly complete picture of how a plant will affect the wholeness of a person.

But plants are of Nature, which is not linear; they don't always fit tidily in our systems of classification and categorization, no matter how refined these systems are. This is where we come to the final doorway, one that reaches into the essence of the plant, its unique identity or spiritual self. This Key is referred to as the "special potency" of the plant, which is a translation of the Ayurvedic concept of *prabhava.* According to Lad and Frawley, "Herbs also possess subtler and more specific qualities that transcend thought and that cannot be placed into a system of energetics. *Prabhava* can be called 'the special potency' of the herb. It is its uniqueness, apart from any general rules about it."[13]

This Key encompasses a plant's qualities, characteristics, and properties that transcend the linearity of classification systems. Within each plant there is something special, something unique, a healing virtue that cannot be placed within the context of taste, affinity, actions, and energetics. *Prabhava* is the part of the system that goes *beyond* the system, the backdoor to escape linear classification. Frawley and Lad explain, "[Ayurveda] understands the value and the limitation of systems, and only uses them as a guide, not a rigid rule. This spiritual orientation, one could say, is the *prabhava* of Ayurveda, the special power which can be learned from it."[14]

The special potency of a plant can exist on a spectrum of influence, ranging from unique abilities they have for the physical body to their subtler psychological, emotional, and spiritual properties. An example of a physical special potency is how Milk Thistle *(Silybum marianum)* contributes to the protection and regeneration of the liver, or how Nettle seed *(Urtica dioica)* restores damaged kidneys.

Another element of physical special potency is what the Eclectic physicians and homeopaths referred to as the "specific indications." These are constellations of physiological and psychological patterns within the body and mind that point toward a particular remedy. This can also include indications found within the pulse or the tongue, such as how Dandelion *(Taraxacum officinale)* is specifically indicated for the "mapped or geographical tongue," or Yellow Dock *(Rumex crispus)* for a ruddy, rusty-colored complexion and tongue.

Essential to the evolutionary herbalism model is the idea that physiological actions of plants are *not separate* from their psycho-spiritual properties. Their influence upon the body is but the densest property of how they influence the soul. The reverse is true as well; their spiritual properties are merely the subtlest aspect of their physical properties. Physical and spiritual properties are ultimately *one and the same*—two sides of the same leaf. To truly understand the holistic plant, we must learn to see how all properties of a plant—physical, energetic, and spiritual—are united within the essential core of the plant. The seemingly different properties of a plant are merely various reflections of one central pattern that is the plant's essence. This essence is what confers its special potency.

Frawley and Lad continue:

> *Prabhava includes the occult properties of plants, their capacity to affect the mind and psyche on a direct and subtle level.... Prabhava includes auric action, astral effect, magnetic effect, and radiation.... Ayurveda investigates the occult and spiritual effects of substances, and is not limited to any materialistic or chemical-based theory.* [15]

This is quite similar to Paracelsus's concept of the *arcana,* said to be the essence of the plant from which all physical characteristics and medicinal properties emerge. It is an invisible spiritual source at the center of the medicinal agent. As such, it operates upon the essence of the person and brings about transformational healing. The entire premise of spagyric alchemy is the extraction and refinement of the *arcana* within a plant.

There are many examples of special potency being reflected in these subtler spiritual properties of plants. Note how Rose flows into our hearts and heals the traumas of past relationships, instilling the courage and trust to love ourselves and others again, to be open-hearted and yet sufficiently protected. The signatures of Calamus restore the physical voice, teach us the power of our word to create our reality, and instill the confidence to use our voices again and translate our inner world to others through communication and self-expression. Cleavers helps us to detangle our relational cords, to let go and surrender our attachments, to have pure and clean relationships. Devil's Club helps us step into our personal power, strength, courage, and confidence through influencing the solar plexus and protecting us from malevolent spiritual forces. These are all examples of the *prabhava* of the plant as it is expressed on the subtler level of being. The goal for the evolutionary herbalist is to learn to see how that subtle influence is a refined expression of what the plant does within the body and become a student of the special potencies within plants.

The Elemental Plant

When this principle of classification is understood, the terminology of the alchemists becomes less recondite and absurd, for it is seen that the classification into Four Elements really refers to four modes of manifestation on the physical plane. This method of classification is of very great value, because it enables the relationship and correspondence between the physical plane and the life-processes behind it to be readily seen. It is especially important in the study of physiology and pathology, and in its practical application it is a most important key to therapeutics.

—DION FORTUNE[1]

Because the Elements form the foundations of the world, we can use them in our understanding of the holistic plant, tracing their patterns to these archetypal forces on various levels. The Elements manifest in plants through their overall structure, habitat, and influence upon the human organism as outlined in the previous chapter: taste, actions, affinities, energetics, and special potency. From leaf edge to root tip, the pattern of the Elements is fused into the entire botanical kingdom.

Note that just because a plant has a particular action, taste, or other trait that relates to a certain Element, that does not mean the *whole plant* corresponds to that Element. We want our Elemental correspondence to a plant to represent its wholeness and essence, not just a single property. Holding this in mind, we will explore each Elemental force and their specific signatures within plants, enabling us to begin to perceive the plants' Elemental architecture.

Earth

Generally, the Earth Element corresponds to the roots of a plant, as the morphological structure that anchors it into the soil. On a more specific level, plants with a strong Earth correspondence tend to be larger in appearance: broad leaves, stout and wide stature, thick, woody stalks, and dense growth patterns. Due to the heavy and sinking quality of Earth, these plants may droop or sag, with a downward movement of their vital force, such as that displayed by Comfrey *(Symphytum officinale)*. They will generally appear strong, sturdy, stiff, rigid, and solid. Red coloration can be indicative of the Earth Element, as it's the slowest wavelength in the color spectrum. In the Vedic tradition red relates to the *manipura chakra* at the base of the spine, which corresponds to the Earth Element.

In Ayurveda the sweet and astringent tastes are associated with Earth. Sweetness nourishes the body, building and strengthening weakened and emaciated tissues (i.e., deficient Earth), as well as moistening dryness. When taken in excess, sweet leads to weight gain and stagnation within the tissues, overbuilding the system with too much physical mass. Astringency binds the Earth together, tightening and tonifying loose, weak, apathetic tissues. This is achieved through tannins, which bind proteins to tightly conjoin the tissues, increasing their stability and strength. We can think of sweet plants nourishing and building the Earth, whereas astringents tighten and bind the Earth together.

In Chinese medicine, Earth correlates to the Stomach as the primary organ responsible for the nourishment of the body. It's paired with the Spleen, which is essentially the digestive system as a whole. In this way, certain bitter remedies that operate upon the stomach and digestion can correlate to the Earth Element. The feelings of worry, anxiety, and nervousness are commonly associated with the Stomach in Chinese medicine, which are notably "ungrounded" feelings and show a deficiency of Earth. When the digestive functions become deficient, it's common for the entire system to be prone to stagnation and toxicity as Earth accumulates in the tissues. This commonly reflects in the skin, which correlates to the Earth as the boundary of the physical body.

From this perspective, the category of bitters and alteratives can generally correlate to the Earth Element. These are important herbal actions for treating Earth Element imbalances, as they stimulate depressed digestive functioning, optimize nourishment (increasing Earth), and cleanse excessive metabolic waste products from the system (decreasing Earth). The latter is achieved by opening up the channels of elimination and cleansing the blood, liver, spleen, lymphatics, kidneys, and digestive system, though alterative plants will have different organ affinities, because this is a broad category. Thus, different alteratives and bitters may have different Elemental correspondences.

Many Earth plants strengthen the skeletal system through the presence of minerals and other nutritive agents, such as the bones, joints, and connective tissues. In this way, nutritive plants, with their large amounts of minerals, amino acids, fats, oils, and vitamins, assist in nourishing and strengthening the Earth Element. These plants often walk the thin line between food and medicine. Vulnerary and astringent properties correspond as they help to heal wounds and regenerate tissues.

Energetically, Earth plants are commonly cooling and drying, with a downward-bearing influence upon the vital force. This would be a sympathetic property. Yet, some are antipathetic in their medicinal actions, helping to warm and disperse excess accumulations of Earth in the body. This is an important point in observing the energetic architecture of a plant, as some remedies will *treat* an excess of an Element within the person (antipathetic), whereas others will *build* and *strengthen* that Element (sympathetic). Therefore, Earth plants can be used to treat the damp/relaxation, dry/atrophy, and damp/stagnation tissue states.

Each plant will manifest different qualities of its Elemental ruler and will thus initiate us into its spiritual teachings in a different way. One attribute of Earth Element plants is they help us feel more grounded and embodied, anchoring the vital force down and in. I also believe that Earth Element plants help us achieve a deeper level of tactile awareness of the world around us, teaching our bodies to become more sensitized to our environments, more in tune with the natural order. They help our minds become clearer, more focused, and less scattered, helping us let go of psychological stagnations in the form of rigid belief systems, outdated values, and conditioning imposed upon us by the external world. They teach our minds and hearts to be solid and strong yet flexible, like a tree that is deeply rooted in the Earth and yet can sway in high winds. Earth plants instill strength, discipline, and boundaries, so we can apply our spirituality with practicality.

These remedies may assist in healing specific traumas that relate to the Earth Element, such as physical abuse, accidents, dissociation from the body, eating disorders, abandonment issues, poor psychological and physical boundaries, and an excessive focus on spiritual practices and beliefs that move the vital force up and out, detaching us from our physical bodies and the Earth.

Burdock *(Arctium lappa)*

Morphologically, Burdock is a large, stout plant, with broad, rigid, rough-textured leaves and a thick taproot that penetrates deep into the soil (this is the part commonly used as medicine). I've seen Burdock roots up to four feet long that went straight down! It contains nutritive constituents that nourish the body in the form of carbohydrates such as inulin, pectin, sugars, and mucilage, giving it an oily, salty, sweet taste. Many of these compounds are strongly healing for the digestive system and provide prebiotic sugars that feed the microbiome of the intestinal tract.

The primary action of Burdock is alterative, with an affinity for the liver, blood, and skin. It's a classic blood purifier, cleansing the liver of excessive metabolic waste products, opening the channels of elimination, and moving stagnation in the lymphatics and blood. This in turn reflects outwardly in the skin. Indeed, one of its primary indications is for chronic skin conditions such as acne, eczema, and boils. These conditions are typically signs of accumulated metabolic waste products, or the Earth Element stagnating and congesting elimination pathways, leading to toxicity and depressed function of the excretory organs, such as the liver and bowels.

The uniqueness of Burdock is its equal application for people with excess Earth, displayed in a *kapha* constitution, or for people deficient in Earth, with a thin frame, dry skin, constipation, and poor absorption of fats and oils (*vata*). For Earth-excess people, Burdock will cleanse their system of accumulated waste products; for Earth-deficient people, it will stimulate digestion, absorption, and distribution of fats, oils, and nutrients. Burdock thus embodies both the sympathetic and the antipathetic aspects of the Earth Element in its medicinal properties.

Its energetic qualities are also unique in that it's not distinctly warming or cooling, but rather neutral. In the short term, it moistens the digestive tissues and skin, as in some instances of constipation, and it increases sebaceous gland secretions in dry skin conditions. But over longer periods of use it can lead to a certain degree of dryness by draining fluids through increasing secretions that ultimately leave the body through the liver, intestines, and urinary tract.

Water

The Water Element expresses in plants predominantly through their stems, which directly connect the roots (Earth) to the leaves (Air). The stems are the rivers that flow through the plant, sending communication between the aerial parts and roots, moving nutrients throughout its entirety.

Water plants will often grow in, around, or near water, and they prefer moist and shady parts of the ecosystem. Morphologically they will be juicy, with saps, mucilage, or a high water content. Their overall structure is often soft, delicate, and graceful in appearance, with cascading or flowing appearances. Their lines will be fluid and smooth, their texture soft, and sometimes the stem will be the predominant part of the plant, such as in Cleavers *(Galium aparine)* and Horsetail *(Equisetum arvense)*, both of which prefer moist habitats. We may see the color orange, as this color relates to the *svadhisthana chakra,* which corresponds to this Element, as seen in Calendula flowers *(Calendula officinalis)*, a notable lymphatic agent. Blues and purples may also correspond, as these are often color signatures for plants that help to remove deep stagnations within the fluids and tissues, such as Blue Flag *(Iris versicolor)* and Poke *(Phytolacca decandra)*.

According to Ayurveda, the two tastes associated with the Water Element are sweet and salty. We saw in the Earth Element that the sweet taste nourishes, but it also moistens, lubricates, and softens tissues that are dry and hard. Two sweet herbs strongly associated with the Water Element are the demulcents Marshmallow *(Althea officinalis)* and Slippery Elm *(Ulmus rubra)*. These contain mucilaginous polysaccharides, chemical constituents that can only be extracted in water.

The salty taste is a sort of crispy, heavy, mineral-like taste, such as is present in Kale or Celery. Table salt leads to water retention, hence the general recommendation to avoid it for people with edema or high blood pressure, but salty plants often indicate the presence of other minerals, as seen in Alfalfa *(Medicago sativa)*, Red Raspberry *(Rubus idaeus)*, Nettles *(Urtica dioica)*, and Horsetail *(Equisetum arvense)*. Minerals determine a great number of physiological processes, but especially kidney function. In contrast to table salt, many salty plants are diuretic, increasing water excretions from the urinary tract.

The primary herbal actions that correspond to the Water Element include diuretic, lymphagogue, demulcent, and the eliminative aspect of alteratives. While we did mention this last action under the Earth Element, it is equally applicable here, as excess Water leads to toxic accumulations of waste products. We can see this as accumulation of both Earth and Water, making it necessary to open the channels of elimination and cleanse the system.

Lymphagogues are a specific type of alterative that cleanse the lymphatic ducts and nodes. During acute and chronic infection, the lymph nodes become swollen with cellular debris, white blood cells, and viral or bacterial wastes. During immunological activity, the body is waging war, and the fields of battle are not often clean; the lymphatic system is responsible for cleaning it all up. When the system gets overworked and can't keep up, these internal waters get congested, and the lymph nodes swell with stagnation. Lymphagogues move this stagnant lymph and purify and filter the blood, and many also stimulate the liver or kidneys to aid in detoxifying the waste products. This reflects the archetypal purifying property of Water.

The stimulation of the kidneys to relieve excess fluids from the body is referred to as diuresis. Yet diuretic remedies don't only act locally on the kidneys; they also act systemically to drain fluids from the tissues, hence their benefit in puffy, swollen arthritic joints or edema. Some diuretics work by directly stimulating kidney activity, while others work more passively through mineral exchange—an action some refer to as "aquaretic." Because this action eliminates fluids from the system, it intuitively makes sense that it bears relationship to the Water Element.

Demulcents are remedies that contain mucilaginous polysaccharides, which act to soothe, moisten, and soften tissues that are dry, weak, and hardened. These constituents have an affinity for the mucosal membranes that line organ systems exposed to the outside world, and their balanced state should be consistently moist. As such, these tissues correlate to the Water Element. Thus, we see a chain of correspondences between medicinal action (demulcent), chemical constituent (mucilage), energetic principle (moistening), and organ affinity (mucosa), the connections of which all come under the dominion of Water. Whereas alteratives, lymphatics, and diuretics are primarily used for an excess of Water, demulcents are applied for Water deficiency or dryness.

Emmenagogues are plants that stimulate menstruation, with a strong affinity for the uterus and blood, relieving fluid stagnation, relaxing tension, and increasing circulation to the pelvic region. The reestablishment of menstrual flow and relieving fluids from the body is a distinctly Water Element quality, although different emmenagogues stimulate menstruation through different mechanisms, such as spasmolytic, circulatory stimulant, or bitter. Different emmenagogues may have different Elemental rulers, but the general action of stimulating menses is under the dominion of Water.

With regard to the energetics of Water plants, we see the dynamic of sympathy and antipathy at play, wherein some are drying through eliminating fluids (antipathetic) and others increase hydration (sympathetic). In their temperature dynamics, many are often cooling, though there are always exceptions to the rule, and some may be warming. This spectrum is represented in how they are used to treat the dry/atrophy and damp/stagnation tissue states.

The evolutionary function of Water plants varies in the same way Water manifests as liquid, gas, or solid, or as snow, hail, rain, lakes, rivers, and oceans. The one universal truth of these plants is their operation through the emotional body, helping us process and express the feeling dimension of our lives in a healthier way. When we feel dried up and atrophied emotionally, they hydrate the soul, allowing us to feel what we feel and accept our emotional reality. When we feel stagnant in emotional patterns, they move those blockages and reestablish the proper flow so we can experience a wider range of emotional expression. When we feel raw and sensitive, boundaryless and open, they contain our internal waters and distinguish self from nonself. They teach us how to navigate our inner emotional tides and how to maintain buoyancy and balance in the expression of feelings.

These remedies can heal traumas that relate to the Water Element, especially those associated with the reproductive system, including sexual abuse, abortion, and miscarriages. They physiologically and spiritually cleanse our internal organs as well as the psychological and emotional patterns generated through these traumatic experiences. Some may help with clearing feelings of shame and regret around past sexual experiences, teaching us to honor our unique sexual identity and to treat our internal sacred waters, as well as those of others, with the utmost respect. In this way many Water Element plants teach us about our relationships, where there may be residual stuck energy in our relational lines, and how to maintain clarity and cleanliness in how we relate with others.

Cleavers *(Galium aparine)*

Cleavers prefers to grow in moist, shady habitats and will avoid areas exposed to too much sun or dry soils. It's incredibly juicy and moist, and it grows in large groups to form lush growth patterns. Morphologically it bends and twists and turns like a river, with whorled leaf patterns and a certain "flowing" appearance. Its most noticeable dynamic is its "clinginess." In fact, Cleavers depends on its relationship to other plants to grow to its full height, a potent signature of its properties.

Within the body, it has a "green," mild, and salty flavor, which is indicative of one of its primary medicinal properties: diuretic. It's gentle yet reliable in its ability to drain stagnant fluids and aid in their elimination from the kidneys. Cleavers is an excellent remedy to flush the urinary tract, and it benefits hot, burning, irritated urinary tract infections (UTIs). At the same time, it's also an invaluable lymphagogue, treating swollen lymph nodes, tonsils, adenoids, lowered immunity, and infections. This combination of both diuretic and lymphagogue shows its strong affinity for the Water Element. This cleansing action is commonly used for chronic skin conditions due to "bad blood" and stagnation of internal fluids. It's cooling and acutely moistening to the mucosa of the urinary tract, making it useful in the treatment of hot, burning UTIs; however, because of its diuretic action, over the long term it will typically dry the constitution.

The special potency of Cleavers is specifically used for "attachment issues" and for people who cling tightly to things, especially other people. In the same way that a patch of Cleavers gets all tangled up in itself, this plant benefits people who get tangled up in unhealthy relational dynamics, ranging from abusive relationships to simply unsuitable partnerships. A Cleavers person has difficulty letting someone go; he or she feels wrapped up in someone else's emotional reality, easily tangled in their world, losing themselves in it. I've used this remedy in a broad range of relationship issues with multiple clients and have seen it work again and again, either by clearing up bad energy and bringing healing to the relationship, or helping the person let go, move on, and return to themselves. This usage was revealed to me directly by the plant itself, but there are many other herbalists who have come to similar conclusions and confirmed this property.

I once had a client who was tangled in an abusive relationship. She wanted out but was afraid of how her partner would respond, especially since he tended toward anger. She had a picture-perfect Cleavers constitution: thin, long limbs; a gentle, deerlike gaze; a soft voice; and a proneness to patches of dry skin. She had dealt with intermittent UTIs for years and corresponding lymphatic congestion in the pelvic region. After I administered three drops of a spagyric essence of Cleavers, she came down with a rather strong UTI that only lasted a few days and soon cleared up, as did her skin. Over a period of time, she felt a renewed courage when she emotionally detached herself from her relationship, as if seeing it from a distance, and realized she needed to get out, which she promptly did. Her chronic UTIs subsided and the dry skin cleared, and she's now in a happy and healthy relationship with someone who respects her.

This shows the multiple layers of signatures and correspondences—the pattern—within the client that correlated not only to the indicated remedy but also to the underlying Elemental force that was influencing her physiologically, energetically, and spiritually. While Cleavers was instrumental in her healing process, the plant was also a vehicle through which the Elemental force of Water flowed through her physical and astral bodies, triggering a transformational healing process that served in her soul's evolution.

Air

The main part of the plant correlating to the Air Element is the leaf, the primary location of gaseous exchange of oxygen and carbon dioxide. It's common in many plants for communication to occur with neighboring botanicals, insects, and animals through the release of volatile compounds from the leaves into the Air, carrying chemical messages to the rest of the ecosystem. In this way leaves are a highly important aspect of plant-to-plant communication.

Morphologically, Air plants tend to grow thin, slender, and angular, with significant amounts of space between their structures. They appear to be light, feathery, hairy, delicate, and gentle in appearance, with a general up and out movement to their vital force and overall form, such as we see with Mullein *(Verbascum thapsus)*. Color expression may range from blue to indigo and violet, which are quite common in plants with affinities for the nervous system, such as Lavender *(Lavandula angustifolia)*, Skullcap *(Scutellaria lateriflora)*, and Blue Vervain *(Verbena hastata)*. Another signature is climbing plants or whirling or spiralic patterns, such as Passionflower *(Passiflora incarnata)*. Their growth patterns may be scattered as opposed to growing in tightly clustered clumps, and some prefer to grow at high elevations. It's common for Air plants to be aromatic, containing volatile compounds that are so lightweight they diffuse into the atmosphere. While many of these are an important part of ecosystem and interspecies communication, most volatile compounds are also medicinal. Fennel *(Foeniculum vulgare)* is a good example, which also has a feathery appearance to its leaves.

According to Ayurveda, the Air Element relates to three tastes: astringent, pungent, and bitter. These are tastes that will typically increase the Air Element, primarily by aggravating dryness within the body. The astringent taste, as we saw in the Earth Element, will bind, tighten, and dry out local tissues. Pungent or spicy plants will increase heat and dryness, driving the vital force upward and outward. Air also moves up and out, so this can be aggravating; but as Air Element constitutions are typically cold, the warmth of pungents can be of benefit. The pungent flavor is also due to the presence of aromatic essential oils with affinities for the respiratory system, intestines, and nervous system, all of which relate to the Air Element.††††

The bitter flavor can aggravate Air because it's often constitutionally cooling and drying. That said, bitters can be of benefit in some situations because they usually move down and in, helping to anchor the vital force. This is why a strong bitter plant sends a shiver down the spine and why they can benefit shock or dissociation. Also, in certain situations of acute dryness they can be of benefit by increasing secretions of the exocrine glands, though it is important to consider that when bitters are used over the long term most of these fluids will eventually leave the body and result in dryness. Many bitter plants, such as Hops *(Humulus lupulus)* and California Poppy *(Eschscholzia californica),* are strongly nervine and antispasmodic as well, which is characteristic of the Air Element.

The corresponding herbal actions include expectorant, nervine, carminative, and spasmolytic. The expectorant action has its primary affinity for the respiratory system, helping to expel excessive mucus and thus making it the primary therapeutic strategy for treating coughs and respiratory infection. There is a wide variety of expectorants, and not all of them correspond to Air; some are warming, aromatic, and stimulating, such as Lomatium *(Lomatium dissectum)* and Elecampane *(Inula helenium);* others are relaxing, such as Lobelia *(Lobelia inflata)* and Skunk Cabbage *(Symplocarpus foetidus);* and still others are moistening, like Licorice *(Glycyrrhiza glabra).* Though based on their general affinity for the lungs, the expectorant category has a relationship to the Air Element.

---

†††† I consider the pungent tastes to be more strongly correspondent with the Fire Element, as they are typically spicy.

Nervines, as the name indicates, affect the nervous system. Like expectorants, there is a wide variety of nervine remedies, with some being stimulant like Coffee *(Coffea arabica)* or Yerba Mate *(Ilex paraguariensis);* others being gently relaxant, such as Chamomile *(Matricaria recutita)* and Lemon Balm *(Melissa officinalis);* still others being strongly hypnotic, like Hops *(Humulus lupulus)* and Passionflower *(Passiflora incarnata);* and some being nourishing and trophorestorative, like Milky Oats *(Avena sativa)*. In herbalism, the therapeutic application of nervines typically focuses on the gentle relaxants, stronger hypnotics, and nutritive trophorestoratives. In a Four-Element model, the Air Element governs the nerves; thus this general action bears correspondence.

Carminatives have their influence on the digestive system, increasing local circulation and relaxing spasm in the gut. These are primarily used to treat an excess of wind, most typically expressed as gas, bloating, tension, and constriction. Both in their affinity for the large intestine and in their treatment of the wind/tension tissue state, carminatives are an important herbal action related to the Air Element.

Along this line we also see the spasmolytics, of which carminatives are a particular type. These remedies operate through the smooth and skeletal muscles, as well as the nerves, providing a relaxant, antispasmodic effect that treats the wind/tension tissue state. Because the nervous system and muscles are systemic in their reach, spasmolytics act throughout a wide variety of organ systems, such as the circulatory system, bronchiole tree, ureters, biliary ducts, intestinal tract, and uterus. Some spasmolytics have systemic effects and can be applied for all manner of cramping and spasm, whereas others will have strong affinities for particular organ systems, such as Skunk Cabbage *(Symplocarpus foetidus)* for the lungs, Wild Yam *(Dioscorea villosa)* for the digestive system, Elderflower

(Sambucus spp.) for the skin, Black Cohosh *(Cimicifuga racemosa)* for the uterus, and Jamaican Dogwood *(Piscidia erythrina)* for the skeletal muscles.

Energetically, Air plants are mostly drying and can be mixed in their warming or cooling properties, although when treating individuals with an Air constitution it's often best to focus on warming agents, as such individuals tend toward cold patterns. The primary energetic property here is *relaxant,* because Air people have a strong predisposition for constriction, both psychologically and physiologically. Many of them will have an up and out movement of their vital force, and Air plants are typically used for the wind/tension tissue state.

Plants that embody the Air Element will embody the initiatic virtues with regard to the healing of our minds and cognition, teaching us our way of seeing the world and how that shapes our experience of life. They detach our awareness from our minds so we can become cognizant of our thoughts and perceptions. To cleanse these perceptions is to decolonize our mind of what is false and conditioned so it can be repatterned with our true essential nature that dwells within the heart, for the healthy mind is one that serves to the heart. In this way our perceptions become holistic, seeing the inner and outer as connected.

Many of these plants also hold important teachings regarding communication, both for how we communicate with ourselves through our thoughts, and for our capacity to translate our inner world to others through language and self-expression. They help us heal our voice, communicate effectively, to reveal who we are to others through our words. They also help us heal ourselves of the lies we tell ourselves, as well as the lies we have been told. By healing our throats, Air plants help us have the courage to speak the truth with compassion.

Mullein *(Verbascum thapsus)*

Mullein is a popular herbal remedy used in the treatment of the lungs and the respiratory system throughout the Western world. It's considered a critically important expectorant with many signatures that point to its relationship to the Air Element. The leaves are broad, lung shaped, and covered in tiny hairs, a common signature for the cilia that line the respiratory system. The basal rosette of leaves grows in a spiralic pattern like a Fibonacci sequence. In its second year of growth, it sends up a thin, tall inflorescence shooting up from the center of the rosette that gets amazingly tall; I've seen some Mulleins towering above me at seven to eight feet in height. This shows the up and outward dynamic of its vital force and indicates a volatile nature. This is reflected in its medicinal action, as it begins in the lungs and gradually moves into the upper respiratory system, sinuses, and head. It also prefers to grow in open, airy spaces and will rarely if ever be seen in the dark parts of the forest.

It's a moistening, demulcent, and relaxant expectorant, benefiting dry, irritated mucous membranes and spasm in the respiratory system. It draws water into dried, hardened tissues, lubricating and enlivening them. It is slightly relaxant, useful when breathing is shallow, irritable, and constricted, opening up the bronchioles and easing tightness. All of this points to its benefit in the treatment of dry/ atrophy and wind/tension in the lungs, our two tissue states generated by an excess of Air.

Another interesting correlation between Mullein and Air is its affinity for the nervous system. The flowers are used in an infused oil for nerve pain within the ears, and the tincture can be used for any type of nerve pain, especially when nerves are inflamed or irritated. After taking Mullein, many feel calmer and more open, not just within their chest, but also within their heads. Mullein is critically indicated for overly intellectual individuals, especially people who are particularly hard on themselves. The core pattern of this remedy is that it softens what has turned hard, which we see in its habitat, respiratory actions, and psychological properties. Mullein people often have tight, restricted thought patterns that turn against themselves in a self-critical manner.

Matthew Wood has this to say about Mullein: "William LeSassier used to say that mullein was for 'intellectuals and hot air people.' I have confirmed this several times. It is for people who think too much and congest the mind, or suffer mental tightness and congestion following difficult projects. Mullein gives such a person a feeling like the mind is opened up to breezes on a fresh spring day."[2] I find it fascinating that the image he uses to describe the action of Mullein evokes its correspondence to the Air Element.

Fire

Just as Fire is dynamic and expressive, representative of our essential nature, so too is the flower of a plant the expression of its true colors, displaying its interior nature to the world through its unique shape and color. Flowers radiate outward like Fire.

Fire plants tend to display medium-sized structures, not being obtuse and dense like Earth plants, thin and delicate like Air plants, or lush and flowing like Water plants. A key signature is the presence of sharpness, such as thorns, prickles, needles, or serrated leaf margins, such with Prickly Ash *(Zanthoxylum clava-herculis)* or Teasel *(Dipsacus sylvestris)*. Fire plants often have a particular intensity and a protective nature, with clearly defined boundaries, dense thickets of growth, or traits that make them unpleasant to touch. As the *pitta dosha* is oily in quality, these plants may also be oily, and because of their volatile nature like Air plants, these oils can be distinctly aromatic and pungent. They have warmer coloration, such as reds, oranges, and yellows, or they have sunlike flowers.

The primary taste attributed to Fire plants is pungent, which is due to the presence of aromatic oils. These compounds often have a spicy flavor that warms the gut, stimulates digestion, and increases circulation of blood. Here we see immediate relationships to the organ systems governed by this Elemental force. Strongly pungent plants drive blood with such force that they dilate capillary beds and open the pores of the skin, promoting sweating, and thus are commonly used in the treatment of fevers. While pungents have a short-term warming effect, they have a net cooling effect over the longer term, as they assist in the removal of internal heat, similar to opening the windows of your house when it gets too hot inside. Many of these aromatic oils are directly antiseptic or immunostimulant as well.

According to Ayurveda, the sour and salty tastes also correspond to the Fire Element. The sour flavor is unique in that it tends to warm the digestive system and stimulate secretions, which is why many people start their day with warm lemon water. And yet in their postdigestive effect, they tend to cool excess heat. Hence during the hot summer months people drink cold lemonade and eat berries. These sour foods contain a high level of antioxidant compounds that reduce inflammation biochemically and strengthen the cardiovascular system, two dynamics correlating with Fire.

The salty taste is said to kindle the digestive fire, with a sharp, cutting quality to it, especially when considering pure salt. Due to its hydrophilic nature and tendency to cause water retention, its excess can lead to blood stagnation and fluid retention, putting excess stress on the heart. In Ayurveda it is considered the least heating of the three abovementioned tastes. Salt burns when rubbed into open wounds.

The primary herbal action for Fire plants is stimulation, which can be provoked through a variety of organ systems. There's a spectrum of stimulants in herbalism, including digestive stimulants, circulatory stimulants, immune stimulants, stimulant diaphoretics, and stimulant expectorants.

Circulatory stimulants have their chief actions upon the heart, blood, and cardiovascular system, all of which are ruled by Fire. These remedies are universally pungent in quality, their spicy aromatic nature warming the gut, dilating peripheral vasculature, and driving the blood into the distant reaches of the system. While they are commonly used for the heart, they are applicable in various conditions, predominantly whenever increased blood flow is desired. Most circulatory stimulants are also carminative, as their aromatic oils stimulate digestion and bring more blood flow to the digestive organs. Some common circulatory stimulants that relate to the Fire Element include Cayenne *(Capsicum annuum)*, Prickly Ash *(Zanthoxylum clava-herculis)*, Ginger *(Zingiber officinale)*, and Garlic *(Allium sativum)*.

Stimulant diaphoretics are particular types of circulatory stimulants that drive blood to the surface of the body and open the pores of the skin, causing you to break a sweat. Even though these pungent, spicy plants initially warm you up, because they open the "vents" of the body and drain internal heat, they ultimately have a constitutional cooling effect. Hence it is common in hot climates for people to eat spicy peppers. These are commonly used to treat fevers, but they also have other applications, such as in chronic skin conditions and circulatory insufficiency to the surface (i.e., paleness). The circulatory stimulants mentioned earlier (Cayenne, Prickly Ash, Ginger, Garlic) also fit into this category.

In conjunction with circulatory stimulants is the general category of plants with a direct affinity for the heart, often referred to as cardiotonics. These remedies directly nourish and strengthen the heart, including its circulation and neural innervation, and they frequently support the strength of the vasculature. The archetypal remedy in this category in Western herbalism is Hawthorn

(Crataegus spp.). Others, such as Motherwort *(Leonurus cardiaca),* have distinct nervine properties, helping to settle a nervous heart, palpitations, and irregular heart patterns.

The adaptogenic category can also apply to the Fire Element, as many stimulate the vital force, especially when taken in higher doses. The general assumption is that these remedies operate upon the hypothalamic-pituitary-adrenal axis and are thus nourishing to the adrenal glands, although the research that supports these claims is questionable. Nonetheless, many adaptogens are quite warming, stimulating to circulation and digestion, and they help replenish a drained vital force from excessive stress, lack of sleep, poor nourishment, and other factors that lead to depletion. Remedies in this category include Asian Ginseng *(Panax ginseng),* Eleuthero *(Eleuth- erococcus senticosus),* Rhodiola *(Rhodiola rosea),* and Ashwagandha *(Withania somnifera).*

Immune stimulants also fit into this category. This can manifest in a variety of ways, from direct acute stimulation, such as with Echinacea (*Echinacea* spp.); strengthening and revitalizing a depleted immune system over time, as with Astragalus *(Astraga- lus membranaceus);* or acting as direct antiseptic, antimicrobial, or antivirals, as in the case of Elder (*Sambucus* spp.), Garlic *(Allium sativum),* and Ginger *(Zingiber officinale).*

Energetically, plants governed by the Fire Element are predominantly warming. Therapeutically speaking, they are applied to disperse stagnations and accumulations prone in Water- and Earth-type people, and to warm up the coldness of Air-type people. This would be an application of antipathy, or using an opposing Elemental force. As for their effects upon moisture, more often than not they are drying due to their innate heat. Typically Fire plants are used to treat cold/depression and damp/stagnation tissue states.

The evolutionary virtues of Fire plants consist in the way they bring us into closer contact with the essential self that dwells in the deepest part of our hearts. Upon activation of our internal fires, the other three Elemental bodies are purified: our minds are calcined of their conditionings, our unconscious emotional patterns are cleansed, and our physical bodies are detoxified and revitalized. Fire removes that which is false, and it not only awakens us to come into synchrony with our true essential nature; it also ignites us to *do something about it,* to shine our own unique spectrum of the Light of Nature out into the world and make a positive difference.

Fire Element plants operate strongly upon the solar plexus, which in the East is referred to as the *manipura chakra,* the center of our willpower, strength, and determination. As our hearts become reinvigorated, it guides our action to be aligned with a larger force than our own self-serving will so we act in accordance with the greater good of all. These remedies help us overcome obstacles to fulfilling our greater purpose in the world, strengthening our sense of self, autonomy, and personal power, and healing past traumas around authority, punishment, shame, and defeat. Anything that makes us think we can't achieve our hopes and dreams, leads us to be hard on ourselves, or value ourselves less than others requires a healing of the inner flame. In this way, Fire plants ignite a renewed sense of confidence, self-esteem, and the personal power to push through anything that holds us back so we can have the strength to shine out into the world the way we were intended to.

Cayenne pepper *(Capsicum annuum)*

This is likely one of the most important remedies in traditional North American herbalism. It was used by a great number of Thomsonian, Physiomedicalist, and Eclectic physicians throughout the nineteenth century and is still widely used by herbalists today. The relationship of Cayenne to the Fire Element is clearly apparent to anyone who has felt its flame on the tongue!

Morphologically, Cayenne displays this Element through its bright-red, flame-shaped fruits, which curve to a sharp tip. The powerful pungency of these peppers makes them one of the hottest plants in the

Western materia medica. Its power is conveyed first to the digestive system, where it warms and increases local circulation to the gut, stimulating digestive fire. This heat radiates outward to the periphery through potent stimulation of circulation. This is achieved by driving the blood, as well as dilating capillary beds and arterial vessels. As the blood travels further outward, it reaches the capillaries under the skin, opens the pores, and promotes sweating. Traditional physicians nicely summarized the primary pattern of this remedy when they said it "equalizes the circulation." It will bring blood to any part of the body where it's lacking.

These effects all point to its incredible benefits for the cardiovascular system. Its medicine is so profound, in fact, that it can save the life of a person having a heart attack by dilating the coronary arteries and driving blood directly into the heart. This indication originally came from Dr. John Christopher. It helps to dissolve phlegmatic accumulations in the blood vessels, maintain their elasticity, reduce oxidative damage, and promote proper distribution of blood throughout the organism. This is why Cayenne is commonly seen in so many herbal formulas; it opens the vessels and helps drive the blood and other herbs to their physiological destinations.

These dynamics are utilized to treat cold/depression and damp/stagnation tissue states, as the Fire Element operating through Cayenne relieves the impurities and lowered functioning associated with these patterns.

The oils contain antiseptic compounds, which treat infection both internally and externally. It's also a useful agent for pain, especially when associated with cold patterns, because it floods the local area with oxygen and nutrient-rich blood, along with warmth. Biochemically, it drains the local area of "substance P," a molecular marker that transmits the pain signal to the brain. Although there's an initial uncomfortable burn as substance P is drained from the local area, this counterirritant effect relieves stiffness in the joints and muscles.[3] This is why it is common to see Cayenne in topical products such as infused oils and salves used for musculoskeletal pain.

Ether

The Ether Element within plants is embodied in the seeds and fruits. Many Western models of plant Elemental morphology don't include this Element, giving fruits and seeds to the Fire Element, as per Rudolf Steiner. Considering that the Quintessence is the perfect harmony of the Four Elements and that the seed contains the roots, stems, leaves, and flowers as latent potentials, it's fitting that fruits and seeds correlate to Ether. The spirit of the seed is that it contains the entire pattern of the plant. In order for the seed's potentiality to become manifest—in order for the Ether of the plant to move down into material form—it must be planted in the Earth and given Water, it must breathe carbon dioxide from the Air, and it must photosynthesize the Fire of the sun to precipitate the next generation of plants.

In a Five-Element model, Ether relates to the nervous system, the brain, and the wind/tension tissue state, whereas in a Four-Element model these associations are under Air. Some herbal actions that correspond include nootropics, spasmolytics, and the nervine category, similar to what we saw under the Air Element. The first action here refers to plants that enhance cognitive function, memory, and acuity of perception. Many increase circulation to the brain and directly operate upon the nervous system in a rejuvenative or stimulating fashion. Spasmolytics and nervines are primary through their affinities for the nerves and influence upon wind/tension.

Psychotropic plants are a primary embodiment of the Ether Element. As Ether corresponds to consciousness and perception, plants that alter our perception and adjust consciousness bear a strong relationship to this Elemental force. Of course, all plants alter perception if we sensitize ourselves to them acutely, but some plants do this in very profound and noticeable ways. Almost every traditional culture around the world has some form of reverential and ceremonial use of intoxicants, many of which were used by traditional healers to enable them with a different perceptual orientation. This allowed them to see the root causes of disease as they exist on a spiritual level, and it helped them acquire a deeper knowledge of Nature through accessing the invisible reality or the archetypal landscape. It's important to note that these plants, mushrooms, and particular preparations were always regarded as *medicines,* not drugs used for escapism or to just get high. Their use in ceremonial and medicinal contexts is central to their appropriate utilization. Psychotropic plants have been on this Earth for a very long time, long before humans, and they perform important ecological functions that exist far beyond the sphere of how they interact with human consciousness.‡‡‡‡

Lobelia *(Lobelia inflata)*

Like Cayenne, Lobelia was an indispensable remedy used throughout North American herbal traditions. The most powerful part of the plant is the seed, though typically all the aerial parts are used as a medicine, including the stems and leaves. This remedy is most simply defined as a *relaxant,* used for treating the wind/tension tissue state, which is generated by an excess of the Ether Element. This relaxant, spasmolytic property is revealed through its distinctly acrid flavor. It relaxes constriction of the smooth and skeletal muscles and is thus used for a wide variety of range and spasm within the body.

While this is a rather simple description, this plant has far-reaching implications. It's considered one of the most "intelligent" of all herbal medicines, in the sense that it will acutely "read" the over-all vital force of a person and orient itself towards the specific organ systems and tissues that require its relaxant effects. From tension in

---

‡‡‡‡ For more information on this fascinating subject, see Stephen Harrod Buhner, *Plant Intelligence and the Imaginal Realm* (Rochester, VT: Inner Traditions, 2014).

the bronchioles in an asthma attack, to the cramping of the ureters when passing a kidney stone or the gallbladder and bile ducts when passing a gallstone, Lobelia has a unique ability to travel to the precise destination where it is most needed. It can be a bit unpredictable and changeable, like wind. Just as it sends itself to where it's most needed, it has the intelligence to direct other plants to where they're needed too. Thus, it's rarely used alone and is considered best in formulation.

These facts all point toward its embodiment of the Ether Element. The blue to purple coloration of the flowers (*Lobelia inflata*) correlates it to the upper energy centers, or *chakras*, of the body. These colors are also often signatures for relaxants and antispasmodics. Its primary effectiveness for wind/tension points toward its benefit in conditions related to *vata*, which is composed of the Air and Ether Elements. As Quintessence relates to intelligence and communication, the way Lobelia orients itself to the individualized needs of the body and tells other plants how to do so in formulation also points towards its embodiment of this final Element in our exploration of Elemental Herbalism.

While plants contain every Elemental force—for they cannot exist without having all of them—each tends to have one or two Elements that are most dominant. These dominant correspondences are determined by assessing the *wholeness of the plant,* not just single aspects of it. The fact that a remedy has spines does not necessarily mean it is ruled by Fire; the fact that a plant is an expectorant does not automatically place it under the dominion of Air. You must look at the entirety of the plant and see which influence is dominant and what force moves through it the strongest. That said, some practitioners will correlate two Elements within a plant; for instance, you could relate one Element to an organ affinity and another to its energetics. An example of this would be Osha (*Ligusticum porteri*), embodying Air and Fire, with its pungent, aromatic, warming essential oils containing a stimulant expectorant property (Fire) with a primary affinity for the respiratory system (Air).

The Elements *never* exist in isolation from one another. While we separate them for the sake of study, life comes into existence only through dynamic interactions between Elemental forces. Perceiving their synergy is the study of life itself, and observing how they interact in natural systems is the best way to understand these patterns. We all know that Fire requires wood from the Earth to burn, that it sends the smoke up into the Air, that fanning the flames with Air makes them grow. If Fire is applied to Water held by the Earth, it will evaporate into the Air, but if the Water comes into direct contact with the flames, the Fire goes out. Water sends Fire into the Earth, and Fire sends Water into the Air. When observing nature—whether in the form of an ecosystem, a plant, or a person—it's critically important to assess how all of the Elemental forces are woven together to understand its core qualities and characteristics. This is important for clearly seeing the medicinal properties of a plant, assessing the organ systems, and developing therapeutic strategies.

15

The Triune Plant

*In wood, stone or herbs there are three things contained, nor
can anything be generated or grow if but one of the three should
be left out. First, there is the power, from which a body comes to
be, whether wood, stone or herbs. After that, there is a sap in that
thing, which is the heart of the thing. Thirdly, there is in it a spring-
ing, flowing power, smell or taste, which is the spirit of the thing,
whereby it groweth and increaseth. Now if any of these three fail,
the thing cannot subsist.*

—JACOB BOEHME[1]

Just as we relate the Five Elements to plants, we can do the same
with the triune pattern of the *doshas* and the Philosophical Principles. As the threefold pattern is born from the Elements, many of the
qualities and characteristics discussed in the previous chapter apply
here, though in a slightly simpler model of organization. Here we will
discuss the process of perceiving the qualities of the Three Principles
and *doshas* within plants, including some of the general therapeutic
strategies for treating with them.

Vata

Plants with *vata* characteristics are similar to those that embody Air and Ether qualities. They are often thin, tall, dry, rough, and hard, with spaciousness between their morphological parts. We often see feathered appearances, such as Cilantro *(Coriandrum sativum)* or Fennel *(Foeniculum vulgare)*, dainty flowers, a small stature, and a general up and outward movement of the vital force. Many *vata* plants are also aromatic in nature, as they diffuse into the Air. Blue Vervain *(Verbena hastata)*, Chamomile *(Matricaria recutita)*, Cleavers *(Galium aparine)*, and Black Cohosh *(Cimicifuga racemosa)* have distinct *vata* morphological characteristics.

Central to the understanding of medicinal substances in Ayurveda is their *rasa,* or taste. Each taste can either pacify or aggravate a particular *dosha.* Accordingly, the bitter, astringent, and pungent tastes are considered aggravating to the *vata dosha,* as they all lead to dryness. That said, pungents can provide a useful therapeutic approach for this constitution because they tend to be cold, and pungents are distinctly warming. It's only when dryness and lightness are prominent that pungents are contraindicated or best used in mild form and for short periods. Herbs that contain these tastes may point toward a correspondence with *vata.* The sweet, salty, and sour flavors are generally considered beneficial for this constitution, as they help to nourish, strengthen, and moisten their weakness and dryness.

As *vata* governs the large intestine and lungs, herbs with an affinity for the respiratory tract (expectorants) and nervous system (nervines) often embody characteristics of this *dosha* because they are united by the Air Element. As *vata* correlates to the overall functioning of the nervous system, plants with this affinity are strongly indicated. Due to its proneness toward tension and cramping, the spasmolytic category proves highly beneficial. Warming carminative agents that increase blood flow and dispel wind from the intestines are useful for *vata's* variable, cold digestion. The overall therapeutic strategy is to bring in warmth, moisture (water and oil), heaviness, and relaxation. Primary affinities include the colon, respiratory system, nerves, and muscles.§§§§

Other useful categories of herbs includes adaptogens, trophorestoratives, demulcents, nutritives, relaxant diaphoretics, and circulatory stimulants. Laxative remedies, when used properly, can treat obstructions of *vata* in the colon, but they must be used with caution. According to Ayurveda the best way to eliminate excess *vata* is through enemas, which clear excess Air from the bowel. This is typically done through specific herbal-infused oils. In terms of our three primal herbal energetics, the astringent/tonics are sympathetic to *vata,* as they increase the tone and tension in the tissues; hence we generally treat its excess with the opposite, relaxants.

This *dosha* is classically difficult to balance, due to its changeable nature. As soon as you try to warm it up, the excess heat provokes dryness. As you attempt to calm and relax its tension, it tends to become overly cold, as many nervines are cold plants. Thus it's best practice to use relatively mild, gentle herbs that don't shift any particular energetic quality too far in one direction or another. This can also be remedied by strategically compounding formulas to balance incongruent energetics in certain indicated herbs.

From the perspective of alchemy, the *vata dosha* closely correlates to the Mercury Principle, which relates to the spirit or alcohol of the plant. Herbs that yield a higher quantity of volatile spirits in the spagyric process are said to have a stronger embodiment of this Philosophical Principle and thus sympathetically target the spirit of the person. This is commonly found in plants with higher quantities of endogenous sugars and starches, which feed the bacteria in the fermentation process and thus yield more alcohol.

---

§§§§ While *vata* generally relates to the lungs through the Air Element, it's worth noting that the lungs are a primary accumulation site for *kapha* via the mucosal membrane.

Some examples of excellent remedies used to treat *vata* constitutions are Marshmallow *(Althea officinalis)*, Licorice *(Glycyrrhiza glabra)*, Fennel *(Foeniculum vulgare)*, Ginger *(Zingiber officinale)*, Ashwagandha *(Withania somnifera)*, Shatavari *(Asparagus racemosus)*, Valerian *(Valeriana officinalis)*, and Tribulus/Gokshura *(Tribulus terrestris)*. It's worth noting that some of these plants will be sympathetic to other *dosha* qualities, as Ayurveda is based on antipathetic medicine. Thus Marshmallow, being soft, lush, soothing, moistening, and cooling, is a distinctly *kapha* plant used to treat the dryness, lightness, and weakness of *vata*.

Kapha

Kapha plants are generally stout in appearance, with thick, broad leaves, a larger stature, and a downward-bearing vital force. They appear lush, soft, juicy, and heavy, and they generally prefer to grow in moist, shady environments due to the fixed qualities of the Earth and Water Elements. Plants such as Burdock *(Arctium lappa)*, Poke *(Phytolacca decandra)*, Comfrey *(Symphytum officinale)*, and Red Root *(Ceanothus* spp.) display distinct *kapha* characteristics.

According to Ayurveda, the sweet, salty, and sour tastes increase the Water Element in the form of mucus, especially sweet and salty. These tastes in excess can lead to *kapha* accumulations in the body, which is balanced by pungent (warming coldness), astringent (drying moisture and tightening laxity), and bitter plants (draining fluids and clearing stagnations).

As *kapha* is the ruler of the stomach and moisture, many bitter tonic and alterative plants bear correspondence with it, as they remove excess waste products and stagnations of fluids, and the bitters stimulate digestion—although we must exercise caution with the coldness of bitters. Due to their damp, relaxed, and cold nature, pungent, aromatic, stimulating, drying, and tonifying remedies prove beneficial for balancing *kapha's* excesses. Therapeutic actions that prove beneficial for *kapha* include astringent, circulatory stimulant, warming, alterative, diuretic, diaphoretic, lymphagogue, and carminative. These are all "reducing" therapies that dry and eliminate.

A major therapeutic strategy is to simply stimulate their system into a greater level of activity, keeping the fluids and organs moving, especially the liver, lymphatics, kidneys, and overall metabolism, and maintaining the digestive flame, which tends to become cold easily. This includes circulatory stimulants, stimulant expectorants, stimulant laxatives, stimulant diaphoretics, and stimulant diuretics. Maintaining proper tissue tone with astringents is also important, to prevent excess laxity or prolapse. According to Ayurveda, the best method for cleansing excess *kapha* is through emetics—clearing it from the stomach—which is its primary site of accumulation.***** Plants that are sweet, demulcent, moistening, relaxing, and cooling are generally contraindicated due to their sympathetic relationship to *kapha,* such as slippery elm *(Ulmus rubra).* In a threefold model of herbal energetics, relaxants most closely correspond to *kapha* because this *dosha* is relaxed in quality, so they are commonly contraindicated. Their opposites, tonic-astringents, are indicated.

In Alchemy the *kapha dosha* most closely correlates to the Salt Principle, which is found in the alkali minerals of plants. These are separated from the plant through a process called calcination, whereby the physical plant is burned down to ash and the minerals are crystallized. Different plants yield varying quantities of alkali salts through this process, although remedies rich in minerals will generally have higher amounts, such as Nettles *(Urtica dioica)* and Horsetail *(Equisetum arvense).* Plants with more alkali salts are rich in this Principle and thus penetrate deeper into the physical body.

***** Most herbalists these days don't administer emetics too often, though most traditional systems of medicine acknowledge their medicinal value. This category of medicines should always be administered with care and knowledge of their proper usage, timing, and indications. Emetics are a central element of Ayurvedic detoxification protocols, called *panchakarma.*

A few remedies considered balancing for an excess of *kapha dosha* are Ginger *(Zingiber officinale)*, Dandelion *(Taraxacum officinale)*, Black Pepper *(Piper nigrum)*, Oak bark *(Quercus alba)*, Horse Chestnut *(Aesculus hippocastanum)*, Osha *(Ligusticum porteri)*, and Oregon Grape *(Mahonia aquifolium)*.

Pitta

Pitta plants, being composed primarily of the Fire Element, evince many similarities to plants under this Elemental correspondence. Much like people, they are generally midsized morphologically, neither stout and thick nor slender and dainty. It's common for them to appear intense, revealed through sharpness, thorns, prickles, and fiery coloration such as oranges, reds, and yellows. They can have a domineering presence. They may be oily as well, as *pitta* is oily in its fluid expression. Some plants that display strong *pitta* qualities include Oregon Grape *(Mahonia aquifolium)*, Cayenne *(Capsicum annuum)*, Nettles *(Urtica dioica)*, Blackberry *(Rubus* spp.), Rose *(Rosa spp.)*, and Prickly Ash *(Zanthoxylum clava-herculis)*. It's worth noting that while all of these plants are *pitta* in their appearance, some of them will increase *pitta* in the body, while others will decrease it. It's important to observe the spectrum of sympathy and antipathy when assessing the energetic architecture of a plant, whether that's according to the *doshas*, the Elements or the Planets.

The distinct quality of *pitta* rests in the embodiment of the Fire Element. Thus, plants that are heating, stimulating, and pungent bear a sympathetic relationship, and are typically contraindicated for people with a *pitta* constitution. The other two tastes in Ayurveda that contain Fire are salty and sour, as salt burns when rubbed in a wound, and strongly sour substances, such as vinegar, distinctly warm the stomach. Yet as mentioned previously, many sour medicines, such as berries, are distinctly cooling to excess heat or *pitta* in the body.

The general therapeutic approach is cooling, soothing, and sedating remedies that relieve excess heat from the body, such as through relaxant diaphoretics. Plants that are antioxidant, sour, bitter, and relaxant often lead to cooling the body. With relaxants this happens because *pitta* tends toward stress and heightened energy levels that need to be calmed. Ayurveda considers bile to be the physical manifestation of Fire in the body, so bitter plants that operate upon the liver and gallbladder are important in *pitta* management, and many bitters are distinctly cooling. Interestingly, in Chinese medicine the liver stores the emotions of anger and frustration, a common psychological tendency for imbalanced *pitta*.

Because Fire breaks things down, the sweet taste is distinctly remedial, as it helps not only to cool excessive heat by providing more Water but also to nourish the system and strengthen weaknesses as a result of heightened metabolic activity and combustion. Plants that operate upon the small intestine, heart, cardiovascular system, and blood may bear correspondence here, especially the latter two, for heat damages the heart and circulatory system more than any other part of the body. When the blood becomes toxic, alteratives help to clear out inflammatory substances and cool irritation. The adrenal glands and immune system are also important considerations for *pitta* plants, making the adaptogen, diaphoretic, and immune stimulant categories pertinent. The corresponding energetic action of the Physiomedicalists is the stimulants, which would certainly be contraindicated for *pitta*-type individuals who are already hot and overstimulated.

According to alchemy, the Sulfur Principle is the equivalent to *pitta*. This Principle is found in the essential oils of the plant, which are considered its soul. In alchemy, Fire is the most volatile of the Four Elements and is thus the first Principle to be released from a plant when it is submitted to distillation. Plants that yield a high amount of essential oils are said to be rich in Sulfur and thus sympathetically have a strong influence upon the human soul.

A few common remedies used to treat excess *pitta dosha* include Lemon Balm *(Melissa officinalis)*, Hawthorn berry *(Crataegus monogyna)*, Rose hips and flowers *(Rosa* spp.), Elderberry *(Sambucus* spp.), Lavender *(Lavandula angustifolia)*, and Yarrow *(Achillea millefolium)*.

The essence of determining constitutions within people is to search for underlying patterns, and the same holds true for herbs. As you observe a plant, it's important to perceive it through the lens of this threefold system, learning to decipher the patterns of the *doshas* within it through not only its physical form but also the underlying patterns in its medicinal properties, organ appropriations, and energetics. This is why the descriptions in this chapter include some general therapeutic strategies for treating the *doshas,* as this is what lends deeper insights into how these forces are imprinted within our remedies and practically applied.

When deciphering the pattern of three within a plant, we should consider the spectrum of sympathy and antipathy, that is, whether the plant will tend to aggravate and increase a particular *dosha,* or whether it will decrease and pacify its excess. Nettles *(Urtica dioica)* illustrates this nicely because it appears particularly *pitta* morphologically, but it's cooling and treats excess heat internally, thus decreasing *pitta.* Other plants are more straightforward, such as Cayenne *(Capsicum annuum),* which also appears very *pitta* with its bright red flame-shaped fruits, and is equally pungent and stimulating in the body, increasing *pitta.*

While the Elements and Principles are intimately related because the latter are generated from the former, it's often true that correlating a single Element or Principle to a plant doesn't fully encompass its wholeness. For example, we may attribute the Water Element to Nettles, based on its diuretic properties and its ability to drain damp/stagnation from the tissues. But this doesn't speak to its rich mineral content or its nutritive or astringent properties, which can be expressed through its strong correlation to the Salt Principle *(kapha)*. Thus we may say that Nettles holds the architecture of the Water Element and the Salt/*kapha* Principle.

Yet even this consideration does not reflect the wholeness of this remedy, which is why the evolutionary herbalism system uses a third pattern of energetics, represented by the Planets. As we progress through the energetic architecture of plants, we begin to see that each pattern is imprinted upon them on various levels. When we apply all three levels of architecture—the Elements, Principles, and Planets—we are able to encompass the wholeness of the remedy and its embodiment of the universal life force.

16

The Celestial Plant

Each plant is in a sympathetic relation with the Macrocosm and consequently also with the microcosm, or, in other words, with Constellation and Organism, and each plant may be considered to be a terrestrial star. Each star in the great firmament and in the firmament of man has its specific influence, and each plant like-wise, and the two correspond together.... In this way, a herbarium spirituale sidereum might be collected.

—PARACELSUS[1]

As with the patterns of the Elements and Principles, the energetic qualities of the Seven Planets correspond with the botanical organism on the multiple scales we have been exploring. In this regard, the Seven Planets, as the harmonic of Nature, form a truly holistic model for understanding plants, revealing their core pattern reflected upon each scale of being. As a translation mechanism, the Planets allow us to see the dotted lines that connect a plant's physiological, psychological, and spiritual properties, as they do with people. In this way, they constitute a holistic universal language that unites people and plants with the pattern of the whole.

As we did with people in chapter 12, the following material will break down the Salt, Mercury, and Sulfur qualities of the Planets as they relate to plants. This encompasses their morphological and environmental qualities (Salt), influences upon the human organism (Mercury), and evolutionary properties for the soul (Sulfur). Many of the environmental and morphological signatures here are derived from the work of Julia Graves and her excellent book *The Language of Plants,* along with my own observations. I derived many of the medicinal signatures myself based on the doctrine of correspondences and on further insights gleaned from Matthew Wood, Judith Hill, and Dr. Samuel Sagan.

The Sun

Salt

Sun plants often favor open fields and southern-facing slopes with optimal amounts of direct sunlight, like Calendula *(Calendula officinalis)* and St. John's Wort *(Hypericum perforatum).* They sometimes follow the pathway of the Sun, such as the heads of Sunflowers *(Helianthus* spp.), or they open in the presence of light and close in its absence, such as California Poppy *(Eschscholzia californica).*

The principle of sympathy and antipathy always applies in our assessment of the energetic architecture of a plant, and this is commonly seen in herbal ecosystems. Thus, warm and dry climates are sympathetic to the Sun, yet many Sun plants grow in cold and damp climates, an antipathetic signature. Angelica *(Angelica archangelica)* seeds can only germinate in cold environments, and they prefer moist and cold habitats, yet its properties are distinctly warming and stimulating to circulation, a particularly solar quality.

Morphologically, a common signature is radiant disclike flowers, yellow-orange in color, such as Calendula, Sunflower, and St. John's Wort mentioned above. Sun plants are not distinctly large or small, but medium in size, with an angular appearance, as we see with Sun people. They appear strong and confident in themselves. The plants may grow individually or in groups, with coloration often being yellow, orange, gold, and possibly white. There's often a general upward and outward movement of the vital force, exhibiting the expansiveness and radiance of the Sun.

Mercury

Sun plants primarily taste pungent, which warms the body, disperses stagnation, expands up and outward to promote sweating, and kindles the digestive Fire. This taste is associated with aromatic volatile oils, resins, or gums, which benefit tissue states and constitutional patterns of cold and damp, a common pattern with Sun deficiency.

The pungent taste corresponds to the primary action of many Sun-ruled plants: circulatory stimulant. This action benefits the heart and vasculature, but also the brain, immunity, and digestive system. If we increase blood flow to the brain, memory will improve. If we increase circulation to the digestive system, we increase nutrition and absorption, and we alleviate a variety of common digestive complaints. And of course, increasing circulation benefits the heart and cardiovascular system by alleviating stagnation within the vasculature, strengthening the tensile strength of veins and arteries, and benefiting literally every cell of the body by increasing oxygen and nutrient delivery and facilitating waste product removal. Many circulatory stimulants raise the core temperature in the *solar* plexus, bringing blood flow to the core, where it's distributed throughout the periphery, bringing warmth to the whole organism. Circulatory stimulants under the dominion of the Sun will often be mildly spicy and aromatic, such as Ginger *(Zingiber officinale)* or Rosemary *(Rosmarinus officinalis),* whereas powerfully hot ones are related to Mars, such as Cayenne *(Capsicum annuum)* or Prickly Ash *(Zanthoxylum clava-herculis).*

Cardiotonics nourish, strengthen, tonify, and have a general affinity for the heart, Hawthorn (*Crataegus* spp.) being the classic example. It's worth noting here that while the Sun rules the physical heart, the emotional and spiritual heart bears relationship to Venus, the archetype of love, harmony, and relationship. There are a number of remedies that operate upon the heart that correlate to Venus, such as Rose *(Rosa* spp.) and Linden *(Tilia europaea)*. Eyebright *(Euphrasia officinalis)* is a classic Sun remedy for its specificity for the eyes, as is Rosemary *(Rosmarinus officinalis)*. Many plants that benefit the eyes do so by operating through circulation.

Adaptogenic herbs build our vital reserve and replenish core energy. Many are immunomodulating, strengthen the adrenal glands, and can be rather stimulating, often giving them a dual rulership with Mars. We will see many similarities between the Sun and Mars, for they both govern the masculine dynamic forces, though each has its specific and distinct qualities. The heat of the Sun is more gentle, constant, and pleasant, while the intense heat of Mars is like inflammation and fever, burning away impurities.

Energetically, solar remedies will be hot and dry and are thus contraindicated in heat/excitation tissue states. And yet we see the interplay of antipathy and sympathy once again, as some Sun herbs are hot and dry, such as Calendula *(Calendula officinalis)*, St. John's Wort *(Hypericum perforatum)*, and Angelica *(Angelica archangelica)*, and others *treat* hot and dry in the body and are thus cooling and soothing, such as the fresh, flowering tops of Chamomile *(Matricaria recutita)*. But the majority of Sun remedies are indeed warming and drying to the constitution. They typically treat the cold/depression and damp/stagnation tissue states, or an excess of *kapha,* and are used for the heart, circulatory system, eyes, heat of digestion, and strengthening our core vitality.

Sulfur

Medicines of the Sun facilitate in connecting to our essential self. They are specific for those whose inner light is dimmed by clouds of self-doubt, who hide from the light of the soul, or who live in accordance with the conditioned self rather than the true self. Solar plants instill confidence, self-worth, and self-esteem, and they help those tending toward depression. By strengthening our abdomen and giving our heart a solid foundation to rest upon, Sun remedies illuminate our being with light, lifting us out of inner darkness to provide clarity, inspiration, and insight into who we truly are, giving us the courage to heal. Through Sun plants, we heal our connection to the center of ourselves and the divine center of Life. Another attribute of Solar plants is that they may support in healing issues with our fathers, as the Sun generally relates to the archetype of the Father,††††† whether we are male or female.

St. John's Wort (Hypericum perforatum)

St. John's Wort flourishes in habitats with full solar exposure, preferring southern-facing slopes. Many times I have driven through the backcountry scouting for St. John's Wort and finding absolutely none ... until I drove around a particular bend in the road and hit the south side of the mountain, where I came upon glorious fields of golden flowers as far as the eye could see. Those golden flowers have the distinct coloration of the Sun, with the pistils radiating from the center being particularly reminiscent of the emanation of light. St. John's Wort has one remarkable signature of the Sun: it starts blooming almost exactly on the summer solstice, the longest day of the year. This identifies it with the feast day of St. John the Baptist, which is the Sunday closest to Midsummer Day.

The taste of St. John's Wort is particularly warming and "balsamic," lending a drying energetic property that disperses stagnation, especially in the liver. The tincture has a blood-red color, a signature for remedies operating in the bloodstream, and St. John's Wort is highly

††††† It's worth noting that issues surrounding the father can also be related to Saturn.

effective for treating blood poisoning and sepsis, especially when caused by puncture wounds and tetanus. While its primary organ correspondence with the nervous system doesn't directly relate to the Sun (this is why I use other layers of energetic architecture that fill in these gaps, in this case, the Air Element), it's the particular *action* upon this organ system that is distinctly solar.

The medicinal effect of St. John's wort is nourishing and strengthening to the nervous system, what is commonly called a nervine trophorestorative. It is suitable for an exhausted, burned-out state that needs to be strengthened and restored, and for the depressed, melancholic person. Both could be seen as a solar deficiency. St. John's Wort directly nourishes and rebuilds a worn-down nervous system, but it also uplifts and mildly stimulates the nerves into a greater level of activity. It's also specific for nerve pain. We can think of it as specific for the cold/depression tissue state, whether afflicting the liver, nerves, or consciousness itself.

For people who feel trapped in their life circumstances—utterly stuck, unable to move forward, and completely disconnected from their true self—St. John's Wort is an effective remedy. It brings a certain quality of light into the heart and mind, illuminating unconscious patterns that we'd rather keep tucked in our interior closets and bringing them to the light of our awareness so we can deal with them. Of course, everyone knows that St. John's Wort is "good for" melancholy and depression, a symptomatic pattern of solar deficiency. In this way it can be likened to a *shen* tonic, uplifting the heart and dispelling inner darkness.

In traditional European folk medicine, it was a highly prized remedy of psychospiritual protection against witchcraft, hexes, curses, and all manner of dark magic. It's said to bring the protection of the angels, surrounding us in a shielding field of light. From my perspective, it does not necessarily work from the outside in, but rather from the inside out, strengthening our connection to the essential solar self so we are empowered and strong—so filled with our own nature there isn't room for anything else to enter. St. John's Wort is said to instill the light of Sun throughout the spirit and soul.

The Moon

Salt

As the Moon relates to the Water Element, plants stamped with a lunar signature often grow in wet or boggy habitats; in, around, or near bodies of Water; or the damp parts of the forest. Naturally, plants containing ample moisture are slimy or produce a mucilaginous substance when mixed with water, such as Marshmallow *(Althea officinalis)*, Slippery Elm *(Ulmus rubra)*, and Chickweed *(Stellaria media)*, and these correlate to the Moon. From an antipathetic perspective, some lunar plants reside in *opposite* habitats from where we might expect, growing in hot and dry environments. A perfect example is Aloe *(Aloe vera)*, a cooling, moistening plant growing in the hot-dry desert. I often think of this as the plant embodying the opposite qualities of the ecosystem, providing balance for people who live in that region.

Many lunar plants express a certain silvery coloration, similar to the color of the Moon. This is commonly seen in the genus *Artemisia* (which is named after Artemis, the Greek goddess attributed to the Moon), in plants such as Mugwort *(Artemisia vulgaris)*, Wormwood *(Artemisia absinthium)*, and Sweet Annie *(Artemisia annua)*. Wormwood is traditionally attributed to Mars and Mugwort to Venus (though I question these correspondences). As a generality, the Artemisias belong to the Moon.

Another color pattern is white, seen in the milky latex exuded from fresh Milky Oat seeds *(Avena sativa)* and in most of the mucilages. The softer colors of purple and blue are also common signatures for many nervine remedies that calm the nervous system and are beneficial for sleep, such as Skullcap *(Scutellaria lateriflora)*, Passionflower *(Passiflora incarnata)*, and Borage *(Borago officinalis)*. Many plants ruled by the Moon will be delicate, juicy, smooth, and soft, with rounded, curved, flowing, graceful forms.

Mercury

The primary tastes of lunar plants are mucilaginous, bland or sweet, and bitter. Healing by sympathy, the mucilaginous property of Aloe *(Aloe vera)*, Marshmallow *(Althea officinalis)*, and Slippery Elm *(Ulmus rubra)* moisturize the mucosal membranes of the urinary, digestive, and respiratory tracts. The mucosa are ruled by the Moon. The sweet taste assists in strengthening weakness and emaciation, and moistening dryness, embodying the nourishing and wet qualities of the Moon. Remember, though, that "sweet" in herbalism indicates more of a bland taste than anything else, such as starches. True sweet-tasting substances are usually attributed to Venus. The bitters provoke secretions from the mucosa, often have a systemic cooling effect, and are excellent for strengthening the digestive capacity of the stomach, calming the nerves, and draining excessive fluid accumulations. Examples are the bitter mints, like Skullcap *(Scutellaria lateriflora)*.

This leads us into our first two actions, demulcent and emollient, which correlate to the mucilaginous polysaccharides contained in the herbs mentioned above. These are essentially indicated for moistening dryness and softening hardness, specific in their application for the dry/atrophy tissue state (Moon deficiency). Many actions that work on our inner Waters have a correspondence to the Moon, such as diuretics (draining fluids), lymphagogues (moving stagnation from the lymphatics), and galactagogues (increasing lactation).

Although nervine remedies that directly sedate, calm, and nourish the nervous system are not traditionally associated with the Moon, I believe they fit under her rulership. This is based on their action upon the brain and their benefit for inducing sleep. There's a spectrum of influence with nervines, from mild sedatives to strong hypnotics and nutritive trophorestoratives. There is also a

wide variety of nervine remedies, and some fit under other Planetary rulers, most notably Venus (who relaxes), Mercury (who rules
aspects of the nervous system), and Uranus (who governs constriction and tension).

Due to the influence of emmenagogue plants upon the uterus,
which is ruled by the Moon, some may correlate through stimulating menstruation. The female reproductive system as a whole is
governed by Venus, and many emmenagogues are under her dominion as well. It is common to see certain degrees of overlap between
lunar and Venusian plants, just as Mars and the Sun sometimes
crossover.

Energetically, lunar plants are moistening and cooling. The
category of moistening plants is relatively limited, however, and
we cannot base lunar correspondences simply on a moistening
property because there are lunar remedies that are energetically
drying, such as the Artemesias. They generally will have an affinity
for the stomach, uterus, fluids, lymphatics, mucosal membranes,
brain, and nerves.

Sulfur

Lunar plants facilitate the development of sensitivity, empathy, and
our overall receptive nature. This requires a purification process
that cleanses the emotional body of traumas, habits, and repeating
past mistakes that hold us in old patterns of emotional behavior.
These remedies tend to dredge up the subconscious patterns we
stuff into the attics of our lives, enabling us to deal with the parts of
the self we hid there. For us to truly reflect the light of the Sun, we
have to face the shadow it casts.

This is where we see the psychological actions of the Artemisias. Mugwort *(A. vulgaris)* has long been used to increase access
to dreamtime. The late Australian herbalist Dorothy Hall used it
as a "brain remedy" for people with unusual or difficult thinking

patterns. Matthew Wood discusses this aspect of the Artemisias in *Seven Herbs, Plants as Teachers.* In addition, many of these plants are worm and parasite remedies, as if physical parasites are analogous to the psychological burdens we pick up along the path of life. Herbalist Sean Donahue calls Wormwood "psychotherapy in a bottle."

These plants teach us to cultivate or return to emotional buoyancy and maturity by dealing with our emotional reality. This involves developing sensitivity, both with ourselves and with others. To generate compassion for all life requires us to develop an emotional connection to it, allowing what's "out there" to enter "in here," and letting the world touch and move us. Lunar remedies teach us to *surrender.*

Moon plants are highly indicated within our masculine-dominant yang culture, bringing in the slowness, receptivity, and magnetic qualities that balance the excessive volatility of the Western world. In these times when our energy is spread thinly and dispersed outward, Moon remedies bring us back home to ourselves and encourage us to take the time to reflect upon our inner nature. This is a potent teaching of the Moon, for it is through these deep emotions that we start to feel the interweaving of the external and the internal. With the Sun, we see the Light of Nature externally; with the Moon we feel it internally.

In a time when imagination and dreams have been reduced to mere coincidences or fantasy, Moon remedies couldn't be more indicated. Through the Moon we connect to the power of the imaginal realm and the power it holds for physical manifestation. These remedies teach us to dream again, not in the Jupiterian sense of life dreams but in a spiritual sense, opening up our imaginal faculties as a valid mode of perception and cognition. As the Moon generally relates to the archetype of the Mother, some lunar remedies may help with supporting issues with our mothers.

Marshmallow Root *(Althea officinalis)*

Lunar signatures are stamped in Marshmallow's soft, delicate leaves and beautiful white flowers fading to serene purple in the center, along with the white roots that are incredibly moist and mucilaginous. The plant as a whole has a lush, gentle appearance and loves growing in moist soils.

The taste is bland and slightly sweet, indicating its nourishing, moistening property. Mucilaginous polysaccharides are responsible for this sweet flavor and for its demulcent action, which moistens dry mucosal membranes in the digestive, respiratory, and urinary systems. Interestingly, these constituents cannot be extracted in any menstruum other than Water. This form of medicine, achieved through a room-temperature water infusion of the roots, yields a thick, mucilaginous substance that hydrates dry tissues. When tissues become dry, they harden and have difficulty receiving oxygen and nutrients, which Water delivers to the cells, so the moistening action of Marshmallow helps to rebuild, strengthen, and nourish weakened and emaciated tissues.

It's one of the most indicated remedies for the dry/atrophy tissue state, a lunar deficiency. While it's specifically used for constipation due to a dry colon, dry coughs, and urinary tract infections, it can be applied any time there's dryness. In Chinese medicine, this is referred to as yin deficiency.

This dryness can also move into the psychological and emotional spheres. The Marshmallow person often feels emotionally dry and hard, unable to flow with their feeling nature and emotional expression. Just like the fluids, the emotions become dry, stuck, and hardened within the emotional body. This pattern reflected in the mind can also lead to difficulty with cognition, thinking, and even nervousness and tension, as the nervous system experiences dryness and becomes functionally impaired. Thinking is not fluid and graceful, communication bogs down, and memory can be impaired, as the Moon relates to memory.

Mars

Salt

Mars plants express through various embodiments of intensity, such as serrated and jagged leaf margins, or any sharp and pointed structures, such as prickles, thorns, or needles. We see this in the leaves of Oregon Grape *(Mahonia aquifolium)* as well as our classic Mars plant, Nettle *(Urtica dioica)*. Plants with a dominating presence, towering over the rest, or growing in aggressive patterns that take over the ecosystem can relate to Mars, like Blackberry (*Rubus* spp.), which has sharp thorns and serrated leaf margins, yet its berries are cooling and anti-inflammatory. We see this reversed action with Nettle as well: it's topically inflammatory and irritating, yet internally it's cooling, anti-inflammatory, and soothing for excess *pitta*. The patterns of sympathy and antipathy express in the signatures of these two plants because they exhibit Mars qualities externally, yet their medicinal virtues help to decrease an excess of Mars internally.

Another physical signature is red or purple coloration, the latter signifying blood stagnation and a need for stimulation. Many alterative and immune activating herbs bear this signature, such as Echinacea (*Echinacea* spp.), whose cone-shaped, prickly flower is a Martian expression. Mars plants are sometimes red, indicating fever, but intensity is a better indicator. As a plant goes into the purple color there is more sepsis with inflammation. Here we see the relationship between Aries and Scorpio, both ruled by Mars, representing fever and septic infection. In modern astrology, Pluto, the ruler of Scorpio, is associated with sepsis and putrefaction. Plants with indigo or purple are antiseptics, like Wild Indigo *(Baptisia tinctoria)*, Echinacea (*Echinacea* spp.), and Poke *(Phytolacca decandra)*. The latter plant is both red and dark purple, yet it has a lazy look and is associated with lymphatics (Moon). Matthew Wood adds:

Burgundy colored plants like beet root (Beta vulgaris), sumac berry (Rhus typhina, R. aromatica), cooked Rehmannia root (Rehmannia glutinosa), and the rusty-burgundy yellow dock root (Rumex crispus) increase blood count in many different ways. I always wondered why this was the case. After twenty years I realized that the bone marrow and liver, which manufacture and store hemoglobin, are grey/burgundy in color.[2]

Iron, the chemical element of the blood and hemoglobin, is ruled by Mars, of course.

Mars plants may like to be in warm and dry habitats, a sympathetic signature, or they may antipathetically prefer cold-damp areas, bringing a warming and drying quality to remain in balance with their environment. The Pacific Northwest has multiple species of Mars plants, such as Devil's Club *(Oplopanax horridus),* but the environment is typically opposite to Mars.

Mercury

The primary taste is pungent, like the Sun, though Mars is more intensely heating than the Sun. These plants strongly move the blood and is intensely stimulating. A subcategory of pungent remedies are the "diffusives," which stimulate innervation and peripheral circulation. Because of this they leave a highly active, tingly sensation on the tongue. This is exhibited by Spilanthes *(Spilanthes oleracea)* and Echinacea (*Echinacea* spp.), which is not just an immune tonic, as advertised in fad herbalism; it is also a stimulant to the venous circulation and lymphatics, through which the immune system operates. The bitter taste also corresponds to the red planet. Many bitter substances have a strong action on the gallbladder, provoking digestion and increasing digestive Fire. Yet most bitters have a constitutionally cooling effect and are strongly indicated for states of heat/excitation, inflammation, and pain. The sour flavor can bear Mars correspondences, as most are cooling to the constitution, decreasing heat, inflammation, and oxidative damage to the tissues, especially the blood vessels.

The bitter taste leads us to our first action for Mars, which is alterative. Now, this is a very general correspondence, for there are many types of alteratives with different planetary correspondences. In general, alteratives help to purify the blood, which has a powerful impact on the whole body, for the blood touches every part of us. People who benefit from alteratives are damp and stagnant, needing Martian stimulation. Most alteratives facilitate general detoxification and the catabolic side of metabolism, but the ones with the strongest affinity for the blood will relate to Mars, with Nettle *(Urtica dioica)* and Echinacea *(Echinacea angustifolia)* being prime examples. The bitter flavor also relates to an action upon the gallbladder, the organ commonly correlated with willpower. Some systems of medical astrology relate the gallbladder to Mars, while others place it under Saturn.

Another primary action of Mars is the stimulant action. This general action has its affinity with our immune, circulatory, and nervous systems. Coffee *(Coffea arabica)* is a stimulant to the nerves, and Echinacea *(Echinacea angustifolia)* is a stimulant to the blood and immunity. Cayenne *(Capsicum annuum)* is a stimulant to the circulation. Another type of stimulant is the category of diaphoretics, with their capacity to help break fevers and general benefits for acute fever and immune deficiency. Stimulant diaphoretics work by actively circulating the blood to the periphery, raising the core body temperature, and opening the pores of the skin to relieve excess internal heat. These are most useful for fevers where the individual is cold, sluggish, and groggy (Mars deficient).

Adaptogens bear correspondence (along with Jupiter) in the way they support the body's overall adaptive response to stress. Many are considered rejuvenative tonics that help to rebuild and restore core vitality (hence they also relate to the Sun), but many are quite stimulating and are commonly believed to help "rebuild" atrophied adrenal glands. (The adrenals are also classically attributed to the signs of Aries and Libra.)

Again we see the sympathetic and antipathetic principle apply to the energetics of Mars plants, as many are distinctly warming and stimulating, whereas others will in fact be cooling and sedative to excess heat patterns. Thus, it's critical to select the appropriate remedy by assessing the tissue states and making sure the chosen Mars plant will either warm its deficiency or cool its excess, achieved by observing the temperature quality. They will generally influence the blood and circulation, adrenals, inflammation, immunity, and gallbladder.

Sulfur

The evolutionary virtues of Mars plants initiate us into reclaiming our strength and personal power, imbuing a warrior spirit. I often think of these remedies as "power plants" for physical and spiritual protection. These plants reintegrate parts of the self that were lost due to trauma, such as accidents, physical abuse, domineering relationships, or other situations where we felt powerless or unable to exert control. This reclamation of our personal power increases our decisiveness, courage, and ability to take action. By harmonizing our egoic will with the divine will of our spirit, Mars plants teach us how to enter a state of spiritual congruency, aligning our actions with the truth that dwells in our hearts. In this way these remedies connect us to the "cosmic fire," which is the divine will in action. They also support imbalanced Martian psychological qualities such as anger and frustration.

Nettles *(Urtica dioica)*

This was one of the first remedies that clearly indicated to me the multilayered relationships between plants and Planets. The patterns of signature and correspondence are nothing short of stunning—an excellent example of the clear connections between above and below.

The leaves have sharp, serrated margins and can develop a reddish-purple coloration, indicating an affinity for the blood and remedial action upon fluid stagnation. The most distinct Mars signature in Nettles is the sharp, formic-acid needles that stud the entire plant. When touched, these glass-like needles shatter, spilling formic acid onto the skin and leading to the classic urticaria response of the Nettle sting. The skin becomes red, inflamed, irritated, and itchy. While some see this as a toxic response, herbalists across the world view it as a unique therapeutic property, using it to stimulate blood circulation, relieve fluid stagnation, and treat dull, achy muscular pain.

Biochemically, Nettles is rich in iron, the metal of Mars. This mineral is highly concentrated in the blood, which is one of the primary affinities of Nettle leaf, which cleanses the blood through its alterative action and nourishes it through its nutritive properties. It's commonly used for "bad blood syndrome," which the Chinese refer to as damp/heat, whereby the tissues are drained of excess fluids, stimulated to relieve stagnation, and cooled of excessive inflammation and irritation. Nettles shows the spectrum of sympathy and antipathy toward Mars, with such strong embodiments in its morphology and affinity; yet it will treat Mars excess in the body through its cooling nature.

Another common use of Nettle leaf is the treatment of histaminic allergies, rhinitis, and hay fever, which provoke inflammatory processes. Just as Nettles creates this response when you touch it, internally it treats the same pattern. It drains fluids, astringes leaky mucosal membranes (i.e., a runny nose), and reduces local inflammation in the upper respiratory tract. Most people experience hay-fever symptoms in the spring, when pollens are excreted into the Air (thus affecting our internal Air Element through the respiratory system), which the body responds to as foreign, igniting an immunological response. Depending on where you live, this is typically the time Nettle leaf is in its prime and is best harvested. The early spring relates to Aries, which is ruled by Mars and in medical astrology is associated with the head. Thus we can think of Mars in Aries being excess heat in the head, or the sinuses, expressed as rhinitis and hay fever. This is precisely the pattern Nettle leaf treats during the season when it is preferably harvested.

The seeds are a valuable remedy, which come into fruition in the beginning of autumn, during Libra, the opposite sign to Aries. Libra rules the kidneys, and Aries rules the adrenal glands that sit atop them. The seeds of Nettles are kidney trophorestoratives that also influence the adrenal glands, which are ruled by Mars. Thus the pattern deepens as Nettles embodies the axis of influence represented by the Aries-Libra polarity and the operations of Mars and Venus. (Venus rules the urinary tract, and Nettles is particularly diuretic).

The roots of Nettles treat the male reproductive system. Like the seeds, the roots are best harvested in autumn, after the vital force of the plant has descended from the aerial parts into the roots. The ideal time to harvest Nettle roots is in the sign of Scorpio, the second sign of the zodiac associated with Mars and the ruler of the male reproductive system.

Spiritually, Nettles is an effective remedy for an excess of Mars, expressed as psychological frustration and irritability, an underlying aggravation in the personality that is easily triggered or "nettled." Like the plant, Nettles people are highly sensitive and easily triggered, always on the edge of boiling over. This can occur either from excessive energy flowing through their vital force that needs to be cooled off, or by being burned out, fatigued, and overly depleted from pushing themselves too hard. This remedy is unique in its ability to both cleanse and strengthen the Martian pattern within a person.

Thus we see a highly complex tapestry of the celestial influence of Mars impressed upon this highly regarded medicinal plant, not only through its morphology or medicinal properties, but also in the different parts of the plant used, their unique affinities in the body, and the seasonal timing for when they are ideally harvested. This example clearly illustrates how planetary correspondences not only influence plants on all levels, but more specifically, how they reflect the core essential pattern that imprints itself upon every form and function of the plant. But as we will see later, Mars on its own does not encompass the wholeness of Nettles. For this, we require seeing into its entire architecture by relating it to the Elements and Principles as well.

Venus

Salt

Venusian plants often have a delicacy and daintiness to them, a graceful, soft, feminine appearance. Some can be tall, slender, and angular, and others can be lush and full, with bright, showy flowers and pale hues of green. Pasqueflower *(Anemone pulsatilla)* and the Rose (*Rosa* spp.) are beautiful examples of Venus plants with showy flowers. It's common to see fernlike leaf structures or feathered appearances, like that seen in Yarrow *(Achillea millefolium)* or Chamomile (*Matricaria recutita)* leaves. Venusian plants may also have sweet fruits.

Often the softer colors of blue, purple, and white will be more prominent in Venusian plants. It is common for many of them to be relatively aromatic and contain volatile essential oils, often floral and "perfumey" in their aromas, as is the case with the Damiana *(Turnera diffusa)*. As Venus has a relationship to the spiritual heart, we may see heart signatures on the plant itself. Their habitats will often be lush, moist, and beautiful, with a certain magic in the air. Venusian plants are a wonder to behold.

Mercury

One of the main tastes/actions that balance Venusian influences is astringents, a property used to treat the damp/relaxation tissue state. Astringents knit together proteins to bring more tone and structure to the tissues, especially the skin, veins, and connective tissues. Horse Chestnut *(Aesculus hippocastanum)*, Witch Hazel *(Hamamelis virginiana)*, and Yarrow *(Achillea millefolium)* are all used to increase tone and structural integrity in cases of hemorrhoids, varicose veins, and other cases of tissue laxity. Many astringents are used topically on the face to tone the skin and enhance beauty, a notably Venusian application.

While excess Venus generally produces relaxation in a person, her medicinal influence in plants may also generate relaxation. Thus

Venusian plants are commonly nervine and antispasmodic, which correlates nicely with her traditional association with being anodyne, or relieving pain. These remedies relax the nervous system and muscles to ease spasm, tension, and cramping, and to bring about a state of openness and calm. Thus, Venus plants can treat an excess of wind/tension or *vata*. A few antispasmodic/nervine remedies associated with Venus include Pasqueflower *(Anemone pulsatilla)*, Motherwort *(Leonurus cardiaca)*, Lavender *(Lavandula angustifolia)*, and Blue Vervain *(Verbena hastata)*.

Considering Venus to be the opposite of Mars, we see interesting parallels in their actions. With Mars, we see fevers being treated sympathetically through the use of stimulant diaphoretics that increase circulation to the periphery. The relaxant Venus, on the other hand, works antipathetically to a fever through what are called relaxant diaphoretics, which function by relaxing peripheral tension in the neuromuscular junctions of the blood vessels, dilating them to bring blood to the surface. It's as if they unkink the hose to allow the fluids to flow more easily and distribute heat to the surface. Then they relax the pores (controlled by tiny muscles) to release the cooling waters of perspiration. In this regard, Venus is cooling. Yet, by astringing and closing pores, Venus prepares us for winter by being mildly warming. "In Venus these mild properties are not contradictory," explains Judith Hill, "because the purpose of Venus is to make us comfortable, whatever form that may take."[3]

As Venus relates to all things sweet, some remedies have a strong sweet taste, such as Licorice *(Glycyrrhiza glabra)* and Fenugreek *(Trigonella foenum-graecum)*, and others, such as Gymnema *(Gymnema sylvestre)*, operate on blood sugar levels. Licorice is an interesting remedy in its relationship to Venus due to its incredibly strong sweet flavor, moistening energetics, cortisol-sparing effects, and strong inflammation-modulating property (Venus balancing Mars excess), as well as its use in traditional medicine to "harmonize a formula." This is fitting, as Venus personifies the principle of harmony. The

sweet taste often indicates demulcents, which are cooling and hydrat-
ing in quality and can correspond to either the Moon or Venus.

Diuretics are important with Venus, as they operate upon the kidneys and urinary tract. But diuretics don't just have their effect on
the kidneys; they affect the Water Element as a whole, purging fluids
from the tissues. Hence, they relieve edema in the ankles, swollen
arthritic joints, or other swellings, draining fluids from the extra cellular space and moving it toward the kidneys for elimination. Therefore the diuretic category has a general correspondence to Venus, as
do remedies that are kidney trophorestoratives and tonics. Manzanita
(Arbutus manzanita) is an excellent example of a Venusian diuretic,
with its soft, evergreen leaves, lush appearance, and delicate, pink
flowers. Eastern and European herbalists will use its cousin Uva-Ursi
(Arctostaphylos uva-ursi) as an astringent diuretic.

Female reproductive actions are ruled by Venus, such as emme-
nagogues and uterine tonics. This latter action is typically associ-
ated with astringents with a specific uterine affinity, such as Lady's
Mantle *(Alchemilla vulgaris)*, Red Raspberry *(Rubus idaeus)*, Yarrow
(Achillea millefolium), Black Haw *(Viburnum prunifolium)*, and Rose
(Rosa spp.). Emmenagogues often have a strong relationship to
Venus through their ability to relieve blood stagnation and stimulate menses. Some are astringent for relaxation, such as Red
Raspberry, while others are relaxants for tension, such as Motherwort *(Leonurus cardiaca)*, and still others are bitter and circulatory
stimulant, like Yarrow. Many spasmolytic and nervine remedies fit
in here, as the female reproductive system is prone to spasm and
cramping, which require the relaxing influence of Venus.

Sulfur

Venusian plants have unique abilities to heal our emotional and
spiritual hearts, especially the wounds they harbor associated with
current or past relationships. These plants help untangle our relational cords, the energetic connections we form with people, when

they get intertwined and messy. If we lack honorable closure with a relationship that has ended, a part of our vital force is still connected to that person, especially when we harbor blame, judgment, or other negative emotions for them (or they harbor such feelings toward us). Venusian remedies untie these old knots and help us forgive both ourselves and the other. A central thematic element of Venusian plants is their support in integrating the lessons presented by these initiatic relationships.

Her influence also applies to the sphere of sexual trauma. Venusian plants restore the spiritual integrity of a reproductive system that has been adversely affected by rape, abortion, or miscarriage, cleansing the organs physically and energetically to restore their purity.

In their highest manifestation, Venus plants teach us to love ourselves so we can learn to love others and clear everything that gets in the way of achieving that most noble pursuit. As Venus purifies our hearts, teaches us to open again, and helps us put our trust and faith in the love that binds everything together, we enter into a new level of relationship, not only with our loved ones, families, and communities, but with all of Creation and ourselves. Venus teaches us to be in co-creative relationships with all of Nature and to see ourselves reflected in the natural world. Through Venus we touch the Earth, and the Earth touches us back, entering the great council of relations on Mother Earth. And through that relationship, we learn to love again.

Rose *(Rosa spp.)*

As a universal symbol for love, no plant relates to Venus more strongly than Rose. We see her signatures in the velvety smooth, delicate texture of the petals, their sweet, aromatic perfume, and their beautiful unfolding. Wild Roses often prefer to grow in open spaces and in communal patches in relationship with one another. But she is not all soft, as the intense thorns display the opposite quality of Mars or the Fire

Element. Interestingly enough, both the petals and fruit sedate excess heat and inflammation in the blood and vasculature—an instance of Venus treating Mars.

Medicinally, Rose petals are astringents for relaxed tissues, especially for the veins and female reproductive system, tightening and tonifying tissues that are loose and lackadaisical (an indication of excess Venus). She is also used topically to tighten the skin and reduce inflammatory skin conditions. Rose hips are quite high in vitamin C, which strengthens capillary beds and provides oxidative protection. These properties all point to Rose as an antipathetic remedy to balance the heat of Mars, or as a sympathetic remedy to treat Venusian relaxation.

Psychologically and spiritually, Rose powerfully influences the emotional and spiritual heart.[#####] She has a physiological affinity for the heart proper, nurturing and strengthening the heart and vasculature, as well as a gentle nervine quality to settle a nervous heart; yet on a deeper level she heals the emotional and spiritual heart. This is especially true in regard to relationships. Rose teaches us how to maintain an open, full, strong, clear heart—just like the flowers—and yet to maintain a proper boundary of protection around our essence, like her sharp thorns. I've seen many cases where Rose helps to integrate lessons presented in past relationships so we can move forward and enter new relationships in accordance with our essential nature. I consider it specific for people who seem to complain about getting in the same kinds of relationships over and over again, and the other is always at fault. She is a plant of forgiveness, both of the self and the other, opening places of closure, strengthening places of weakness, and softening the hardened walls we unconsciously build to protect ourselves. She heals through love, and she ultimately teaches that our *true heart can never be broken.*

[#####] Although the heart is traditionally under dominion of the Sun, I propose that Venus also displays heart properties, as it is the energy center attributed to love. I've found many Venusian plants to operate upon the physical, emotional, and spiritual heart. These seem to be signatures rooted in Venus reflecting the light of the Sun more brightly than any other Planet.

Jupiter

Salt

Jupiter plants are often large, broad-leaved, thick, and oily. They have a strong presence, with their vital force expanding up and out, appearing plump and full. The potential habitats associated with Jupiter are wide-open spaces because they often don't like being suppressed or crowded. They want to be "the king." Due to its association with the liver, the yellow-orange color often corresponds to Jupiter plants as a common signature for bile, which we see in Dandelion flowers *(Taraxacum officinale)*, Oregon Grape roots and flowers *(Mahonia aquifolium)*, and Greater Celandine flowers and latex *(Chelidonium majus)*. The seeds of Dandelion are a notable Jupiter signature, as a radiant orb of lightweight, airborne seeds that travel long distances to repopulate themselves (long-distance travel relates to Sagittarius, a Jupiter-ruled sign).

Because Jupiter relates to fats, plants with oily or resinous qualities signify the kingly planet. A good example of an oily Jupiter plant is Burdock *(Arctium lappa)* or Lomatium *(Lomatium dissectum)*. This is true of fixed oils that are nutritive, but it also applies to aromatic oils. Essential oils are qualitatively expansive, radiating themselves beyond the physical body of the plant, a unique signature of the boundaryless property of Jupiter. Many of these oils act as carminatives that help to expel gas and wind from the gastrointestinal tract—a notable feature for the gas Planet!

Mercury

When Jupiter people eat too much heavy, meaty, rich, greasy, or sugary food, they benefit from one primary taste and herbal action: bitter. As mentioned in earlier sections, the bitter taste helps purify the blood, lymph, gallbladder, and digestive system, but most notably bitters influence the liver, which is a primary organ governed by Jupiter. The bitter action stimulates the body to increase bile secretions from the liver and gallbladder, hydrochloric acid secretions in the stomach, and pancreatic enzyme secretions to the small intestine. These actions assist with the anabolic side of metabolism by enhancing digestion and with the catabolic side by supporting elimination. This latter action of bitters is reflected in alteratives, which open the channels of elimination and detoxification. This is the essential action used for damp/stagnation tissue states. Through both sympathy and antipathy, bitters can increase Jupiter by enhancing anabolism and nutrition, and they decrease excess Jupiter by enhancing catabolism or detoxification. Through increasing bile, they support fat and oil absorption, both of which are attributed to Jupiter.

Many bitter alteratives, though not all, have a general cooling, draining, downward-moving, and drying effect that benefits individuals tending toward Jupiter energetics, which is warm, moist, and upward-moving. This correlates to the pattern in Chinese medicine referred to as damp/heat, which manifests as inflamed, weeping eczema; puffy, swollen arthritic joints; and the overall "bad blood" pattern in Western herbalism. When the liver becomes toxic in this manner, the toxicity radiates out into the blood, lymphatics, kidneys, and ultimately the skin. Alterative plants correct this pattern by cleansing the body from the inside out, with their root in the liver, thus treating Jupiter excesses. Many bitter alteratives with a strong affinity for the liver correspond to Jupiter, such as Dandelion root *(Taraxacum officinale)*, Greater Celandine *(Chelidonium majus)*, and Oregon Grape *(Mahonia aquifolium)*.

Nutritive tonics are sympathetic to Jupiter because they build, strengthen, and nourish the body. A weak Jupiter may be deficient in nutrients, with impaired digestion and absorption, and these plants—especially those with heavy, fixed oils—help to strengthen these constitutions. A plump, ripe Avocado is a great example of an oily Jupiter plant. Digestive carminatives may also correlate to Jupiter, as the gas Planet can produce gas in the gastrointestinal tract, especially when the liver is sluggish and digestive secretions are low. The aromatic property of carminatives reflects the gaseousness of Jupiter, as does the expansive upward and outward movement of their volatile oils.

Sulfur

Jupiter plants expand our consciousness, lift up our spirit, and instill faith into our hearts and minds. When Jupiter is deficient, consciousness becomes depressed, moving down and in, with restriction and limitation. Remedies of the gas giant expand us beyond these boundaries, to raise our minds above the haze so we can see beyond our self-imposed limitations. Through their initiations, these remedies help us to transcend the ego, see the grand pattern of our lives, and connect with our greater purpose. In this way, Jupiter helps to provide the level of clarity needed to help us to get unstuck and move forward in accordance with what we are meant to do with our lives. Jupiter remedies can help us to simply be happy by uplifting our hearts and minds.

This initiation into our life's work involves coming into our strength, power, and confidence, reflecting Jupiter's connection with Mars and the Sun. Jupiter bestows a vision of our future so we can see where we are going and what paths we must take to reach our destiny. Through Jupiter plants, we cultivate faith and belief in what we are shown, even if it doesn't rationally make sense, even if we can't see the ultimate goal yet. Jupiter, like all the Planets, works in mysterious ways, and through his connection to the ethereal plane we are often shown things that are outside of our models of reality. But if we remain flexible, stay open to the outcome, and trust in what we receive, good things will come so one day we can look back and see that our life mattered.

Lemon Balm *(Melissa officinalis)*

I was confused when I first learned of Lemon Balm's classic association with Jupiter. From my understanding of this remedy, with its gentle, calming nervine effect, cooling action for heat and irritation, and carminative support for the digestive system, I had thought it must be associated with the Moon or Venus. I thought plants ruled by Jupiter had to work through the liver because that's Jupiter's primary organ affinity. But as I came to understand this plant on a deeper level, it began to open itself to me in ways that revealed its pattern of relationship to Jupiter. This plant taught me a critical lesson in determining planetary correspondences in plants, which is that you cannot base them on one property of the plant. In the plant-to-Planet relationship, the Planet relates to the *core essence of the plant* and how that essence relates to the pattern within the person.

As we have seen, Jupiter is the principle of expansion, lifting us up to see beyond our current limitations. The core nature of Lemon Balm embodies this uplifting quality, especially around the heart. Its aromatic nature raises the vital force upward, volatilizing up into the nervous system and out into the capillary beds, where it relaxes. Hence, it's a primary remedy used in depression, for times when we feel like the walls are caving in around us, our consciousness is low, and we cannot see beyond our struggles and limitations. The essence of Lemon Balm lifts us out of these dark times, instilling a happiness unlike any other plant. It's the perfect combination in that it uplifts the spirit while inducing a calm state of consciousness. In Chinese terminology, we might refer to it as a *shen* tonic. Fresh Lemon Balm has more volatile oils, which are gently relaxing, but as the plant dries it becomes slightly bitter and takes on the properties of a mild bitter, increasing digestive activity and moving through the liver.

Morphologically, we see Jupiter signatures in the leaf pattern, which has a certain cloudlike, plumped-up appearance, and in its aromatic property. These aromatic oils are digestive carminatives, dispersing an excess of Jupiter manifesting as gas, bloating, and abdominal distension. Some carminatives, especially those with a nervine action, also act as "liver relaxants," used when the liver is hot, tense, and stagnant—a pattern very common with excess Jupiter types. This liver tension can manifest as hot, full headaches with a red face, as well as irritability, frustration, and anger. Lemon balm assists in cooling this heat and equalizing the distribution of the vital force by relaxing tension in the liver. Not many herbalists speak of Lemon Balm as a liver remedy, but is quite effective as a liver relaxant.

Lemon Balm is considered a specific medicine for hyperthyroidism. This state can be seen as Mars overstimulating Jupiter, or excessive activity of the thyroid leading to an accelerated metabolic rate. Hyperthyroidism leads to rapid cellular breakdown, patterns of heat and irritation in the tissues, and the vital force radiating out to the periphery, leading to elevated heart rate, sweating, and nervousness. It's common for there to be physical wasting, emaciation, and weakness, with overstimulation at the same time. This pattern leads to a weak Jupiter. Because of this excessive metabolism and cellular functioning, there is a high amount of waste products for the liver to process, which can lead to the liver pattern mentioned above. Lemon Balm helps to settle this symptomatic constellation and to directly calm excessive thyroid function.

Saturn

Salt

Saturnian plants can be slender and tall in stature, with dense, angular, rigid forms, like Boneset *(Eupatorium perfoliatum)*. Saturn rules hardness and structure, so these plants will likely be strong, fibrous, rough, dry, and tough. Because Saturn constricts, these remedies may be stiff and inflexible. Boneset snaps like a broken bone. The overall movement of energy is down and in, whereas with Jupiter we see expansive upward and outward movement. This signature is strong within Comfrey *(Symphytum officinale)*, which has such density that it falls to the ground when it grows too tall and is very dry and rough to the touch.

A second signature is prominent joints in the plant, for Saturn is the ruler of bones and joints. We see this in Smartweed *(Polygonum* spp.), the Latin name for which means "many joints"; in Boneset *(Eupatorium perfoliatum)*, whose leaves are pierced by the stems at every joint; Gentian *(Gentiana lutea)*, which puts out flowers at the joints; and Solomon's Seal *(Polygonatum* spp.), which unifies the Moon (mucilage, nourishment, white flowers) with Saturn (the joints).

A third signature in remedies of the ringed planet is the presence of circles, whorls, or rings, which is evident in Horsetail *(Equisetum arvense);* Mullein (*Verbascum thapsus);* Plantain *(Plantago* spp.), a mucilaginous astringent (Saturn-Moon); and Blessed Thistle *(Cnicus benedictus)*. The latter two are poison antidotes, an important Saturnian function.

A plant that is tall and angular and has prominent joints and a flower that blooms in a circle is Teasel *(Dipsacus sylvetris)*. The Chinese name for this plant means "to restore what is broken," and it is an admirable remedy for bone, joint, and muscle trauma. As Matthew Wood notes: "A tall teasel looks like a skeleton hanging in a medical dissection laboratory, balefully looking down at the miseries of life."[4]

White coloration is possible, as are black and red. Red relates to the *muladhara* or root *chakra,* which is the most fixed and material aspect of creation; and yet, Saturn is also the most distant visible Planet in the solar system, so it is also sometimes correlated with the *sahasrara chakra,* or the crown, giving it color correspondences of white or purple. Many times Saturnian remedies will prefer dry, hard, rocky, harsh, or cold environments, as seen with Mullein *(Verbascum thapsus)*.

Because of Saturn's relationship to death, many toxic plants come under his rulership, along with intense appearances or even a spooky feeling when in their presence—a nebulous sensation of being connected closely to another world. Sometimes the smell will be sickening, like something rotting or putrefying, perhaps masked by a superficial sweetness. We see this in Poison Hemlock *(Conium maculatum)* and Datura *(Datura stramonium)*, plants that are so deeply connected to the other world that they can kill you. This is symbolic of Saturn resting at the border of the visible and invisible worlds.

Mercury

A key signature for Saturn plants is astringency, which contracts tissues and increases their firmness and structural integrity. This ultimately creates stronger boundaries, which is needed in damp/ relaxation, where fluids freely leak due to the tissues' lack of tone. This tissue state commonly afflicts the connective tissues, which can lose their tension, leading to organ prolapse or joint hyperextension. Astringents are also drying and thus can be used for fluid accumulation and excessive moisture, such as sweating, urination, or a runny nose.

While astringency is sympathetic to Saturn, some Saturnian plants may work in an opposite fashion, most notably through acrid spasmolytics like Black Cohosh *(Cimicifuga racemosa)*, which is also indicated for a dark, heavy, Saturnian depression. When Saturn is tromping through our lives, we commonly experience stress and tension; thus, the acrids can be thought of as antipathetic remedies to relax excess Saturnian constriction.

The salty taste indicates minerals that provide bulk nourishment to the physical body, strengthening deficient *vata*, building the bones and connective tissues, and nourish weakness in the structural elements of the body. These operate on the atrophic side of the dry/atrophy tissue state. The classic remedy here is Horsetail *(Equisetum arvense)*.

Bitter plants relate to Saturn in their direct action upon the gall-bladder (co-ruled by Mars) as well as the downward movement of the vital force in response to them. This is why a really strong bitter plant sends a shiver down your spine as it activates the manifesting current that Saturn represents. As such they anchor the spirit more deeply in the body, which is why many strong bitters are helpful in states of shock, such as Gentian *(Gentiana lutea)*. Because Saturn is cold and dry, these remedies are beneficial for treating patterns of dampness and heat, astringing flaccid tissues, drying fluid accumulations, and sedating heat and irritation. This damp/heat pattern is common in arthritis.

In essence, the medicinal influence of Saturnian plants will be cooling, drying, and constricting or astringent, affecting the structural tissues of the body. While Saturn is typically considered "malevolent" and the cause of many diseases, it also treats most diseases: the cooling property treats excesses of the Sun and Mars, the drying influence treats excesses of the Moon, Jupiter, and Venus, and the constricting aspect treats excesses of Venus and Jupiter.

Saturnian medicines act on calcium deposition, distribution, and use, which lends to treatment of the bones, joints, and cartilage. We see this in Horsetail, Comfrey, Boneset, Teasel, Solomon's Seal, and even Mullein, a plant increasingly coming into use as a lubricating remedy for the spine and joints. We also see this in the antilithics (remedies used to remove stones and calcifications). Examples include Boneset's cousin, Gravel root *(Eupatorium purpureum)*, and Smartweed *(Polygonum* spp.). Both of these plants remove stones and decalcify stiff joints.

Matthew Wood observes, "One Saturnian niche in the environment is the edge of water and solid, where so many of these plants—horsetail, boneset, gravel root, smartweed—and other antilithics like to grow. This teaches us something about Saturn: it isn't just for drying, it is for balancing water and solid."[5]

Sulfur

Saturnian plants assist the mind in developing discipline, giving our lives a structure and foundation to help us grow. The establishment of psychological and emotional boundaries protects us from unwanted psychic influences and brings a solidity to the auric field. As a teacher, Saturn assists us in learning and integrating the lessons life presents to us.

Those lessons are not always easy, so Saturn plants can be intense, to say the least. They provide some of the deepest initiations of the soul, breaking down the structures and illusions that are discordant with our true nature.

As they unwind the karmic imprints of our past, Saturn plants help us establish a clearer understanding of our essential nature by removing everything misaligned to our spiritual core. It's interesting that in the West, Saturn relates to karma, and in the East they say karma is stored in the bones—and Saturn governs our bones, medically speaking. Thus we see a universal truth about the influence of ancestral patterns, past lives, or the expression of the DNA as governed by our epigenetic structure (which are different ways of speaking about the Eastern concept of karma). Regardless of the model we use to explain this phenomenon, the fact remains that Saturn plants bring about the deepest level of healing possible by clearing these deep-seated residues that lead us to repeat old patterns and prevent us from progressing on our evolutionary path.

By restructuring our bones (physically and spiritually), Saturn imprints the pattern of the universe within our astral body, revealing to us the grand pattern of Nature as it exists within us. This is because he sits the farthest away from us and thus has the highest, most distant perspective of all the celestial forces. At the border between the known and unknown worlds, Saturn looks over the physical universe, gazing upon the other Planetary powers, understanding them, and patterning their influences. As the Cosmic

Mother, Saturn gives birth to all of form, and in this way we understand the *pattern behind forms*.

For Saturn to be expressed to its fullest capacity, it must be balanced with the qualities of Jupiter; indeed, they need one another to
reach their highest expressions. Through Jupiter we break through
the limiting structures placed upon us by Saturn, but it is only
through Saturn that we can practically implement and integrate
the visions we receive from Jupiter. Without Jupiter, we are forever
limited in our life, and without Saturn, we never gain a foothold
in this practical world to make anything happen in a tangible way.
Vision must be balanced with practice, and practice must always
be guided by vision; thus we see the dynamic balance between the
expansive and contractive forces represented by the gaseous king
and the ringed Planet.

Horsetail *(Equisetum arvense)*

We see the signatures of Saturn imprinted upon Horsetail, with the
rings that move up the central stalk and the whorled leaf patterns
that radiate around it. The plant is particularly stiff and rigid in its
appearance and rough to the touch, which is why it was used as a
brush to scrub pots and pans and was called "scouring rush." It also
bears the signature of growing at the edge of waterways, showing its
relationship to fluids and solids.

Biochemically Horsetail has one of the highest concentrations of
silicic acid, or silica, a mineral that strengthens the structural tissues
of the body: hair, skin, nails, bones, and connective tissues. The presence of these minerals is indicated by its mineral-earthen-salty flavor,
which relates to Saturn, as well as its influence on these primary organ
rulerships. Horsetail revitalizes atrophied structural tissues, which can
occur from malabsorption or poor diet and can manifest as brittle
hair and nails, poor wound healing, and connective tissue weakness.

Horsetail is also excellent for relaxation, as one of its primary properties is astringent. It tightens overly loose connective tissues, which can lead to organ prolapse or hyperextension of the joints. This astringency potently influences the urinary tract, another main organ of influence (hence its Elemental ruler of Water). Here it treats relaxation of the kidneys and bladder, excessive urination, and bleeding from UTIs, and it dries excess fluid accumulation and dispels stagnation. It acts on many of the tissue states by reestablishing structural integrity, the great medical gift of Saturn.

The Horsetails are one of the oldest forms of plant life to exist on Earth. In fact, the first Horsetails were the size of trees. These are ancient plants, and their morphogenetic field has seen most of the evolution of life on Earth. Thus they have witnessed most of the radical transformations that have occurred on our planet for millions of years. This relationship with time is an important signature for Horsetail, as Saturn is none other than the archetype of Father Time. There is an ancient memory stored within these plants, and alchemically it's said to operate upon old karmic patterns lodged deep within the psyche, manifesting through the bones.

Mercury

Salt

An intriguing signature of Mercury plants is hollowness, which relates to the staff of Hermes and the *sushumna* channel that runs from the base of the spine to the crown, thus identifying Mercury with the nervous system. In several shamanic traditions, hollow tubes in plants are looked upon as signatures for remedies that guide us to the other world. We see this hollowness in plants such as Osha *(Ligusticum porteri)*, which has an affinity for the respiratory tract, one of the primary systems that corresponds to Mercury. We also see this in its cousin Angelica *(Angelica archangelica),* a sha-manic plant of northern Scandinavia. Herbalist Sean Donahue often observes that Osha helps us go down into the underworld and Angelica up into the upper world.

Another signature here is a relatively balanced appearance between the above- and below-ground parts, representing the prin-ciple of "as above, so below." We see this reflection of balance in size and shape with the leaves of Ginkgo *(Ginkgo biloba)* as well, signi-fying the hemispheres of the brain. Of course, Ginkgo is renowned for its actions on circulation to the brain and increased cognitive function, all of which relate to Mercury.

Folds can represent Mercury by signifying the folds of the brain, the digestive system, and the larynx, as well as the overlap-ping of worlds, as seen in Lungwort *(Pulmonaria officinalis),* Cala-mus *(Acorus calamus),* and Blue Flag *(Iris versicolor).*

Another important signature is the presence and aromatic quality of volatile oils, which were mentioned under Jupiter as well. Aromatic plants essentially exist in two places at once: they reside within their physical bodies but they also occupy the space around it through the exudation of compounds into the atmosphere. Mercury, as an alchemical Principle, rules volatility, dispersion, and rarification.

Because of his swift and airy nature, Mercury plants can embody a *vata*-like quality: thin, delicate, slender, feathered, or finely divided appearances, with lots of space in and around them, a good example of which is Fennel *(Foeniculum vulgare).* Some may form patterns that resemble neural networks, like Usnea *(Usnea* spp.), another respiratory remedy, with branching patterns that resemble the bronchiole tree.

Mercury

As mentioned above, the primary taste of Mercury plants is aromatic, which indicates volatile oils. Volatile oils are important because they have an affinity for the nervous system (which is coated in oils), the respiratory system, and the digestive system. Because volatile oils are lightweight and airy, many go straight to the lungs, where they are excreted through the breath. Volatile oils also operate on the digestive system as carminatives, helping to relieve cramping and tension or the excessive wind conditions that Mercury can generate. The intestines are sometimes correlated to Mercury through its ruling sign, Virgo. A good example of an aromatic carminative governed by Mercury is Fennel *(Foeniculum vulgare)*.

The primary actions we see with Mercury are expectorant, spasmolytic, nervine, and carminative. Many of these properties are sympathetic to Mercury. The expectorant action has an affinity for the lungs and respiratory tract, facilitating the expulsion of stagnant mucus from the mucosa. There are many different types of expectorants, from pungent, aromatic, irritating, stimulant ones to moistening and demulcent ones, as well as those that help relax tension in the bronchioles. For this reason, different expectorants may have different planetary associations, but in general, based on their affinity for the lungs the overall category of expectorants is particularly Mercurial. (While expectorants relate to Mercury through association with the lungs, Judith Hill notes that the general function of throwing materials out of the body is Mars.)[6] The relaxant expectorants are particularly Mercurial, as this planet generates tension and constriction.

The antispasmodic action crosses over with a few aforementioned actions. Many expectorants are also antispasmodic because they help relax the bronchioles and ease excessive, nonproductive coughing, such as Lobelia *(Lobelia inflata)*, a distinctly Mercurial plant. Carminatives are also antispasmodic with a specific tropism for the digestive system. Because Mercury is considered one of the tense Planets, through sympathy his plants may correct these types of conditions, specifically the wind/tension tissue state.

Some nervines will also fall under this category for their overall influence upon the nervous system. We looked briefly at the relationship between the Moon and Mercury in their rulership over the brain and nervous system in chapter 12; nervines will often will rest in one of these categories, or with Venus, as she embodies the overall state of relaxation. The difference is that remedies of the Moon will most likely be sedating and make you sleepy, such as Hops *(Humulus lupulus)* or Skullcap *(Scutellaria lateriflora)*. Mercury remedies increase cognitive functions, such as Ginkgo *(Ginkgo biloba)* and Gotu Kola *(Centella asiatica)*. Many of these increase blood circulation to the brain and gently calm the nerves.

Because Mercury is so unpredictable and quick to change, the energetics can vary from person to person and plant to plant. Generally speaking, they will tend to be dry and can manifest either as warm or cold.

Sulfur

A primary evolutionary function of Mercurial plants involves helping us understand the nature of our minds by cultivating an awareness of thoughts. As the mind is primarily composed of the memories of our past and our projections into the future, Mercury teaches us to dwell in the center of the two: this present moment. These remedies teach us to consciously use the mind as the tool it is designed to be, rather than being slave to the wandering monkey mind. Mercury cultivates a detached awareness and shows us the "tapes" that play in our minds and how to consciously respond from the present moment, rather than repeating the past. In this way Mercury plants assist in the development of psychological clarity and intelligence.

One of the primary initiations through Mercury involves reclaiming our voices. Many go through traumatic experiences that cause us to "lose our voice." Maybe as a child we were told to shut up or that our opinions didn't matter. There are many ways we can learn to distrust our words or suppress our self-expression. Through Mercurial plants, we have the capacity to reclaim our power to speak and to trust that we have a voice and that it should be heard. By reintegrating our capacity to express ourselves through language, we come to a deeper understanding that *everything* has a language, even if it doesn't use the medium of words. This connects us to what the alchemists called the "Language of the Birds" or the "green tongue," which is none other than the intelligence of Nature. We are better able to read the language of the body, the subtle communications of the plants, and the symbolic nature of life.

Ultimately, Mercury plants have the ability to strengthen not just the mind but also the *consciousness that uses the mind.* In that way we don't mistake the messenger for the message, the tool for the user of the tool. This places the mind back in its rightful place as the humble servant of the essential self. The healthy place for Mercury is to be so close to the Sun that it becomes its perfect reflection, so that our minds are congruous with the natural order of the heart.

Calamus *(Acorus calamus)*

Calamus is one of my favorite Mercurial plants. Its signature is in the structure of the roots, which precisely resemble the vocal cords and the throat. Interestingly, in Ayurveda the name for this plant is *vacha*, which translates to "the power of the word or voice." Medicinally, Calamus is an aromatic bitter, a unique combination of essential oils and bitter compounds, which indicates its affinity for the digestive system. The carminative action helps to relieve gas, bloating, and indigestion, and the bitters help to stimulate gastric secretions and optimize absorption. Its influence on the intestines is notably Mercurial through a relationship to Virgo.

These properties also influence the upper respiratory system and the mucosal membranes. The combination of the warming aromatic property and the draining bitter property indicates its benefit in treating damp/stagnation tissue states where mucus has accumulated and become stuck. This can manifest as phlegmatic coughs or stagnation in the gastrointestinal tract impeding absorption. This is reflected in how Calamus grows in swampy, boggy environments; it treats a tissue state that mirrors the ecosystem where it grows. Thus, I generally relate it to the Water Element as well.

The third main site of action of Calamus is upon the nervous system and perception, a distinctly Mercurial pattern. It's specifically indicated for people with brain fog, poor concentration and cognition, speech issues, and an overall sensation of "cotton balls in the mind." These would be Mercury deficiencies. The Calamus person isn't necessarily spaced out and ungrounded, but they feel the damp/stagnation tissue state in their mind and perception. I once shared a Calamus spagyric preparation with Matthew Wood, and after he took a few drops he perked up immediately and said, "I feel like it just scraped all the mucus out of my brain!" This is a nice description of how Calamus cleanses the mind and perception.

In Ayurveda, *vacha* is said to open the *sahasrara chakra*, or the crown, allowing it to bring in a greater level of vital force that moves through the *nadis* (the Ayurvedic equivalent of meridians), cleansing them of stagnations. It also operates through the *udana vayu*, or the upward-moving Airs of exhalation. In alchemy this would be seen as a purification of the astral body or of the subtle energetic channels that connect our psyche and body—a connection that is distinctly Mercurial. In this way it purifies us physically as an alterative, and psychologically as a nootropic, clarifying perception and enhancing cognition.

The Vedic translation of *vacha* also points to its unique *prabhava*, whereby Calamus harmonizes the solar plexus and the throat—the power of the word. This is expressed through its bitter-carminative and expectorant properties. This plant is the ultimate teacher of communication, healing traumas and wounding where we have been programmed to suppress our thoughts, to shut up and not speak our minds. Calamus helps us find our voice and instills the power to share it with the world with clarity and confidence.

In texts that speak of planetary correspondences with plants, it's common to simply give long lists of plants that correlate to a particular planetary force, without much description of why and how those correspondences are made. I believe there is a significant amount of refinement to be made in this area of study, and the correspondences and signatures presented above are intended to provide a starting point. This is by no means an exhaustive treatise on the vast subject of plant-to-Planet connections, but hopefully it provides some clarity regarding how you can start to see planetary patterns in plants for yourself, based on the multifaceted signatures and correspondences of an herbal medicine.

These connections between plants and Planets form the foundation of the practice of spagyrics, or herbal alchemy. As we see the spectrum of a Planet within a plant and understand its correspondences through the signatures and patterns of influence, we hold the secret key that enables us to unlock the latent potencies of the plant through the art and practice of alchemy. These unique forms of medicine concentrate the physical, energetic, and spiritual virtues of the Planets within the plants, ultimately supporting the evolutionary journey of the soul and rejuvenation of the physiological and psychological self.

The Energetic Architecture
of People and Plants

There is, furthermore, a great sympathy existing between the planets
and stars and the organs of the human body. Such a sympathy exists
between the stars and the plants, between stars and stars, between
plants and plants, and between the plants and the organs of the
human body, in consequence of which relationship each body may
produce certain changes in the activity of life in another body that is
in sympathy with the former. Thus may the action of certain specific
medicines in certain diseases be explained.

—FRANZ HARTMANN[1]

The energetic architecture model is a map representing the holistic
pattern of the natural world, giving us a universal philosophy that
unites the physical, energetic, and spiritual qualities of people and
plants. The spectrum of correspondences and signatures between
macrocosm and microcosm enables us to connect seemingly disparate
parts in a cohesive whole, uniting the science, medicine, and spirituality of herbal medicine.

The correspondences among the Planets, Elements, and Principles together constitute a model I have worked with and further

developed based on my experience in clinical practice, preparing spagyric medicines, and studying the holistic properties of medicinal plants. I propose that future research can draw upon this model to map the connections between the virtues of people and plants on the one hand and these archetypal forces of the macrocosm on the other. The ultimate goal is to develop and implement a sound therapeutic model that facilitates physical, mental, emotional, and spiritual rejuvenation and health.

The three layers of energetic architecture (Seven Planets, Five Elements, and Three Principles) correlate to the pattern of the Three Principles, opening up a new layer of this fractal pattern. This is revealed through the relative volatile and fixed signatures of each layer, with the Principles considered the earthliest manifestation, the Planets the subtlest, and the Elements mediating between the two. This understanding aligns with the doctrines of emanations and correspondences outlined in chapter 4, which reveal the gradual progression of the Source down into the physical plane.

The Planets relate to the Sulfur Principle because they are the most volatile expression of energetics. A Planetary correspondence within a plant or a person thus relates to their soul essence. Just as the Planets are the farthest out in the sky in the macrocosm, the reverse is true in the microcosm, in that they are the deepest parts of the self internally.

The Elements correspond to the Mercury Principle, as they are the primal substances that come together to shape physical matter, and yet they exist just behind the physical world. As you will see, in the alchemical tradition it's through the Elements that the Three Principles of plants are volatilized up into the Heavens to collect the celestial forces of the Planets and then fixed back down into the Earth. In this way, the Elements are the mediators between above and below, giving them a Mercurial quality.

This correspondence is confirmed by Paracelsus:

In order to further delineate philosophus, let it be known that he is under-
stood in two ways: one of the heavens, the other of the earth. Accordingly,
each sphere gives rise to an aspect of the physician; and both of them are
still not a complete physician. He is a philosophus who has knowledge of
the Lower Sphere; he an astronomus who knows the Upper Sphere. And
yet the two together embody a single sense and art. Subject to these two are
the mysteria of the four elements. For one aspect coincides with knowing
about mercurius; the other with knowing about Aquilatus. [2]

A footnote in the text defines *Aquilatus* as an adjective derived from
the constellation *Aquila,* which Paracelsus designated as equivalent
to the earthly *mercurius.*

Lastly, we have the Three Principles corresponding to the Salt
level, which relates to this three-dimensional, substantial world. As
we have seen, the Elements recombine in different ratios to form
the Three Principles, their combinations giving rise to the primal
substances that shape and mold every physical being.

Although we can relate the Planets to Sulfur, the Elements to
Mercury, and the Principles to Salt, it's important not to become
too rigid in our systems of metaphysics. We must remember that
the Planetary correspondence of a plant will not only relate to the
soul qualities of the herb but will also manifest in its physical and
energetic qualities. In a similar way, the Principle or *dosha* governing a plant will not only reflect its physiological virtues but will
also relate to the plant's subtler influences upon the mind and
consciousness. That said, when we relate a Planet to a plant, in my
opinion, it *should* bear relationship to the soul of the herb, just as
the Principle *should* relate to the physical properties of the plant.
Seeing this "energetic architecture of energetic architecture" gives
us a vision of this pattern and a way of seeing how it is reflected in
the macrocosm and microcosm.

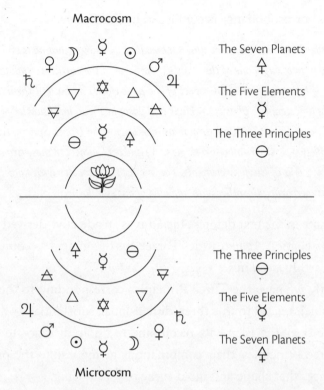

Figure 23. The energetic architecture within macrocosm and microcosm

Figure 23 reveals these three layers of energetic architecture and their relative degrees of volatility and fixity, along with their correspondences to Sulfur, Mercury, and Salt in the macrocosm and the microcosm. Note that the pattern reverses itself within the microcosm; as we cross the barrier between above and below, we shift dimensions, and thus the pattern mirrors itself. The further out into the macrocosm you go from the Principles up to the Planets, the deeper into the microcosm you go. Each of the forces of energetic architecture is in orbit as the energetics of time and space change throughout the daily, seasonal, and astrological cycles (this is explored more in chapter 19).

The work of the evolutionary herbalist is to determine the energetic architecture of the remedies we work with and the people we serve. The above pattern can be a helpful way of delineating which layer of energetics corresponds to which facet of the self. Thus, when we are considering the evolutionary process of the soul, we consider the Planets. When looking into psychology and emotional dynamics, the Elements provide valuable insight. And when we consider the general constitutional patterns of the body, the Principles are an excellent pattern to work with.

To restate, we do not want to get too rigid in this application. *Each layer of energetic architecture has its soul, spirit, and body correspondences.* Hence, the system is, in fact, quite flexible.

In the previous chapters we have analyzed each of these forces separately in significant detail for the sake of study, but it's crucial to remember that they are not disconnected from one another; they all come together within plants and people. Each being has a unique constellation of these forces that they embody most strongly. Another way to conceptualize this is to think of them as constitutional patterns. We typically only think of constitutions as relating to people, but plants also have their particular constitutional expressions. We can think of every person and plant as having a specific constitution for its soul, spirit, and body, which will *generally* relate to a Planet, Element, and Principle, respectively.

It's common to see only one layer of these correspondences applied in the alchemical, Ayurvedic, or astrological traditions, such as Nettles being ruled by Mars or relating specifically to *pitta*. I'd like to propose that we use the full spectrum of energetic architecture as it applies to plants. This is important because a singular Planetary or Elemental ruler simply does not encompass the wholeness of a plant.

Following our Nettles example, we see the Mars correspondence in its intensity of appearance and the serrated leaves and sharp needles that sting and inflame the skin. We also see Mars in its affinity for the blood, the way it builds and cleanses blood, its inflammation-modulating properties, and its overall stimulant nature. The seed's affinities for the adrenals and the root's affinity for the prostate gland also indicate Mars. But these correspondences with Mars do not encompass other critically important properties of this plant. Mars does not speak to its diuretic action, its affinity for the uterus and kidneys, or its nutritive properties. While I believe Mars does indeed encompass the soul essence or archetypal form of Nettles, there are other aspects of its nature that are not Martian. Thus, to grasp its wholeness we need to incorporate other patterns of energetic architecture, relating it not only to a Planet but also to an Element and a Principle.

Through this approach we can see that Nettles relates strongly to the Water Element in its preference for moist habitats, strong diuretic action, and affinity for the kidneys, urinary tract, and uterus, as well as its overall cleansing alterative action for damp and stagnant tissue states.

Furthermore, we can relate Nettles to the Salt Principle. This is expressed in its rich mineral and nutrient content that nourishes the body, strengthening structural elements such as bones, hair, skin, nails, and connective tissues. Nettles is also astringent, tightening and tonifying the Earth Element, and it treats damp/relaxation tissue states, which can be thought of as Earth deficiency. Its alterative actions benefit *kapha* constitutions, which is the Ayurvedic equivalent of the Salt Principle. Thus we could say that the energetic architecture of Nettles is Mars-Water-Salt, which I feel encompasses the wholeness of this plant more completely than merely assigning one Planetary ruler.§§§§§

---

§§§§§ One could also assign correspondences to Nettles based strictly on a single layer of energetic architecture. For example, some might say Nettles also relates to Venus, governing the diuretic and kidney tropism, as well as Saturn, governing the nutritive, mineral-rich, structural components. We could also consider Nettles tri-*doshic* in that it cleanses excess fluids *(kapha)*, reduces heat and irritation *(pitta)*, and strengthens weakness *(vata)*. We could also say it relates to the Fire, Air, and Earth Elements. These are all different ways of expressing essentially the same things.

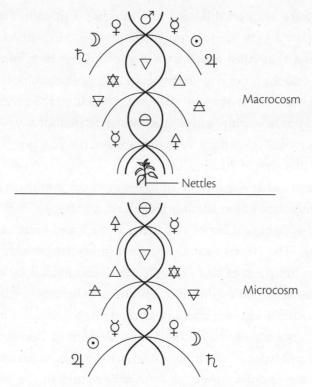

Figure 24. The energetic architecture of Nettles (Urtica dioica)

Figure 24 shows how the forces in the macrocosm are sympathetically aligned to the corresponding forces within the plant as microcosm. As we will explore in a future chapter, the practice of spagyrics, or herbal alchemy, is the art of harvesting and preparing herbal medicines in alignment with its unique energetic architecture. We understand the forces in the macrocosm, see them in the microcosm of the plant, and craft a living medicine to concentrate this specific constellation within it. It is precisely these forms of medicine that lead to transformational levels of healing.

We can use the entire energetic architecture model in our understanding of people as well. In the case history I described in chapter 14, the benefit of this system became starkly clear to me. A client came to me with a primary complaint of chronic UTIs, where the

tissues were irritated, inflamed, and burning with pain. The lymphatic glands in her pelvic region were tender, sore, and enlarged.
She had a thin constitution with dryness of the skin, joints, and
tongue, and she tended toward a nervous disposition. Upon deeper
investigation, it turned out that she was currently in a rather
unhealthy relationship with a man who was emotionally—and, at
times, physically—abusive. And this was not the first time she had
been in this type of relationship.

We can use this information to begin to see into the underlying architecture of her situation. The first archetype that is clearly
present is Venus, ruler of the urinary tract and intimate relationships. The abuses visited upon her in her relationships indicated an affliction of this Planet, further exemplified by chronic
UTIs, as Venus rules this system. The urinary tract imbalance,
along with the chronic swelling of the lymph nodes, indicated a
systemic imbalance within the Water Element of her body. Her
thin, dry, nervous disposition was clearly an indication of a predominance of *vata* in her constitution, relating to the Mercury
Principle. Thus we could say her energetic architecture was
Venus-Water-Mercury/*vata*.

These would all be considered sympathetic correspondences
with her overall architecture, though I often find it helpful to dig
a little deeper and see the full spectrum of influence, integrating
antipathetic principles as well. This perspective would allow us to
see this situation from a few different angles. The excessive inflammation, irritation, and infection in the urinary tract could be seen
either as an excess of the Fire Element within Venus or as an excess
of Mars within the Water Element. Regardless of how we look at it,
we can see that the combination of an Element and a Planet points
to the specific tissue state within the afflicted organ system. This
indicates that we would want a remedy that will balance Fire or
Mars (heat/excitation tissue state) and have a specific orientation
toward Venus or Water (urinary tract). This translates into a plant

with a soothing, cooling, sedative, diuretic action with a primary affinity for the urinary tract.

I treated her with a simple remedy, one whose energetic architecture perfectly matched hers: Cleavers *(Galium aparine)*. As a reliable diuretic and lymphagogue that prefers to grow in moist habitats and contains a high water content, it nicely embodies the Water Element. Its strong affinity for the urinary tract and kidneys relates it to Venus, as does its "clingy" signature. Its cooling, soothing property was perfectly matched for the irritation in the tissues of the urinary tract (Venus treating Mars or Fire), and yet the alterative property for the lymph helped to clear the damp accumulation and stagnation there (Water). The daintiness of Cleavers is particularly *vata* in appearance, and its gentle effects on the nervous system matched the *vata* constitutional quality of this client.

After we administered a spagyric essence of this remedy in low doses of three drops three times a day, the irritation in her urinary tract cleared quite quickly, and the lymphatic stagnation was reduced. While all of her physiological symptoms subsided, what occurred in her psyche was the most notable response. She saw the underlying Venusian pattern in her life in how she repeatedly entered unhealthy, abusive relationships, getting tangled up in other people's lives as she tried to rescue them. Venus was trying to wake her up and get her attention so it could be separated, purified, and evolved in a higher expression.

As Cleavers connected her to the archetype of Venus, it repatterned this force within her inner energetic architecture, transforming it from its lower embodiment into its more evolved, virtuous expression. She soon got out of the relationship, and instead of jumping right into another one, as she had done in the past, she took time to be alone and connect with herself, to find out who she really is and what kind of person she wanted to be with. She hasn't gotten a UTI in years, and she is now happily partnered with a person who loves, cherishes, and respects her.

A typical approach to this case might have been to give herbs "good for" a urinary tract infection, such as Uva-Ursi *(Arctostaphylos uva-ursi)*, Juniper *(Juniperus communis)*, or Pipsissewa *(Chimaphila umbellata)*. This may have helped the acute situation, but it doesn't get to the roots of the problem. The latter two remedies indeed could have been aggravating due to their warming and stimulating nature. In this particular situation, what was occurring in her physical body was a condensed manifestation of an archetypal pattern playing out in her life, influencing her mind, emotions, actions, and body. The Venusian force was stamped upon her constitution, patterning her life experiences in an effort to facilitate her soul's development. Cleavers was simply a mirror image of this same constellation of forces, which targeted the corresponding parts of her internal energetic architecture and gradually opened, purified, healed, and transformed those parts of herself. This is what we might refer to as finding a *specific medicine,* one where the pattern in the plant matches the pattern in the person and the whole plant addresses the wholeness of the person, because it is aligned with the wholeness of life itself.

This quick example demonstrates the process of seeing the energetic architecture in both the plant and the person and then matching their patterns together. This type of thinking, based on correspondences, signatures, patterns, and archetypes, may seem difficult to follow, as it is not necessarily a linear process. While this approach involves study of the correspondences, qualities, and characteristics of plants and people, it must not be overlooked that the heart as an organ of perception is central to this process—for therein lies the intuitive faculty where these relationships come to life. Once a practitioner has mastered even part of a system of correspondences, the hidden, internal relationships of physiology, psychology, life circumstances, and herbal treatment automatically shine through and guide one's intuition. Each part magically falls into place and assembles into a cohesive *pattern of wholeness,* uniting plant and person with underlying archetypal influences. This orientation is quite different from a reductionist approach to selecting herbal remedies but is not contrary to it, for we can rationally show why the remedy is appropriate for the person. Yet within this approach there lies a deeper connection to the formative patterns of creation itself, which ultimately leads to transformational levels of healing.

PART IV

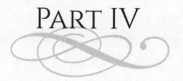

Transformational
Medicine

The physician is only the servant of nature, not her master. Therefore it behooves medicine to follow the will of nature. He who would be a good physician must find his faith in the rational light of nature, he must work with it, and not undertake anything without it.

—PARACELSUS[1]

The first three pillars of evolutionary herbalism—the Light of Nature, Energetic Architecture, and Universal Herbalism—constitute a philosophical foundation for the practice of transformational medicine, which grounds these principles in a holistic therapeutic model. This approach to herbalism uses plants to facilitate the soul's evolution without ignoring the health of the body, for the evolutionary herbalist sees the two as inseparable. True healing must reach into our essence, and from there radiate outward and touch upon every facet of the self.

Plants are embodiments of transformational cycles. They germinate and sprout in the Earth; receive the light of the Sun, Moon, and stars; and absorb Water and Air, transforming the Elemental forces into a new form. From the spreading of their leaves, opening of their flowers, and generation of fruits and seeds to their ultimate death and return to the Earth, plants move through distinct processes of transformation. These life cycles are reflections of not only the transformational cycles of Nature but also our own life cycles, each one rich with symbolic meaning reflecting the archetypal forces of life itself.

The practice of evolutionary herbalism harnesses the healing virtues of the plants, along with their embodiments of these transformational processes, which are in turn integrated into our lives. Through this cycle, the plants both heal us and teach us, transforming us into the humans we are designed to become. The fertile soil of our true nature is sown with seeds gathered from the heart of the Earth, where they sprout, grow, and flower within us. *An inner forest begins to grow as we become a part of the Earth again, cracking through the concrete shell of our worldly conditioned self.*

The deeper we enter into these transformational cycles, the more clearly we see the underlying blueprint of Nature imprinted within ourselves and the botanical kingdom. We see how we live in ways incongruous to Nature internally and externally, seeking to reestablish our connection to our unique energetic architecture and harness the power of the plants through their distinct connection to the archetypal landscape of the macrocosm. It is this realm of the archetypes reflected in people and plants that elevates our practice of herbalism to become transformationally healing. In this model of healing, the plants aren't the only ones healing us; they act as bridges to these universal forces that touch every part of our lives.

Transformational medicine involves matching the energetic architecture of plants with the constellation of forces within the person, interweaving their healing intelligence into the fabric of someone's life. *They mirror an essential part of who we are back to us.* There is something in the plant that is similar—*sympathetic*—to our own Nature, to the architecture of our souls, spirits, and bodies, that they reflect back to us. Each plant reclaims these essential parts of the self, teaching us to express the highest virtues of each archetypal force—retrieving parts of our souls, making our minds natural again, rejuvenating our bodies, putting us on the path we are destined to walk. For this process of transformation to be complete, it must weave throughout the warp and weft of our entire being, stitching the various parts of the self into a cohesive wholeness. We are not only whole unto ourselves, but deeply integrated with the order of creation, rejoining the microcosm of our being to the macrocosm of life. This level of healing directly influences the evolution of consciousness.

To do this, we must know how to properly assess people holistically and to see how the forces of Nature specifically affect them on the physical, psychological, and spiritual levels. We must have a therapeutic strategy that sees beyond symptoms and into the underlying archetypal forces generating them, so that same power can be transformed into its highest virtues.

And if we are to be truly holistic, we must not only consider the wholeness of the person and the plant; the prepared medicine must also be an embodiment of that wholeness. It must not only contain the plant, but the Planetary, Elemental, and Principle powers that it embodies. Our herbal pharmacy must equally concentrate the chemistry, energetics, and soul of the plants so it will affect the corresponding levels in the person. We achieve this through spagyric methods of preparation outlined in the alchemical tradition, which provides a model of medicine-making that harnesses and embodies the energetic architecture of the plants. When we assess the imbalanced forces within the person and prepare a medicine that embodies those forces, we are able to weave the healing intelligence of the macrocosm within plants into the person, ultimately turning our trauma into transformation.

Therapeutic Strategies:
Tending to the Inner Cosmos

*He who wants to know man must look upon him as a whole and
not as a patched-up piece of work. If he finds a part of the human
body diseased, he must look for the causes which produce the disease, and not merely treat the external effects. Philosophy—IE the
true perception and understanding of cause and effect is the mother
of the physician, and explains the origin of all his diseases. In this
understanding rests the indication of the true remedy, and he who is
not able to understand will accomplish nothing.*

—PARACELSUS[1]

Therapeutic strategies are our guideposts for finding the appropriate
herbal remedies that match our clients' physical, mental, emotional,
and spiritual needs. The goal is to look beyond administering herbs
for symptoms alone and to address primary root causes that reside
on an archetypal level. This involves assessing our clients holistically, as the precision of our remedy selection is based solely on how
acutely we are able to draw out the right information from our clients, whether that takes place through our words, our senses, or our
hearts. In the evolutionary model, assessment and therapeutics focus

on deciphering the pattern of energetic architecture in the person and in the remedies we administer, so the whole medicine will heal the whole person.

Holistic Evaluation: Searching for the Pattern

Diagnostic methods in modern biomedicine have become increasingly reliant upon technology. These discoveries give us potent ways of seeing into the body and deciphering molecular imbalances, but they often tend to disconnect the practitioner from the patient because the machines do all the work, not to mention the fact that they completely ignore the spirit and soul. This disconnection between practitioner and patient can unfortunately lead to a distancing of empathy and compassion within the physician as they look into screens and test results rather than the eyes and heart of the person desperately seeking their help. Traditional physicians used a more ancient technology to assess their clients: their senses.

Yet holistic assessment need not replace conventional biomedical diagnosis; the two methods can work alongside each other to provide a more complete explanation for the presenting symptoms. An herbalist can be greatly helped by a biomedicine report, and conversely, holistic examination can catch underlying patterns overlooked in conventional medicine. The combination of two different viewpoints is often more insightful than one by itself. As herbalists, our goal is not to search for the name of a particular disease but rather to arrive at an energetic description that points toward the root causes and indicates an appropriate therapeutic strategy. The evolutionary herbalist takes it a step further by seeing the macrocosmic forces influencing the whole person. And we already possess all the technology we need for this task within our senses, words, hearts, and minds.

There are a variety of methods for holistic assessment, though the most important is the interview and intake process. This is likely the main approach herbalists use, though it often isn't used with an underlying strategy that guides questioning to extract the information needed to choose the right plants. A lot of beginning herbalists quickly get lost in an interview and don't know which questions to ask or which information is important (or unimportant).

There is an art to conducting an effective interview. The focus is getting the information we need, but it's also an opportunity to earn the trust of the client. *Developing this trust is an essential part of the process.* As trust grows, the client gradually opens up and shares deeper parts of their lives. Often these recesses of the self are the critical pieces of the puzzle that allow to you to see the roots of the problem, but they won't share these parts of themselves if they don't trust you.

The first step is to note the entry complaint. This opening phase is an opportunity for the client to express everything bothering them that they want to address. The *only* thing you do here is listen attentively, emptying yourself to receive whatever they need to express, for they need to know that you will listen to them. At this stage, I don't ask clarifying questions, and I never make recommendations. I only ask, "Anything else?" until they finally say "no."

At this point the next phase begins, which goes into detail on each primary complaint. This method can be outlined by the mnemonic OPQRST, a model used by conventional and alternative health practitioners to assess chief complaints, signs, and symptoms.

- **Onset:** when the problem first manifested and what was going on in their lives at that time.

- **Palliate/Provoke:** anything that brings symptomatic relief or aggravates the symptoms, such as weather or seasonal changes, foods, drugs, herbs, activities, etc. This clarifies the energetics of the condition.

- **Quality:** a characteristic description of the symptoms and how they actually *feel* to the client.

- **Radiation:** where the symptom is located and how it affects other parts of the body or their life, such as pain leading to difficulty sleeping.

- **Severity (Symptom Score):** assesses how serious the problem is from the client's perspective, on a scale of 1–10 (1 being minor, 10 being significant). This component is critical because it allows you to track improvement during follow-ups.

- **Timing:** time of day or year when symptoms improve or get worse, or when they manifest. This can also point toward whether the symptom is occasional, infrequent, frequent, or constant, which can be another way of assessing severity.

OPQRST is used for each primary complaint. It gathers a wealth of understanding from your client and lends insight into the underlying patterns behind the symptoms. This model of intake can be used for acute or chronic disease, as well as for psychological and emotional issues. This framework will be enhanced by eliciting further insights into health history, traumas, surgeries, current medications, and other relevant information.

But there are limitations to words. An interview requires the person to translate their experience into language, and it requires us to understand them. Critical information might get lost in translation. This is why the crux of most traditional methods of assessment turn directly to the body and let it speak for itself.

In both Eastern and Western holistic medicine, assessment of the tongue and pulse form the foundation of diagnostic skills. Just as the human organism is a microcosm of Nature, a part reflecting the whole, this is also true on a smaller scale: the wholeness of the body is reflected within a part of the body. This is the case with the tongue and pulse, both of which mirror the whole body.

Through them you can see the inner workings of the organ systems and tissues, assess constitutional patterns, observe relative excesses and deficiencies, and get further clarity on appropriate therapeutic protocols.

Observation of the tongue typically looks at four primary characteristics: 1) the shape of the tongue body, 2) the color of the tongue body, 3) the nature of the coating, and 4) the overall moisture. We can apply our understanding of energetic architecture to assessment of the tongue, seeing the patterns of the *doshas,* Elements, and Planets present within these patterns. Further detail can be obtained by looking at specific locations on the tongue, which represent organ systems and further clarify their specific patterns.

Pulse assessment is a significantly subtler and subjective process, requiring years of experience reading thousands of pulses to perfect. Most traditions acknowledge three pulse positions: the distal, medial, and proximal areas on the wrist, on the superficial and deep levels. When counting both wrists, this gives a total of twelve pulse positions, which correlate to the twelve meridians of Chinese medicine and the twelve signs of the zodiac. There are many different qualitative factors to assess within the pulse, such as time (rapid, slow, irregular, even), tone (tense, relaxed, tight, loose, full, empty), and power (strong, weak, firm, flat, hidden, faint), among many others. The pulse expresses pressure waves within the blood, which touches every part of the body, giving the ability to peer into the state of the internal organs and constitution through the tips of our fingers. The best book on Western pulse assessment in print at the time of this writing is *Traditional Western Herbalism, Pulse Evaluation, a Conversation,* by Matthew Wood, Francis Bonaldo, and Phyllis Light (2016).

Another method focuses on evaluation of the facial lines, the complexion, and tone of the skin. This method (along with many others) is described by herbalist Margi Flint in her highly recommended text *The Practicing Herbalist.*

Medical astrology is also an incredibly precise tool for assessment. The birth chart holds a key to the wholeness of the individual and the connections between the body, mind, and soul. Just as the tongue and the pulse can further refine the intake process, so too can an evaluation of someone's birth chart, especially alongside the effects of transiting Planets (where they currently reside in relationship to the natal chart). The beauty of medical astrology is that it's not nearly as subjective as pulse and tongue assessment. In fact, it's quite mechanical in the way it works. Each part of the chart represents certain parts of the body and energetic qualities that fit together like pieces of a puzzle based on what the person is going through. The chart not only reveals the underlying patterns of disease but also informs the best therapeutic strategies to help the client find balance, whether it be in the body, the mind, or the soul. The chart shows the disease, but it also shows the cure. A simpler form of medical astrology, taught by Robin Murphy, ND, focuses on the Seven Planets alone, based on the planetary hours and days. In this method we look at the specific day and time of birth to find the ruling Planets for the Salt, Mercury, and Sulfur levels of being.

There's also a more nonlinear approach to evaluation wherein we move into the heart as an organ of perception. Described by Stephen Buhner in *The Secret Teachings of Plants*, "depth-diagnostics" involves entraining our heart field with the person and their imbalanced organ systems using a method similar to that described for plants in chapter 3. This invisible component of the intake process allows the organs to communicate to us directly, as they are indeed intelligent organisms unto themselves. As we envelop organs with our heart field, we receive nonlinear communications from them that unravel the deeper layers of meaning beneath the surface of the symptom. As we are attuned to our inner forest, the correct medicines that will heal those deeper patterns can emerge within our imaginal vision.

Each method of assessment gives us a certain angle, a piece of the puzzle, a perspective that unlocks a layer of the client's life so we can help them. Cultivating a spectrum of assessment and evaluation skills enables us to understand their constitutional dynamics, the afflicted organ systems, and their tissue states, and it can also be used for any psychological, emotional, or spiritual concerns. Throughout this process we are constantly *searching for the pattern* within the person and the archetypal forces associated with it, so we can see their underlying energetic architecture, which ultimately guides us to appropriate remedy selection.

Selecting the Right Remedies

In order to select the right remedies, we must first refine our organizational systems of herbal medicines beyond simply what symptoms they treat and understand them according to their medicinal patterns. If an herbalist is treating someone with a cough, they often think in terms of a single aspect of a plant's medicine, such as using an expectorant. So they turn to their expectorant section in a book and see the massive list of plants with this action, select a few (or many) herbs, throw them in a bottle, and hope it will work. But we don't want to be "hope herbalists"; we want to be strategic holistic herbalists who consider the wholeness of plants and people.

Simply integrating the element of energetics in our assessment of people and classification of plants gets us significantly closer to finding more specific remedies. The massive list of expectorants can become much more precise by dividing it into expectorants that are warming and drying, relaxing, or moistening. A list of forty herbs can get organized into three subcategories, making it much easier to find the most effective plant. This also reduces the potential of aggravating symptoms and causing further constitutional imbalances.

The art of remedy selection requires translating what you learn from holistic assessment into finding the appropriate herbs. A simple way of doing this is to draw five columns on a piece of paper, each with the heading of one of the Five Keys to plant properties (tastes, affinities, actions, energetics, specific indications). As you review your case notes, make note of the primary qualities you want your herbs to have. Here's a list of questions to guide this process:

- **Affinities:** What are the main imbalanced organs, systems, or tissues? Is there one tissue type or organ at the root of their various symptoms? For example, if someone has nervousness, uterine cramping, a stiff lower back, and high blood pressure, it's quite possible that the nerves and muscles are the primary affinities, rather than thinking in terms of the brain, the uterus, the back, and the cardiovascular system. **This guides you to the primary parts of the body** your herbs should act upon.

- **Actions:** What are the main physiological processes imbalanced within the person? This often looks similar to the above question, but here we aren't just looking at *where* the problem is in the body but rather *how* that part is expressing the problem. For example, with high blood pressure, we see from the first question that the main affinity is the heart and cardiovascular system, but we want to see precisely *how* that system is imbalanced. Does the client have cold extremities and poor circulation? Is there an excess of stress and nervousness putting strain on the heart? Is there an accumulation of toxins within the tissues? **This guides you to the primary actions** that will best support the organ systems, such as circulatory stimulants, nervines, or alteratives in this example.

- **Energetics:** What are the specific tissue states of the afflicted parts of the body? What are their temperature, moisture, and tonal qualities? Are the tissues irritated, red, and hypermetabolic, or are they pale, poorly functioning, and cold? Is there fluid stagnation and toxicity, or are the tissues dried out and hardened? Do they seem too tense and spasmodic, or are they overly loose and lacking tone? For example, if the person with high blood pressure seems overweight, has edema in their ankles and varicose veins, looks pale, and feels cold all the time, we can assume that they have a combination of cold, damp, and relaxation within their tissues. **This will point you toward the primary herbal energetics needed.**

- **Specific indications:** What is the state of someone's mind and emotions? Do they have a primary pattern of expression dominating their lives and connected to their main physiological complaints? Was there a particular experience they went through that is connected to their problems? For example, the person with high blood pressure notes that this problem started after she divorced her spouse, and she notices that she is exhibiting patterns similar to her parents. This lends insight into any particular ways the mind and heart need to be tended to and can point to specific indications for a certain remedy. This helps to whittle down the possible options for plants into a small handful of specific herbs. **This further refines remedy selection.**

- **Tastes:** Are there any tastes that seem beneficial in supporting the person's primary complaints? For example, if someone has chronic digestive insufficiency, he would be supported by bitters, or if someone else has chronic tension and nervousness, she would benefit from the acrid flavor. This is also important from the perspective of compliance, especially for infusions and decoctions, as strongly bitter, acrid, or other unpleasant-tasting plants can be difficult to consume.

Let's put this together in an example. Say a middle-aged woman comes to you with the following primary complaints: uterine cramping, lack of menses, high blood pressure, nervousness and anxiety, heart palpitations, hyperthyroidism, digestive bloating, and constipation. Her skin appears red and flushed; her pulse is superficial, rapid, and intermittent; and her tongue body is dry, the coating slight, and the color carmine pink. You note in her astrological chart that she has Leo ruling her sixth house of health, with Saturn, Uranus, and the South Node present there, all indicating a state of constriction and weakness in the heart. Her North Node is in Aquarius, adding to her nervous disposition. She also has many hard aspects to Venus. These forces all point to issues around the heart, relational challenges, and overall tension.

During the consultation, the client notes that these patterns started to emerge during her divorce, and she explains that throughout the divorce process she felt disempowered, didn't hold strongly to her own heart, and lacked the courage to say what she needed to say. Ever since then she has felt weak. As you sit and envelop her being with the care of your heart field and move deeper into her heart, her nerves, her womb, you begin to feel shut down, closed, dishonored in some way. You experience a visual flash of a scared little girl in a corner being screamed at by her mother.

Following the light of our Five Keys, we could get a list that looks like this:

- **Tastes:** bitter, sour, acrid (cooling, relaxant, digestive stimulating)

- **Affinities:** uterus, heart, nerves, digestion, smooth muscles

- **Actions:** emmenagogue, bitter tonic, carminative, spasmolytic, nervine, circulatory/cardiovascular tonic

- **Energetics:** cooling, relaxant, moistening

- **Special potency/specific indications:** childhood trauma associated with the mother, closure of the heart, unresolved relational issues, confidence and courage within the heart

If we approached this situation from an allopathic perspective, we would simply choose herbs that are good for these different symptoms and turn it into a "kitchen sink" formula. Perhaps we'd give some Crampbark *(Viburnum opulus)* for her uterine cramping, a bit of Valerian *(Valeriana officinalis)* for her nervousness, some Hawthorn *(Crataegus monogyna)* and Cayenne *(Capsicum annum)* for her heart, and some Ginger *(Zingiber officinale)* for her digestive bloating, maybe with a little Cascara *(Rhamnus purshiana)* for the constipation. While this formula might help to a certain extent, it will only go so far, because it's merely addressing the superficial symptom rather than the root causes. It's also a quite warming formula (Valerian, Cayenne, Ginger), and this client is notably hot.

From a holistic standpoint, our first question should be, "Is there a single remedy that contains this pattern of tastes, actions, energetics, affinities, and special potency?" If you can find one remedy that matches the pattern within the person, you have found what the Eclectic physicians called the "specific medicine." In this situation, there's one remedy specifically indicated for this constellation of symptoms: Motherwort *(Leonurus cardiaca)*.

This plant tastes bitter and acrid, is cooling and relaxant energetically, and has bitter tonic, nervine sedative, spasmolytic, cardiovascular tonic, emmenagogue, and slightly carminative actions. It has powerful affinities for the liver, heart and cardiovascular, nervous, female reproductive, and digestive systems. The bitterness and carminative properties will stimulate digestive secretions and relieve constipation and bloating; the spasmolytic and nervine actions will calm the stress and anxiety felt within the heart, as well as relax tension in the vasculature and help lower blood pressure; the emmenagogue action will promote menses; and the cardiovascular tonic actions will help to strengthen the blood vessels and heart itself. It is also a specifically indicated remedy for hyperthyroidism. In short, from a physiological standpoint, this plant hits every element of what is needed.

On a deeper level, Motherwort embodies the psychological, emotional, and spiritual support that best suits our client. This plant is classically attributed to Venus and Leo (ruled by the Sun), pointing to its affinities for female health and the heart. Motherwort operates upon patterns around our hearts where the fire has been dimmed, expressed as a lack of courage, strength, and personal power emanating from our hearts, resulting in weakness and closed-heartedness. This plant commonly heals ancestral patterns around the female side of our lineage and helps us step into a place of empowerment, strength, and confidence. Just as the Latin name indicates, this plant is the "lion-hearted" (*Leonurus cardiaca*). Thus we can see that this remedy not only matches the physiological side of the client but also addresses the underlying energetic architecture of her issues, in this situation Venus and the Sun (which is associated with Leo).

There is one aspect of Motherwort that is contraindicated, which is its drying energetics. This is a common aspect of herbal therapeutics because many herbs are drying. That's why it's common to see the addition of moistening agents in herbal formulas, such as Licorice root (*Glycyrrhiza glabra*). The "harmonizing" quality of a plant like Licorice is largely due to its moistening humoral quality, which balances the dryness of other plants in a formula. However, Licorice is contraindicated in this particular situation because it can increase blood pressure.

To remedy this, a secondary plant could be given, and I would suggest a powder or decoction of Marshmallow root *(Althea officinalis)*, which will moisten the mucous membrane in the digestive system and support in healing constipation, along with her constitutional dryness, which is likely due in part to the excessive heat in the system "cooking off" fluids.

While this example uses a single remedy that matches the pattern in the person, it's common for many herbalists to put multiple herbs together in a compound. This leads to a much larger question in the area of therapeutics: whether to simple or to formulate.

Simples vs. Formulas

The archaic term "simpler" refers to an Old World village herbalist who used "simples" or individual plants (usually few in number) for specific symptoms or conditions. These practitioners were contrasted with the educated doctors who had access to theories about formulation or compounding. Simplers were seen as inferior to the educated doctors, yet Paracelsus notes, "The ways of nature are simple and she does not require any complicated prescriptions."[2] In the nineteenth century, the informal doctrines of simpling—use of one or a few remedies for specific indications based on experience—were worked into a medical system called "specific medication," a branch of the Eclectic medical movement innovated by Dr. John M. Scudder.

Traditionally, homeopaths and Eclectic physicians focused on understanding the overarching pattern of symptomatic expression and the single remedy, while the Physiomedicalists preferred to combine multiple herbs together, forming a wholly unique compound that was specifically tailored to match the needs of the patient and was considered greater than the sum of its parts. The vast majority of modern herbalists formulate; a few simple. Sometimes the reason is doctrine; sometimes it's simply "what works" for the individual practitioner. This was in fact the attitude of Scudder himself, who, though he introduced specific medicine, did not advocate it as an exclusive system. Simples and formulas both have their place in the practice of herbalism.

The art of simpling rests on a foundation of knowing your remedies and holistically assessing the client with incredible precision. To select a single plant, you must understand its holistic nature and its total global influence on the human organism. This involves seeing the fundamental pattern in the person and matching it to the fundamental pattern in the plant. There is a precision to simpling that requires the herbalist to be acutely attuned to both person and plant for it to be truly effective.

It's far more common in modern herbalism to practice formulation. While it's essential to understand the wholeness of both person and plant in simpling, *this is also true in formulation,* though formulation does leave more flexibility in remedy selection. Compounding formulas can be slightly more forgiving, as you can use other plants to fill in gaps when you can't find the single remedy that addresses the whole person. That said, there's an art and strategy to formulation that goes beyond the idea that throwing together a bunch of herbs suited to a disease constitutes a "formula." The evolutionary herbalist doesn't just compound "shotgun" or kitchen-sink formulas that lack an underlying strategy, precision, or focus. Each plant is chosen for a very specific purpose that addresses particular needs to heal the whole person. Indeed, formulas can be compounded in highly specific ways based on the nature of someone's astrological chart.

The Elements provide a useful framework for delineating the different purposes of the various parts of a formula. The Ether Element consists of the lead or chief herbs in a formula. This is the primary herb(s) that provides the majority of the properties required to heal the person. These lead herbs should *always* address the primary complaint of the person and ideally should provide most, if not all, of the actions, affinities, and energetics required to regain balance. How much of the formula this part takes up differs from herbalist to herbalist, though it usually constitutes the bulk of the formula.

The Air Element represents supportive remedies that back up the lead component. These can provide secondary actions or affinities that support the effects of the lead, such as attending to juxtaposed organs, systems, or tissues, or providing another action the lead doesn't contain. This part of the formula fills in gaps the chief herbs don't address or support other parts of the body that attend to the primary complaint.

The Fire Element represents driving herbs. These remedies are navigators that orient, or "drive," the formula into the desired parts of the body. These are often circulatory stimulants that dilate the vasculature and move the blood to deliver the herbs where they need to go. Sometimes relaxant remedies are used as drivers as well, for if there is excess constriction or tension (i.e., kinks in the hose), then delivery will be difficult. This is why many classic North American formulas contain small amounts of Cayenne *(Capsicum annum)* and Lobelia *(Lobelia inflata),* a simple yet powerful pair consisting of a circulatory stimulant and a relaxant to open up the body and deliver the rest of the formula. Drivers are not always necessary, but they can be important to consider. They are typically used in small amounts. In addition, they increase the innate heat of the formula and can thus be contraindicated for excessively hot constitutions.

The Water Element represents synergists. This portion corrects or balances the net effects of the formula built so far, especially in terms of energetics. Thus, these can be warming herbs if the formula seems too cold, cooling herbs if it seems too hot, drying herbs if the formula is too moist, or moistening herbs if the formula is too dry. This latter property is how synergists are often used, as mentioned previously; many herbs are drying energetically and require the synergy of a moistening agent to balance the whole formula.

Another way this is described is as "corrigents," derived from the Latin *corrigere,* which means "correct." In modern herbalism corrigents are usually discussed as adding pleasant-tasting herbs to make the formula more palatable and thus increase compliance. While this can certainly be one element of a corrigent, the truer understanding of this term is in correcting the properties of the overall formula. John Mumford Swan notes in his *Prescription Writing and Formulary* (1910), "The *corrigent* is a drug which is added to correct or modify the base."[3]

The Earth Element represents the specific form of administration for the medicine or delivery mechanism. Will it be delivered as an infusion, a decoction, or a powder? A tincture or a vinegar? A spagyric essence or plant stone? This is important to consider because certain herbs do not extract well in alcohol, and others extract poorly in water. This necessitates knowing how each herb is best prepared and making sure you are compounding it in an appropriate form. A good example of this is how demulcents rich in mucilaginous polysaccharides, such as Marshmallow *(Althea officinalis)* and Slippery Elm *(Ulmus rubra)* are not best extracted in alcohol and are preferably given as powders, capsules, or infusions. Selecting ideal extraction menstruums requires knowing some pharmacognosy, or plant chemistry, along with preferred solubility ranges. Finally, the Earth Element represents what the particular ratios of each remedy will be in the formula, calculated either in parts or percentages, as well as what the dosage and frequency of use will be for the client.

Herbal formulation is an art as well as a science: the empty bottle is your canvas, each plant a color on your palette, each combination a particular brushstroke. Every Element of a formula is a particular technique for creating your art, the final work being the transformational healing of the person you are helping—the revival of Nature within them.

Spagyrics: The Art of
Spiritual Pharmacy

Whatever appears in the world must divide if it is to appear at all. What has divided seeks itself again, can return to itself and reunite.... In the reunion of the intensified halves it will produce a third thing, something new, higher, unexpected.

—GOETHE[1]

For the seed of transformational healing to sprout, the medicines we use must not only contain the wholeness of the plant but must embody the wholeness of Nature as well. The holistic medicine is prepared in accordance with the universal principles of life and the cosmology of Nature, and it carries the influence of the archetypal landscape through its energetic architecture. These forms of medicine facilitate the evolution of consciousness by touching the Earth and Heavens within a person. These are the medicines crafted through the art of plant alchemy or spagyrics: *one medicine* that equally operates upon the body, spirit, and soul.

People are commonly treated separately, the body one way and the mind and soul another. The same separation is seen in the sphere of herbal pharmacy. It's customary to think of different preparations used to strictly treat the body (such as infusions, tinctures, powders, and capsules), and entirely different forms of medicine to address the psychological and emotional territory (such as homeopathics, flower essences, or plant-spirit healing). While these are all valid and powerful forms of medicine, many modern herbalists are unaware of the advanced methods of herbal pharmacy carried down through the alchemical and spagyric traditions that integrate the physiological, psychological, and spiritual plant.

My primary teacher in alchemy, Robert Bartlett, commonly defined alchemy as the practice of "consciously assisted evolution,"[2] whereby natural substances—such as plants, minerals, and metals—are prepared into medicines in accordance with their energetic architecture and the steps of Creation itself. The alchemist consciously assists the evolution of the medicine, which in turn consciously assists our evolution when ingested, completing the cycle of "as above, so below." The alchemical tradition is not just a system of symbolism, psychological allegory, or "primitive chemistry," but rather a refined system of spiritual pharmacy.

The term *spagyrics* refers to a branch of alchemy that focuses on the preparation of botanical medicines. The word was coined by Paracelsus to refer to his particular methods of extraction and purification of plants. Derived from two Greek words, *spao* and *ageiro*, it is commonly translated as "to separate and recombine," because the Three Principles of plants are separated, purified, and recombined to produce their rarefied essence, or what Paracelsus called *arcanum*.[3] The parts are always recombined back into wholeness. A more precise translation of the term, "to separate and reawaken,"[4] presents the spagyric process as a cycle of death and rebirth, whereby the plant dies and is reborn anew, transformed into its essence. This death and rebirth process is precisely how spagyric medicines heal: separating and purifying the nonessential parts within us, and rebirthing us into accordance with our essential self.

Spagyric pharmacy is founded upon the pattern of transformation everything goes through in Nature. From the changing of the seasons, the life cycle of plants, and the formation of metals and minerals in the Earth's molten core, to the conception and birth of the human being, everything goes through specific steps of change throughout the course of its birth, life, and death. This order, this *pattern* of Nature, forms the basis of the spagyric method and the art of alchemy, and as such, the medicines carry the innate process of life transformation itself. The alchemists of old didn't simply make up their system of pharmacy; they observed it within Nature first and carried that knowledge gleaned from the Light of Nature into the laboratory.

Paracelsus was the founder of pharmacy and pharmacological science. He introduced separation of constituent parts through distillation, chemical change or combustion, and precipitation. These methods are still used in pharmacology, and until the early part of the twentieth century they were the main methods used to prepare botanical medicines. However, pharmacy never attempted to "put the pieces back together" as alchemy does, and increasingly, pharmacology has isolated organic molecules that do not represent the whole plant. As our worldview became more mechanistic, alchemy gradually degraded into chemistry as the meaning was stripped from the system.

Today the phytopharmaceutical industry focuses on isolated plant constituents and the standardization of extracts, reducing the medicinal virtues of plants to artificially precise fractions of their biochemical profiles. These medicines are beginning to look (and act) more like drugs. While these standardized extracts are often better options than over-the-counter or prescription drugs, they are created with the same reductionist mindset of biomedicine that separates mind from body, part from whole. Plants are prepared and administered allopathically, like drugs. But they don't fit into this mold: they are whole beings that heal whole beings.

Truly holistic herbalism isn't just understanding the wholeness of plants and people; *it uses medicines that contain the plant's wholeness.*

Even the best conventional methods of herbal pharmacy throw away (or hopefully compost) the physical plant material once the constituents have been extracted. Alchemy uses all of it, wasting nothing. This wholeness of the plant is represented in spagyric medicines by concentrating their chemical, energetic, and spiritual properties.

When I worked in the herbal medicine-making lab at Bastyr University, I always hated throwing away the extracted plant material. I wanted to make the most powerful herbal medicines possible. I'd make a tincture as concentrated as I could, press it out, extract it with vinegar, extract it with water, put it all together, and concentrate it. I'd put a little of the flower essence in there for good measure. But no matter what, at the end those leaves, roots, and flowers ended up in the compost bin, and I felt guilty about it. I felt a nagging sense that there was still medicine trapped within the plant. I just didn't know how to extract it.

It turns out I was right. The spagyric process shows specifically how to extract the critically important principles missing in almost all forms of herbal extracts available today. An *immense* amount of credit is due to Robert Bartlett****** for his teachings on alchemy and spagyrics, along with the work of the late Manfred Junius and Frater Albertus, Mark Stavish, Dennis William Hauck, Israel Regardie, and Clare Goodrick-Clarke.

The Three Philosophical Principles in Plants

To fully grasp what spagyric preparations are and how they are crafted, we begin with our triune pattern of energetic architecture: Salt, Mercury, and Sulfur. These are the primary functional units within plants that are separated, purified, and recombined in

---

****** I highly recommend both of Robert's most recent works, *Real Alchemy* (2007) and *The Way of the Crucible* (2008), for further explorations of alchemy and spagyrics.

spagyric works. As the Three Principles are the most fixed, or physical, layer of energetic architecture (Salt), they represent the tangible materials we can work with in laboratory alchemy.

Sulfur represents the plant's soul, which manifests in the material plane as the essential oils. This is the most volatile portion of a plant, evaporating into the air with the slightest exposure to heat. They are typically pungent in nature. These properties show how the volatile oils embody the Air and Fire Elements, which are the Elements that form the Sulfur Principle. It's interesting to note that these are referred to as *essential* oils, indicating that they represent the essence of the plant, a property of the soul and thus Sulfur. In the spagyric process, Sulfur is separated through hydro-distillation or steam distillation. Just as all human beings have a distinct and individual soul, so too do the essential oils of plants have their own distinct properties and character, as Lavender is quite different from Rosemary or Angelica.

Mercury represents the spirit of the plant, present in its alcohol and water-soluble chemistry. From a traditional perspective, Mercury is the alcohol within the plant, separated through fermentation or putrefaction. If *any plant* is placed in a vessel, covered with water, and allowed to ferment, it *always yields* ethyl alcohol. The alchemists saw the signature of alcohol as the universal spirit of the botanical kingdom, just as Mercury is the one spirit that flows through all things, or the vital force. Hence we refer to distilled alcohol as "spirits." In modern terminology, the Mercury within plants is their chemical constituents extracted through an alcohol menstruum, such as through tincturing processes. These refined substances, isolated through distillation, preserve that part of the plant through which its intelligence operates; the chemistry is merely a vehicle for its life force.

Salt is the body of the plant. This is the primary missing component in most modern herbal preparations, as the physical plant is discarded after extraction. Just as Sulfur manifests as the essential oils and Mercury manifests as the alcohol-soluble chemistry, Salt has a specific physical manifestation of its own: the alkali minerals.

These minerals are separated through calcination and dissolution, whereby the physical plant is burned to ash, purified, and crystallized to form beautiful crystalline mineral salts. Just as our own body is the vessel through which our spirit and soul manifest in this world, so do the alkali mineral salts in plants form the vehicle through which Mercury and Sulfur influence this physical plane.

Because most forms of modern herbal medicine, such as tinctures, discard the physical plant after extraction, they are missing the all-important Salt Principle. Most tinctures contain the Sulfur and Mercury of the plant, but because they are missing the purified body, they do not have as strong an affinity for the physical body. Generally speaking, the Sulfur of the plant acts on the Sulfur of the person, the Mercury of the plant works on the Mercury of the person, and the Salt of the plant operates on the Salt of the person.

In this way, standard herbal tinctures can be considered "disembodied medicine" due to the lack of presence of the mineral salts. Herbal medicines containing the purified Salt carry the Mercury (intelligence) and Sulfur (consciousness) deeper into the physical organs, systems, and tissues of the body, for the body of the plant is within the medicine. They have their specialized vehicle through which they influence our physiology. This is not to say that standard herbal tinctures are ineffective, but they are likely to be less effective, efficient, and potent than remedies that contain these alkali minerals. Not only does the Salt operate upon the physical organs; because they carry the Mercury and Sulfur, it influences their intelligence and archetypal forms.

Matthew Wood notes:

> In the "cell salt" method of healing, the important alkaline salts that control cellular life are homeopathically prepared and used as powerful healing substances. This testifies to the importance of the Salt Principle of the plant. If these cell salts can alone cure, how much more so the alkaline salts in plants, in their original balance, associated with their original constituents and essential oils. [5]

Spagyric Processes

Each step in the spagyric process signifies a stage in Nature's grand cycles of transformation. The ancient alchemists were astute students of the natural world, observing the patterns of change occurring within the Earth and Cosmos, and applying those patterns in their crafting of medicine. In this way, each step in the spagyric method is a signature for a natural cycle and is rich with symbolic meaning, both externally within the glassware and internally within the vessel of our being. Below is a brief overview of the primary processes used in spagyrics.

Distillation

Nature is distilling around us all the time. The water cycle shows us the universality of distillation: as the Sun warms Water, it evaporates into the sky as vapor, where it cools and condenses into liquid and rains down upon the Earth. This natural cycle is reflected within the confines of glassware in the distillation process, which contains each of the Elemental forces that occur in Nature. Earth is the physical plant material, Fire is the heating apparatus (whether it be open flame, a mantle, hot plate, etc.), the boiling flask is filled with Water, and the vapors rise into the Air.

In the distillation apparatus we see the vertical axis of the three worlds represented: lower (boiling flask, collection flask), middle (ascending columns, condenser), and upper (still head). Thus the entire macrocosm is represented within distillation. This is similar to the "triple burner" of Chinese medicine, as noted by Matthew Wood:

> *Chinese herbal medicine was originally alchemical, so the body is looked upon as analogous to a distillation unit. The "lower burner," dominated by the kidneys and bladder, held the liquids, the "middle burner," consisting primarily of the digestive and metabolic viscera, was like the rivulets of water running down the side of a distillation still, while the "upper burner" (in*

which the air and blood were "misted" by the lungs and heart, for distribu-
tion around the body) was like the mist or vapor in the still.

> *The upper burner, containing the heart and upper part of the body, cor-*
> *responds to the intelligence, so we can see how the shen, "mind" or "spirit"*
> *stored in the heart, also corresponds to the Mercury, while the salts then*
> *control the water in the kidneys and in the interstitial fluids in the matrix*
> *around the cells. This is the Salt Principle. The fire of life burns in the center,*
> *like the agni of Ayurveda, the source of the digestive and metabolic fire.*
> *This is the Sulfur Principle.* [6]

Distillation consists of raising the temperature of a liquid to
the point of evaporation. As the vapors rise, they are cooled and
turned back into a liquid, which is collected as the distillate. We
use this process for the separation of Sulfur and purification of
Mercury of the plant, as well as simple distillation of Water for
spagyric works.

As Sulfur is considered the most volatile portion of the plant, it's
often the first to be separated. As water is boiled, the steam passes
through the plant material and attaches itself to the essential oils,
elevating them to the upper world of the still, which represents the
cosmos. As these invisible vapors are gradually cooled with a condenser, they progress from a volatile steam into droplets of liquid
collected in a flask. During this time, the medicine is highly sensitive and is imprinted with the energetic qualities flowing through
the cosmos of the macrocosm, as well as the consciousness of the
operator. On a technical level, we are distilling the essential oils from
the plant, but from an alchemical perspective, we are separating the
soul of the plant from its body, liberating it from its material form.
It is the symbolic death of the plant and the beginning of its cycle
of transformation.

Distillation is also the process used to purify the plant's Mercury. Starting with the wine of the plant, generated through fermentation, we distill the volatile spirit. Because alcohol is lighter in

weight than water, a gentle heat will gradually separate the alcohol portion of the wine from the watery part, leading to a more concentrated and refined expression of Mercury. As wine is both alcohol and water, we can immediately see how Mercury is the amalgam of the Air (alcohol) and Water (water) Elements. Traditionally, the purification of Mercury is done seven times to represent the harmonic of Nature and often yields a 95 percent pure alcohol—an alcohol that is prepared *from the plant itself.*

Just as distillation separates the Soul of the plant from its body and purifies its Spirit, so too does inner distillation. Our consciousness is freed from the limits and boundaries of our physical body and our daily grind so we can look at our lives from a distant perspective to gain insight and understanding. Distillation help us see further down our road of life, where we are going if we continue the way we are living, and how we might change our orientation if we don't like what we see. I like to think of distillation as achieving a degree of clarity in our lives. In *The Emerald Tablet,* Dennis William Hauck summarizes internal distillation nicely:

> *Psychologically, the white stage of distillation is a repeated separation and recombination of the subtle and the gross aspects of the personality. This process continues until peace and well-being bond to the personality in what would be the corresponding sublimation. In spiritual terms, distillation is a rejuvenating immersion in the womb of the primal forces of the universe that marks the final death of the old ego and the rebirth of the transpersonal self.*[7]

This beautiful process of self-distillation can help us reach clarity within the bigger picture of our lives, and the inspiration and freedom to consciously direct our path in accordance with our purpose. It establishes a direct connection with our soul to receive its guidance and wisdom (Sulfur) and to further refine our true hearts and minds (Mercury) so they are pure, clean, and in congruence with the soul's intent.

Fermentation

After the Sulfur is separated through distillation, the next step is fermentation. The soul has been separated from the body—the latter commonly referred to as the *corpus*—and the plant is now incomplete and in between worlds. As the soul has ascended into the Heavens through purification by Fire (distillation), the spirit must now be separated from the *corpus* through the cleansing of Water. The plant is placed into a vessel, covered with Water, and allowed to slowly putrefy, decompose, and ferment as the spirit releases its grip on the physical form. This gradual decomposition opens the *corpus* to the spirit of the Water, lifting it up through the progressive transformation of the plant's endogenous sugars and yeasts into alcohol, which rises to the surface. In essence, a wine is prepared from the distilled plant material.

Through fermentation we see how Mercury is composed of Air and Water, as the plant is essentially "drowned" in Water and actively bubbles and off-gasses into the Air as alcohol is generated. Yet all of the Elements are contained: Earth in the sugars, Fire in the yeast, Water (or the hydrosol from Sulfur distillation), and Air as the soulless plant itself, whose intelligence is being extracted in the process.

Whereas distillation is the ascent into the upper world of the Heavens, fermentation is the descent into the lower world of the Earth. Although the epiphanies, inspirations, and clarity we receive through distillation are profound as we come into contact with our soul, when we come back we are left with the realities of our minds and emotions (Air and Water), which don't always reflect what we see in our Sulfur. We have residue to deal with, old parts of the self that require purification. In fermentation we become aware of the ways in which our lives are discordant with the higher self we encountered through distillation. In short, we have work to do.

The first phase of fermentation involves the body of the plant breaking open, decaying, surrendering its mind and heart to the Water, and making a "journey into the underworld" where it "faces its shadow"—the patterns buried deep in the unconscious parts of the self. This process can be likened to the "dark night of the soul," where we confront our demons and the parts of ourselves that we push into the closets of our being. When those repressed parts are not attended to and integrated, they decompose within us, get angry, and start to percolate up to get our attention—usually not in the most pleasant ways.

The second phase of fermentation represents the dawn, the light at the end of the tunnel, as the spirit rises up from the depths and reenters the middle world, just as the alcohol rises to the surface of the ferment. This process is a period of self-reflection when we confront our shadow, shine the light of our consciousness upon it, and ultimately integrate it into our essence.

This is why fermentation is best achieved in a dark room and a hermetically sealed vessel—that is, protected from outside influences—where Air doesn't enter the container but can escape it. These are signatures for our inward journey into the underworld and the ability of suppressed parts of the self to consciously percolate up. This process is not achieved overnight; it typically takes forty days and nights, demonstrating that lasting change requires disciplined focus and patience to separate the true from the false.

Yet the spirit formed through fermentation is still intermixed with the shadow side, separated from the body but not yet pure unto itself. Hence the next phase requires distillation of the wine to purify the spirit by separating the alcohol from the water. We move from the lower world back into the upper world, the inner result being a liberation of our true spirit, the freeing of our minds and hearts from the dross of our past.

Calcination

Distillation and fermentation separate and purify the Sulfur and Mercury through the power of Fire and Water. We continue to work with these Elemental forces to separate and purify the Salt, or body, of the plant. This is achieved through calcination, whereby the spent plant is dried and incinerated to an ash. This ash is further purified by the Earth Element—the physical action of grinding the ashes to reduce the particle size, followed by subsequent burning. This cycle of burning and grinding continues to purify the plant's body until the ash has a smooth, soft consistency and white to light gray coloration.

Physically, calcination burns the structural components of the plant, such as cellulose and fibers, reducing it to the alkali minerals. On an esoteric level, calcination liberates physical impurities that are not essential to its form, reducing it down to the mineral matrix that is the material foundation of the plant—the essence of the body.

Within our transformational cycles, calcination purifies our lives through the rawness of Fire, stripping away elements of the self that are not true to our essential nature. The fermentation process helps us face our shadow and separate our true mind and heart from it (Mercury), although there is residue left over. These residues represent our old patterns of thinking and feeling, the conditioned self, or what we might refer to as the ego. We are not necessarily destroying the ego but rather its aberrant self-rule. This is what we are calcining, and those fires, like all fires, can indeed burn.

Often the inner calcination process is marked by flames raging through us internally and externally, stripping away what is no longer serving us, removing the conditioned layers of the self. Just as the Fire Element resides within the heart, I like to think of the heart fire purifying everything in our lives not in accordance with it. And letting go isn't always easy.

Dennis William Hauck has this to say about calcination:

> There is no escape from the fires of Calcination until we are able to identify with what psychologists call the transpersonal Self, which in alchemy is known as the Philosopher's Stone. Only the Stone can survive the Dragon's Breath, the fires of the hell we all make for ourselves. There is no room for two rulers of the personality, and only by destroying the ego can the Stone manifest itself. Calcination is truly the "death of the profane," the sacrifice of specious ego concerns for a higher level of being that is a necessary

*condition for spiritual advancement and understanding. During this initial
stage of personal alchemy, the extravagances and illusions we have built up
over the course of lives are eliminated.*[8]

Calcination reflects the purification our bodies need to go
through, removing stagnations and impurities lodged within us,
impeding the flow of vitality. Often these impurities arise through
improper digestion of foods from a weak digestive fire and metabolism. Just as calcination purifies the material elements of the plant,
so too does the inner alchemical furnace, or the digestive fire, purify
the raw materials of the foods we consume and the impurities we
accumulate (both physically and psychologically). We can thus liken
the flames of calcination to the flames that exist within our guts and
the necessity to strengthen that fire internally so we can reach an
optimal level of physical purification.

Dissolution

After calcination, we have a small pile of smooth, soft, white ash
that has been effectively purified by the Fire and Earth. Dissolution
involves dissolving this ash in water to separate the water-soluble
minerals from the insoluble minerals, which precipitate out of solution. These insoluble, ashen minerals are called the *caput mortuum,* or
the "death's head," which represent the plant's impurities. This tiny
fraction of the original starting materials is typically the only portion
of the plant that is discarded,[††††††] for it represents the "dark side"
or the "ego" of the plant. In alchemy, everything is evolving toward
oneness, which involves the purification of "imperfections." In short,
plants, just like people, have their "stuff" to deal with, and the *caput
mortuum* is the extracted material from the plant not true to its essential being. In this way, I like to think of the spagyric process as actually providing a healing for the archetype, or spirit, of the plant itself.

[††††††] While the *caput mortuum* is typically discarded, there are other spagyric works
where it's further purified, transformed, and integrated into a particular form
of medicine, such as the "alixir."

After dissolving the purified ash in water, the precipitated *caput mortuum* is filtered from the solution containing the water-soluble minerals. The liquid containing the water-soluble salts is slowly evaporated to reveal the final crystalline minerals, which are considered the true and pure Salt principle of the plant used in the final preparation.

The crystalline nature of the Salt is transparent—you can see through it—yet it is physical. It is there, and yet in a certain way, it is not. In this way we see that the body has become "spiritualized," both visible and invisible, and is thus the ideal receptacle for the spirit and soul embodied by the Mercury (alcohol) and Sulfur (oils). The body is thus prepared to be reunited with its intelligence and consciousness so it can be reborn whole and complete, yet transformed.

Some practitioners use the unpurified ash in their spagyric extract, but I personally don't agree with this approach for both philosophical and practical reasons. The unpurified ash may contain mineral elements unsuitable for ingestion and may cause certain health issues; as they are dissolved into alcohol, they may leach more than just water-soluble minerals into the final extract. On a physiological level, we generally do not want minerals precipitating out of the aqueous cellular matrix, preferring them to be soluble and dissolved. From a philosophical standpoint, the Sulfur and Mercury Principles are extracted through a combination of Fire and Water, and so it should be with the body. Just as the Earth Element contains Fire, Water, and Air, so too should it be purified with all of the Elements. Thus, the dissolution process represents cleansing the plant's body through the Water Element and completing its cycle of transformation.

Until this point, we have come into contact with our soul essence through distillation of Sulfur, faced our internal darkness through fermentation, and liberated our true spirit as we purified Mercury. But there is still the "dross" of what's left over after these two processes, the residues of our purification. What calcination does not purify through the action of Fire, dissolution completes through Water, signifying the cleansing of the emotional body. Although the pure spirit and soul are critically important in our personal development, they mean nothing unless they are integrated back into our bodies, into our daily lives. Our spirituality and practicality must unite, in the same way that the above and below within the plant are recombined.

Cohobation

The final step is cohobation, where Sulfur, Mercury, and Salt are recombined. This process can be performed in a variety of ways to produce different forms of spagyric medicines. Slower cohobations can form solid, fixed medicines such as the plant stone or the quintessence. Faster cohobations form liquid, volatile medicines such as the spagyric essence.

Regardless, cohobation is the reuniting of the purified soul, spirit, and body of the plant, and as such represents its rebirth. Here the plant enters a new phase in its evolution, as the spagyric represents its "true form" or a reflection of its rarefied essence as its soul, spirit, and body come into perfect balance—the *prima materia* of the plant. The spagyric contains the essential, archetypal medicinal form of the plant, a concentrated embodiment of its unique constellation of energetic architecture. Cohobation is often represented in alchemical symbolism by the marriage of the Sun and Moon, the union of the Heavens and the Earth, or the integration of our inner dynamic and magnetic natures.

Within us, cohobation represents integration, where we take our lessons, healing, inspiration, and insight, and live them every day, walking our spiritual path with practical feet. Cohobation is when our essential soul, clarified spirit, and purified body unite, freed from what was cleansed through this transformational process. This is where it all comes together and brings about lasting change, reflected in how we choose to live our lives on a daily basis. We move forward in a good way, cleansed of our past. Without this step in the process, the transformational cycle is not complete; it remains an ethereal dream. In order for it to become *real,* it must be integrated, the soul and spirit embodied.

These are the universal processes utilized to prepare different forms of spagyric medicines, though there are certainly others, such as various methods of extraction, digestion, circulation, etc. Each of these stages of purification have chemical attributes that concentrate the medicinal potency of the plant, as well as their archetypal expressions, or spiritual signatures, that represent cycles of transformation within the natural world. In this way, there is a practical aspect of preparing spagyrics, as well as a philosophical or spiritual aspect to the medicine-making process—an external and an internal component. Both sides must always be attended to. While the act of preparing medicines in this way holds the innate power of transformation, there is an essential element in crafting true spagyrics that further refines the energetic and spiritual potency of the medicine, which can only be achieved through astrology.

Astral Pharmacy

As we have seen, the astrological pattern holistically illustrates the virtues of people and plants. It can also be used as an integral part of preparing our medicines holistically. This is achieved through specific timing mechanisms whereby certain planetary forces are harvested during their peak influence and captured within the medicine to magnify their innate power. One of the unique potencies of astrology is that it not only describes the underlying energetics of Nature but also connects them to cyclical patterns of time. In this regard, it enables us to see the energetic qualities—*the spirit*—of time as it flows through a specific place. This is an important facet of both alchemy and the esoteric traditions of the West.

Energetic understandings of time are expressed throughout spiritual and medical traditions across the world. In Ayurveda, the three *doshas* have particular seasonal qualities as well as influences during times of the day. Chinese medicine divides time into corresponding meridians, organ systems, and Elements. Often it's thought that an energetic understanding of time is unique to Eastern traditions, yet few realize that we have a precise system in Western astrology for calculating the energetics of time. In fact, the Western system is often considered *more* precise than the sometimes rigid patterns developed in the East, as astral timing mechanisms change from day to day, season to season, and even location to location. This enables one to get very precise snapshots of Planetary influences within their particular bioregion.

While standard herbal pharmacy extracts and concentrates the physical properties of plants, spagyrics takes it a step further by "harvesting" the underlying planetary ruler of the plant and concentrating it into the medicine. *Herbalism harvests plants; alchemy harvests planets.* Our medicine is "prepared in the stars" so that they become an integral part of the medicine. And because the medicine is prepared astrologically, they will operate upon and develop the "astral body"—our inner starry sky.

There are two divisions of planetary time used in spagyrics: days of the week and hours. The planetary days are the energetic qualities governing a particular day, a sort of generalized influence, whereas the planetary hours are specific qualities of energy that flow throughout the changing day. The days are like a generalized ray, whereas the hours are like focused lasers. The days of the week correspond to the Seven Planets as follows:

Sunday	Sun
Monday	Moon
Tuesday	Mars
Wednesday	Mercury
Thursday	Jupiter

Friday   Venus

Saturday   Saturn

There's still a residue of these correspondences within our language, as *Sun*-day is ruled by the Sun, *Satur*-day by Saturn, *Mon*-day by the Moon, and so on. Many of the romance languages are even more explicit in this relationship. In Spanish, Monday is *lunes,* Tuesday is *martes,* Wednesday is *miercoles,* and so forth. The days in Italian and French are similar to the planetary names. English substituted the names of the Old English gods for the Latin: Tiew (Mars), Woden (Mercury), Frigga (Venus). The correspondences of the Seven Planets to the seven days of the week are an old pattern based an understanding of time that goes back to ancient Egypt.

Planetary hours are where it gets a little more complicated. There are multiple systems for calculating planetary hours, but they're generally divided into fixed and flexible systems. The fixed planetary hour system divides the day into seven planetary "hours" of approximately three hours and twenty-five minutes each. Thus there's an "hour" from midnight to 3:25 a.m., another from 3:26 a.m. to 6:51 a.m., and so on. This second planetary "hour" is considered the ruling hour for that particular day of the week, since it's assumed the Sun will rise around this time. Thus, 3:26 a.m. to 6:51 a.m. on Wednesday is ruled by Mercury, on Thursday Jupiter, on Saturday Saturn, and so on.

I do not subscribe to this planetary hour system, primarily because a fixed system doesn't accurately represent Nature, which is far from fixed! The way the morning *feels* at 3:26–6:51 a.m. in January is distinctly different from the way the morning feels during the same time in June. The whole purpose of planetary hour systems is to accurately describe the energetic quality of time, but natural time changes with the seasons based on the relationship between the Earth and the Sun. Indeed, where I'm from, in the Pacific Northwest, the Sun doesn't rise in the winter until well after

6:51 a.m.! Thus, in my opinion the flexible timing systems are more appropriate as a reflection of the "spirit of time."

In the flexible system, the day and night are divided into twelve unequal planetary "hours" based on the specific time of sunrise and sunset for a particular location. This method takes the time from sunrise to sunset and calculates the number of minutes of daylight. This is divided by twelve to get the length of the daytime planetary "hour." In the spring and summer these hours will be more than sixty minutes, as there is more daylight than darkness, whereas in the autumn and winter they will be less than sixty minutes, as the nights are longer than the days. From there you take the number of minutes of daylight and subtract it from 1,440 (how many minutes there are in a day). This number is then divided by 12 to get the length of the nighttime planetary "hour." Thus you have twelve daylight "hours" and twelve nighttime "hours."

Say for example the sun rises at 5:44 a.m. and sets at 8:24 p.m. This means there are fourteen hours and forty minutes of daylight. We multiply 14 hours by 60 minutes and add that to 40 minutes, giving us 880 minutes of daylight. Dividing this by 12 gives us a daytime planetary hour of 73.33 minutes. Then we subtract 880 from 1,440, which gives us 560 minutes of night. Dividing that by 12 gives us a nighttime "hour" of 46.67 minutes.

This gives you all the information you need to start determining the planetary hours for the day. The general rule is that the moment of sunrise and the following "hour" are ruled by the Planet that governs that day of the week. The order of the Planets progresses in a particular order based on the Ptolemaic vision of the world, with the Earth being surrounded by seven celestial bodies, the Moon being the closest, and Saturn being the farthest. This also follows the Qabalistic Tree of Life "lightning flash" pattern that dates back to ancient Egypt: Saturn-Jupiter-Mars-Sun-Venus-Mercury-Moon.

So, if today is Thursday, then 5:44–6:58 a.m. (~73 minutes) is ruled by Jupiter, 6:58–8:11 a.m. by Mars, 8:11–9:24 a.m. by the Sun, etc. If your sunrise hour begins with Sun, you just move to the next planet, which would be Venus, then Mercury, then the Moon, and back to Saturn. This is broken down in figure 25.

	HOUR AND TIME	PLANETARY RULER (FOR SATURDAY)
	1- 05:44 a.m. – 06:58 a.m.	Jupiter
	2- 06:58 a.m. – 08:11 a.m.	Mars
	3- 08:11 a.m. – 09:24 a.m.	Sun
	4- 09:24 a.m. – 10:38 a.m.	Venus
	5- 10:38 a.m. – 11:51 a.m.	Mercury
Day Hours (73.33 minutes)	6- 11:51 a.m. – 01:04 p.m.	Moon
	7- 01:04 p.m. – 02:18 p.m.	Saturn
	8- 02:18 p.m. – 03:31 p.m.	Jupiter
	9- 03:31 p.m. – 04:44 p.m.	Mars
	10- 04:44 p.m. – 05:58 p.m.	Sun
	11- 05:58 p.m. – 07:11 p.m.	Venus
	12- 07:11 p.m. – 08:24 p.m.	Mercury
	1- 08:24 p.m. – 09:11 p.m.	Moon
	2- 09:11 p.m. – 09:57 p.m.	Saturn
	3- 09:57 p.m. – 10:44 p.m.	Jupiter
	4- 10:44 p.m. – 11:31 p.m.	Mars
	5- 11:31 a.m. – 12:17 a.m.	Sun
Night Hours (46.67 minutes)	6- 12:17 a.m. – 01:04 a.m.	Venus
	7- 01:04 a.m. – 01:50 a.m.	Mercury
	8- 01:50 a.m. – 02:37 a.m.	Moon
	9- 02:37 a.m. – 03:23 a.m.	Saturn
	10- 03:23 a.m. – 04:10 a.m.	Jupiter
	11- 04:10 a.m. – 04:56 a.m.	Mars
	12- 04:56 a.m. – 05:43 a.m.	Sun

Note: Table based on an example time of sunrise at 5:44 a.m. on Thursday.

Figure 25. Table of planetary hours

Notice how precisely this lines up, as the final night hour from 4:56 a.m. to 5:43 a.m., ruled by the Sun, leads us directly into sunrise of the next day (Friday), ruled by Venus. Thus the first planetary hour of the next day *always* lines up with that particular day of the week.

The pattern of planetary timing is represented by the heptagram, or the seven-pointed star, also known as the "star of the Magi," which shows relationships among the planetary powers. The planets are connected in two different ways: one is by drawing a circle around it, the clockwise order of them representing the "lightning flash" pattern of the Tree of Life and thus the planetary hours; the other is the lines that constitute the star, which follow the planetary days of the week.

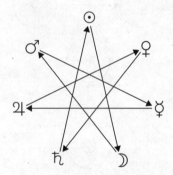

Figure 26. The heptagram, or star of the Magi

Thus, starting from the top of the heptagram and moving clockwise, we see the Sun, followed by Venus, Mercury, the Moon, Saturn, Jupiter, and Mars to the Sun, showing the order of the planetary hours. Starting back at the Sun, we follow the line descending to the right, moving to the Moon, which then touches Mars, to Mercury, Jupiter, then Venus, and finally Saturn, back to the Sun, ordering the days of the week.

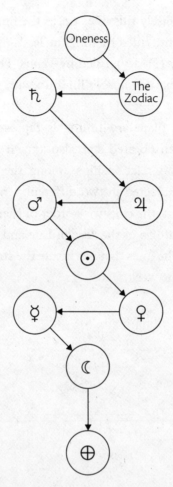

Figure 27. The lightning flash of the Tree of Life

This diagram also indicates interesting qualities in terms of antipathetic energies to the Planets, or which Planets balance the others. The Sun opposes Saturn and the Moon, whose coldness and moisture balance the heat of the Sun. The Moon, being damp, stagnant, and cold, is balanced by the drying heat of Mars and the Sun. We can learn much about planetary signatures and the principle of antipathy by reflecting upon this powerful geometric pattern.

Astral timing mechanisms are incorporated into spagyrics by selecting the correct planetary day and hour of the Planet governing the plant you're working with, and planning the harvesting and all spagyric processes in accordance with those times. In this way, you consciously prepare the medicine in accordance with its celestial rulership and bring that planetary energy directly into the medicine, as all the work is done with that force at its peak influence.

For example, with the distillation process, when the volatile components of the plant are turning into a vapor, they are subtle in their form and delicate in their sensitivity, both to the surrounding environment and to the consciousness of the operator. As the Sulfur or Mercury turns into this invisible, volatile substance and moves into the upper portion of the still, the strongest astrological forces at that moment of time impress themselves upon the medicine, infusing it with their vibrational quality. The still head is the microcosm of the Heavens, and whatever forces are most influential at that time in the macrocosm will directly imprint their energetic signature upon the medicine. The way we harvest the stars into our medicine is one of the primary demonstrations of the alchemical principle of "as above, so below."

The Spagyric Essence

The spagyric essence is said by some to be a "liquid stone," representing the perfect harmony of the Three Principles within the plant. The beauty of this preparation is that it integrates a wide variety of medicine-making practices (such as distillation of essential oils, herbal wine making, etc.) into a single form of medicine. To be clear, there are *many* different forms of spagyric preparations. This example is a good starting place for the new practitioner to get a handle on the different processes, especially before diving into the more involved (and dangerous) mineral and metallic works.

Separation of Sulfur

We begin with fresh plant materials harvested at the appropriate planetary day and hour. After cleaning and garbling (separating the usable parts of the plant from what we don't use, such as pulling leaves off the stems), we submit the plant to distillation to separate the Sulfur, or essential oils. This is typically done through one of two methods: steam distillation for lighter, aerial plant parts such as delicate leaves and flowers, or hydro-distillation for tougher barks, roots, and seeds. In steam distillation, the plant material is placed into a round "bioflask," with a boiling flask placed underneath it. As the water boils, steam passes through the plant's body and grabs the oils, drawing them up and out with the vapors. In hydro-distillation, the plant is placed directly in the boiling flask with the water, as the active boiling opens up woodier, tougher plant parts. This difference is similar to the distinction between infusions and decoctions in standard herbal pharmacy.

The primary parts of a distillation unit are as follows: the boiling flask, holding the water that's boiled into steam to separate the Sulfur (lower world); the "bioflask," holding the plant material in steam distillation or an ascending column for hydro-distillation (middle world); the still head, where steam collects and begins to cool (upper world); the condenser with cold water circulating through it to condense the vapor into liquid (middle world); and the collection flask or separatory funnel (middle world). (See figures 28 and 29.)

As the water boils to separate the Sulfur from the Salt, it rises up as an invisible, vaporous substance, which due to its subtle nature is incredibly sensitive to the surrounding environment as well as the intent of the operator. Keeping a clean and clear inner and outer laboratory is essential to the process, as is the astrological timing so the Sulfur is infused with the proper planetary power.

The distillate contains two primary products: the essential oils and the water that comes over with it, called the hydrosol. This hydrosol is a volatile, distilled water imprinted with the signatures of the plant. There is also the residue: the spent, soulless body of the plant (the marc), and any water left over from the boiling flask, which has essentially become a strong tea of the plant. Distillation is determined to be complete when the volume of Sulfur does not increase over a period of fifteen to thirty minutes, and when the hydrosol tastes inert, less volatile or sharp. The Sulfur is drawn off from the hydrosol, labeled, and placed in a dark space until it is retrieved later for cohobation.

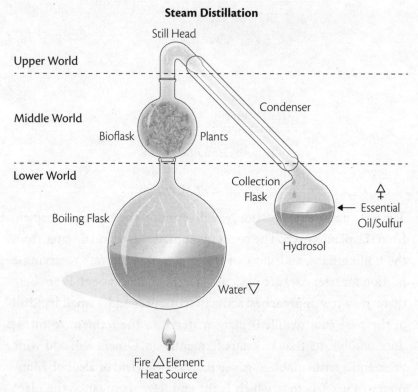

Figure 28. Steam distillation

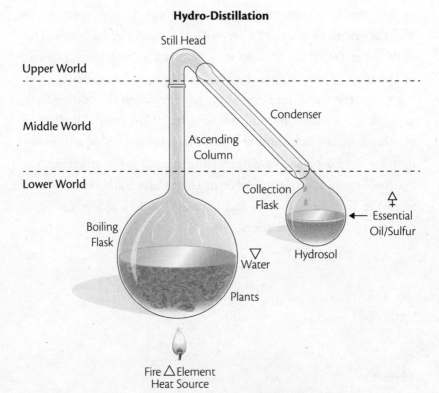

Hydro-Distillation

Still Head

Upper World

- -

Condenser

Middle World

Ascending
Column

- -

Lower World

Collection
Flask

Boiling
Flask

Essential
Oil/Sulfur

▽
Water

Hydrosol

Plants

Fire △ Element
Heat Source

Figure 29. Hydro-Distillation

Separation of Mercury

The next step is fermentation, which separates the Mercury, or spirit, from the plant's body. The spent plant material, residual water from the boiling flask, and most of the hydrosol (I suggest reserving a portion for later use) are placed in a fermentation vessel. From here there are a few approaches: some practitioners add a small handful of the *fresh* (not distilled) plant material to the ferment to introduce wild yeasts that kickstart fermentation. Others will add wine yeast and a fermentable sugar to increase the yield of alcohol. Many prefer to use fructose, which is the endogenous sugar of the plant kingdom and is thus not technically adding something foreign to the fermentation. If there isn't enough residual water and hydrosol to cover the plant, fresh distilled water is added.

From there, the ferment is sealed and an airlock is placed on the lid to allow air to escape but prevent any from entering. The temperature should be kept around 70 degrees Fahrenheit and stored in a darkened room as the plant "journeys into the underworld." The fermentation process is complete once the airlock finishes off-gassing and producing bubbles. Upon removal of the lid there should be a distinct alcoholic smell. This process is best done for forty days and nights, an "alchemical month." This separates the Mercury from the plant's body.

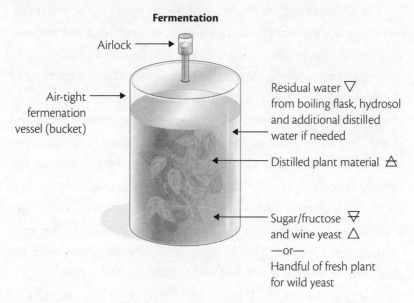

Figure 30. The Elements of fermentation

Purification of Mercury

The next step is to purify the Mercury, that is, to distill the wine to separate the alcohol from the water (Air and Water). To begin, press the plant material from the wine, separating as much liquid from the marc as possible. The wine is then placed in a distillation apparatus and gently heated to separate the alcohol from the water. These can have either ascending columns or expansion chambers above the boiling flask.

This purification can be observed by placing a thermometer in the still head (the glassware the rising vapors come into contact with). Alcohol distills at approximately 78 degrees Celsius and water at 100 degrees Celsius; thus alcohol is lighter, or more volatile, than water and will come over first. As the distillation proceeds, it will usually sit at 78 degrees while pure alcohol is being distilled. As it progresses, the temperature gradually rises as more water is distilled over with the alcohol. Once it reaches 100 degrees Celsius, then we are simply distilling water (referred to as "phlegm") and this stage is complete.

The alchemists of old didn't have fancy glassware or thermometers to read the temperature. Thus, they developed organoleptic methods (sensory observations) to analyze the status of their distillations, as well as distillation trains to separate different fractions of the Mercury. As alcohol is more volatile than water, it tends to be sharp, pungent, and penetrating in taste, whereas water is heavy and bland. Consistently tasting the quality of the distillate can determine the relative amount of water and alcohol being distilled. You can also visually note the quality of the vapors condensing on the glassware. As pure Mercury distills, it's virtually invisible, forming very slight rings around the glassware (if it's perceptible at all), whereas condensing water appears "cloudy" and forms droplets that cling to the glass, similar to what your windshield looks like after a rain.

The purification of Mercury is referred to as "rectification," a process classically repeated up to seven times to yield a pure plant alcohol. Each time the volume of distillate decreases as the alcohol becomes stronger, both in its proof and in its planetary influence, as timing mechanisms are always observed. The initial rectification yields two primary fractions: the distilled Mercury and the leftover "watery wine" in the boiling flask. This residue in the boiling flask contains an important element of the plant's body, referred to as the Salt of Sulfur. Thus we have the separated and purified Mercury through fermentation and rectification, which leaves us with the preparation of the Salts.

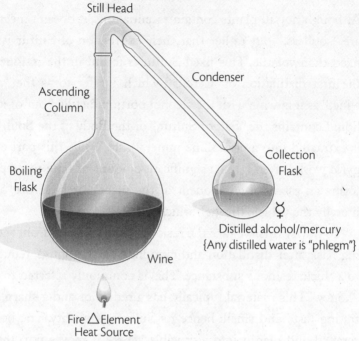

Separation of Mercury

Still Head

Condenser

Ascending
Column

Collection
Flask

Boiling
Flask

☿

Distilled alcohol/mercury
{Any distilled water is "phlegm"}

Wine

Fire △ Element
Heat Source

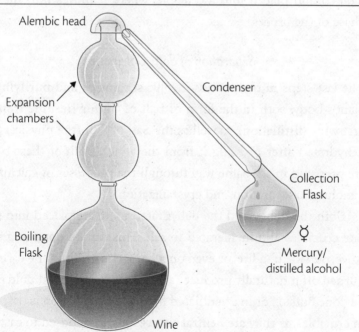

Alembic head

Condenser

Expansion
chambers

Collection
Flask

Boiling
Flask

☿

Mercury/
distilled alcohol

Wine

Figure 31. Distillation, or rectification, of Mercury

Separation of the Salt of Sulfur

Although not all plants contain essential oils, it doesn't mean they are "soulless," but rather that their expression of Sulfur is more fixed than volatile. This fixed Sulfur is found in the residue from the first distillation of Mercury, which I refer to as the "watery wine," as it is wine with the alcohol portion distilled out of it. This liquid contains the "Salt of Sulfur," or the Body of the Soul, which is extracted into a crystalline mineral salt. While this part of spagyric works often takes a significant amount of time to prepare, it forms an essential component of the plant's architecture, as it is literally the vehicle through which the soul manifests.

To purify this, we take the residual "watery wine" from the boiling flask after distillation and evaporate all the liquid, reducing it to a thick, resinous substance. This is commonly referred to as the "honey." This material typically has a red color and a sharp, penetrating taste and smell; hence its Sulfurous quality. The honey is scraped and placed into a crucible, where it moves into the next phase of the process.

Separation of Salt: Calcination

The last steps in the process involve separating and purifying the plant's body, both in the form of Salt of Sulfur (residue from the first wine distillation), as well as the Salt of Salt (the physical plant dehydrated after pressing it from the wine). Both of these bodies are prepared in the same way through the processes of calcination, dissolution, separation, and crystallization.

Both the honey and the dehydrated marc are placed into separate crucibles and incinerated to ash. This can be done in a wood stove, outside in a fire, or even on a barbecue grill! As the carbon is burned off it naturally produces a lot of smoke, so this should either be done outside or in a ventilated fireplace. Calcination is best done in crucibles, as they are neutral clay vessels, as opposed to cast-iron pots, which hold signatures of Mars.

After it has cooled, place the ash into a mortar and grind with a pestle to open the body of the plant and reduce the particle size. While the marc typically burns to an ash quickly, the honey takes on a different form: charcoal. This Salt of Sulfur will usually form large, hardened chunks of black "coal" that can be quite resistant to being ground down to a powder. After grinding, the materials are calcined again. This process of calcining and grinding is done over and over again, until both the Salt of Salt and the Salt of Sulfur form a smooth, soft, white-to-light gray colored ash. If the Salt of Sulfur is difficult to whiten, often a small amount of reserved hydrosol or phlegm can be added while grinding, which will help the materials to volatilize.

Purification of Salt: Dissolution

Next, the ashes are dissolved in distilled water (ideally distilled on the planetary day and hour that rule the plant). In fact, we already have not only a distilled planetary water but one stamped with the innate volatile signatures of the plant: the hydrosol. The ashes are placed into a glass jar, and the hydrosol or distilled water is added in a ratio of three parts liquid to one part ash. This ratio is typically just eyeballed, seeing the level of the ash on the wall of the jar as being one part and then adding three times that amount. This will effectively separate the *caput mortuum* from the water-soluble alkali mineral salts. Gently warming the water often assists in dissolution.

The fluid is separated from the insoluble ash by pouring the contents through a coffee filter, which catches the ash and allows the hydrosol with the dissolved minerals to drip into a fresh jar. From here, the *caput mortuum* left in the coffee filter is discarded in this particular preparation (though as mentioned previously, it's used in other forms of spagyrics). The jar with the dissolved minerals is placed on a *very gentle* heat to evaporate the water. You can use a heating pad or a seed starting mat, or place it covered outside on a hot day to slowly evaporate the water. As this occurs, the dissolved minerals will gradually condense and materialize into crystalline mineral salts. Thus we have separated and purified the Salt Principle.

Cohobation, Rebirth, and Circulation

The final step is cohobation, where the Sulfur, Mercury and Salt are reunited. As we are literally rebirthing the plant into a new, more evolved form, we can determine its specific moment of birth and thus its unique astrological profile. This is usually done by lining up the planetary day and hour, though some practitioners will forecast more specifically. In the latter case, the plant's planetary ruler should be in beneficial aspect with other Planets, the Moon should be in a sign corresponding to the parts of the body the plant is specific for, or the Moon should be conjunct the planetary ruler. As the Moon is the closest celestial body to the Earth, it moves incredibly fast, changing signs every two to three days, and it has powerful influences that both we and the plants can directly feel.

One could indeed get quite precise with this. If you were working with Rosemary, classically a solar remedy, you could cohobate on a Sunday, at the Sun hour, with the Moon in the Sign of Leo, ruler of the heart. Naturally this would take some planning, but we also can't wait for the whole universe to line up to move our work forward. This level of timing precision constitutes an element of alchemical artistry.

The moment of cohobation is precious, for we are reconstituting the wholeness of the plant. As such, we want to observe the way in which life manifests, that is, moving from the most volatile, spiritual qualities down into fixed, physical forms. We begin by ensouling the spirit—adding the Sulfur to the Mercury. This is simply done by adding the essential oils to the distilled alcohol. From there we embody the soul and the spirit by adding in the Salt of Salt and the Salt of Sulfur.

If done properly, the Three Principles will unite into a cohesive, stabilized form, equally distributed among one another. In order to encourage this, the cohobated medicine can be circulated, which involves placing it in a boiling flask with a condenser affixed to its top, submitting it to a very gentle heat, and allowing it to gently rise and fall from the boiling flask to the condenser and back down again. The cohobated material is circulated between the Heavens and the Earth in its new form, and it gathers the celestial forces in its gradual volatilizing and fixing from the above to the below. Some practitioners will gently circulate the cohobated medicine for another alchemical month, or forty days and nights. There are various circulation setups that can be used, such as the classic pelican, as shown in figure 32.

When I was first learning the art and science of alchemy, I once spent months immersed in the works of an incredibly powerful plant, *Lomatium dissectum,* when finally the time came for its cohobation. The purified Sulfur, Mercury, and Salt sat on my lab workbench, affixed atop the planetary seal of Jupiter, as I waited for the moment of the planetary hour to peak. When it came, I added the Sulfur to the Mercury. As I watched, the oil droplets penetrated down into the clear, volatile liquid, and gradually rose to the surface and floated on the top. Not what I was hoping for, as it indicated that, for some reason, the seven-times-distilled spirit was not volatile enough for the oils to equally distribute throughout the menstruum. "It must be too watery," I thought. "At least the Salts should dissolve nicely."

I then added the crystalline Salt of Salt to the ensouled spirit, and my heart sank with disappointment as the minerals sank to the bottom of the jar. It just didn't make any sense! How could the Salt not dissolve in the Mercury when the Sulfur floated on the top? How do you get an essential *oil* to properly mix with *water*-soluble minerals? It seemed like my months of dedicated, diligent, hard work were all for nothing.

Circulation

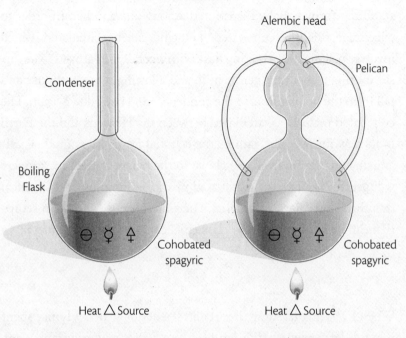

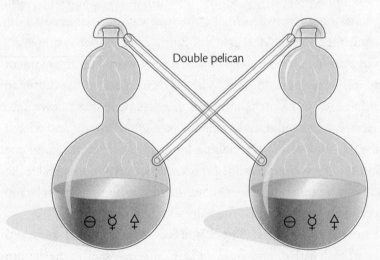

Figure 32. Circulation apparatuses

My confidence in this whole spagyrics idea seriously weakened, I decided to finish the cohobation process and add the Salt of Sulfur. "What's the point?" I wondered. "The medicine isn't right anyway." But as I emptied the crystalline contents into the jar, something wondrous unfolded before my eyes. Tiny crystalline structures gathered atop the oils floating on the surface of the medicine, and they slowly began to descend. As they did, they grabbed tiny droplets of oil as they sank, shining crystals against iridescent oils. They sank to the bottom of the jar and seemed to "pick up" the minerals at the bottom, forming a trinity as the Salt of Sulfur, *the Body of the Soul,* united the volatile Sulfur on the surface and the fixed Salt in the depths.

The mixture became homogenous and the entire spagyric came to life as the crystals and oils expanded and radiated throughout the vessel, refracting light like millions of tiny stars shimmering in the galaxy. And as I witnessed the interweaving of plants and planets, I felt the pulse of Jupiter uplifting my heart and mind, and I understood the power of his influence. I literally perceived the above and the below interwoven within the flask as the soul, spirit, and body of the plant reunited—seeing the stars within the medicine and the medicine within the stars.

Circulation of the Vital Force

As we have discussed throughout this work, the pattern of energetic architecture is universal in its application. Every living thing has its unique signatures of the Planets, Elements, and Principles, which lend insight into its holistic and essential nature. The art of spagyric pharmacy prepares plants in accordance with these energetic forces that operate through them, concentrating and potentizing them in material form. Thus, upon ingestion they target the corresponding forces within the human organism. Because the wholeness of the plant is within the medicine, it operates upon the wholeness of the person. But the spagyric process as a whole also embodies the pattern of energetic architecture.

The Three Philosophical Principles of Sulfur, Mercury, and Salt are the tangible, material properties within plants that are worked with spagyrically, whereas the Elemental forces of Earth, Water, Air, and Fire are the mediums used to separate, purify, and recombine them. The Planets represent the subtle celestial forces harvested by aligning the medicine-making process with the energetics of time and space. In this way, each layer of energetic architecture is present within spagyric works.

As we have seen, the three layers of energetic architecture correspond in their own way to Sulfur, Mercury, and Salt. The Three Principles represent the most physical level, relating to Salt (what we physically work with in the lab). The Planets represent the invisible spiritual forces, relating to Sulfur (the subtle energies flowing through time and space). The Elements are the mediating forces that enable the Three Principles to be carried up into the sphere of the Planets and fixed back down into the Earth, relating to Mercury. Spagyric pharmacy uses the Elements to extract the Three Principles, volatilize them into the realm of the Planets, and fixate their energies back down into the Earth. This process is commonly referred to as circulation, as the vital force ascends and descends from the celestial to the terrestrial worlds.

Figure 33 illustrates the energetic architecture of the plant, as shown within the central channel in the lower half of the chart. In this example, the plant has the architecture of Mercury (Planet), Quintessence (Element), and Mercury (Principle). All spagyric works are done when those same forces in the macrocosm are aligned through astral timing mechanisms.

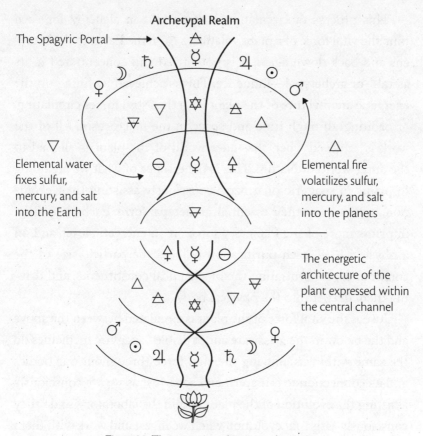

Figure 33. The energetic architecture of spagyrics

The vital force can only ascend into the Heavens through the dynamic operations of Fire, considered the most important Elemental force in all alchemical works, for it's only through Fire that Sulfur, Mercury, and Salt can be volatilized into the Heavens and impressed by the Planets. Conversely, the Water Element draws the vital force down into the Earth. This is why most distillation processes use water flowing through a condenser to cool and fix the volatile Mercury and Sulfur from vapor back into liquid. Fire and Water are the essential Elements, the channels, that support the circulation of the vital force of the plant between Heaven and Earth.

This process of circulation is important in alchemy, for each time the vital force of a plant volatilizes from the Earth to the Heavens and back down again, it is potentized and concentrated in its astral—or archetypal—influence. This is achieved by lining up the energetic architecture of the plant with the astral forces circulating, or orbiting, through time and space in the macrocosm. All of the work is achieved when the inner world of the plant is aligned to the outer world of Nature. This is the essence of what we are doing to plants in spagyric pharmacy: consciously assisting their evolution, bringing out their essential, archetypal form. Each circulation imprints more of the Planetary force on an energetic level, and on a physical level, each purification reduces the particle size of the compounds, concentrating the biochemical constituents, and driving them deeper into the physical body.

Just as the vital force of the plant is circulated between the above and the below in the glassware and crucibles, spagyric medicines do the same within us, moving the vital force throughout our bodies and its connection to our spirit and soul. Just as we are consciously assisting the evolution of the plant within the laboratory, so do they consciously assist *our* evolution when we ingest and work with them consciously. They separate and purify the essential from the non-essential components of the self, and they recombine us in a more whole, purified state of being.

The spagyric process can be thought of as creating *portals* between the above and the below, through which very specific archetypal forces are able to travel through and imprint themselves upon the medicine. As the medicines circulate throughout our being, they establish our connection to these archetypal forces so we can harmonize with them and embody their highest virtues. These channels of divinity, along with the spagyric processes that reflect Nature's transformational cycles and the integration of the whole plant, are precisely what make spagyric medicines distinct when compared to other forms of herbal extracts. While spagyrics honors the physical constituents within the plant, it also recognizes the plant's innate spiritual force, its unique relationship and embodiment of the macrocosm.

In this way, spagyrics are both biochemical and energetic, the process both science and spirituality, the preparation space both laboratory and temple. Spagyric medicines have a power that reaches beyond the body and touches upon our very consciousness itself, imbuing both healing and an initiatic virtue that catalyzes spiritual transformation.

Transformational Medicine

The "initiatic virtues" of alchemical medicines serve not only to heal disease but also act as initiations that catalyze new levels of spiritual development. The plants are not only healers, but teachers as well. The initiatic process opens a doorway for the person to enter a new stage of development within their spiritual life, reaching heightened self- and collective awareness. But for something new to be stepped into, the old must be separated and purified to create space for the vital force to flow. This is achieved through the unique action spagyrics have upon the astral body.

Because the medicines are prepared astrologically, they operate through the astral, or etheric, body, which is the Western equivalent of the *nadis* and *chakras* of Ayurveda or the meridians of Chinese medicine. While we have our gross physical anatomy, there's also a subtle, energetic anatomy relating our organ systems to the spirit and soul. As we live our lives every day, with our habitual thoughts, feelings, foods, and ways of perceiving, we determine the way the vital force moves through our astral body. Where it is healthy, it flows, and where it is not, it condenses and coagulates. These restrictions are seen as root determinants of disease in alchemical medicine.

Spagyrically prepared medicines orient themselves within the corresponding regions of the astral body sympathetic to the energetic architecture of the plant, gradually purging these stagnations, opening up the channels, and purifying our minds, hearts, and bodies. Because of the sensitive ways they concentrate celestial forces, the operations upon the astral body manifest in unique forms, such as the experience of vivid or lucid dreams, synchronistic patterns in daily life, suppressed memories emerging to the surface, the unlocking of repressed emotions and traumas, and deeper insight into the places within ourselves where we can heal and grow.

The specific ways these experiences occur are dependent upon the archetypal force the plant sympathetically connects us to, based on its correspondences and signatures. For example, when working with a Venusian plant, such as the Rose, it's common for people's relationship troubles to come to a head. The lessons presented from past relationships may become more deeply integrated but also perhaps more externally manifested, such as bumping into an ex with whom there was unresolved conflict. Someone with a closed heart gains insight into the patterns behind it. Perhaps when working with a Mars plant such as Nettles, our anger issues may rise to the surface, memories of past experiences when we felt disempowered, and deeper insight into why we don't feel strong and confident in ourselves. Each plant has unique ways in which it embodies a planetary pattern, which determines the specific way it will flow through the astral body and bring up different layers of the healing process surrounding the pattern of that archetype.

As we ingest spagyric remedies, the planetary and elemental forces of the plant flow through the astral body, establishing the resonant pattern of our energy field, or what we can think of as the frequency of our electromagnetic emissions. Our entire being becomes attuned, or *sympathetic,* to the archetypal force we are working with. As we begin to "vibrate" in coherence with the force of Mars or Venus or any of the other Planets, we attract situations in the outer world and experiences in our inner world that are sympathetic to their influence. *We directly see and understand these archetypal forces* with our own eyes, as they manifest immediately in our experience. This is how alchemical medicines are essentially magical: they not only change the environment of our bodies but also transform the external environment of our experience. This brings our study of energetic architecture to a whole new level, beyond that of books (even this one) and into the sphere of our direct experience, which is really the only way to truly understand it.

As the vital force flows and clears these blockages in our bodies, hearts and minds, it flows closer to our essence. On a physical level, it enters deeper into the organs, systems, and tissues of the body, down to the cellular level. I believe spagyrics have an ability to directly affect our DNA by adjusting the epigenetic structure, which is commonly associated with changes in fundamental belief patterns, thoughts, and feelings. As the epigenetic structure shifts, so does DNA-RNA gene transcription. The healing process triggered by spagyric medicines goes very deep indeed, as they reach into our essence. And what is DNA but the physiological essence, or *blueprint*, of our being? It is also interesting that research has been conducted on the influence of specific mineral elements upon the genetic structure.[9] When considering that spagyrically prepared plants contain a broad spectrum of these minerals, we have the beginnings of scientific proof of the transformational level of healing alchemical medicines provide—confirming what the ancients have said for a very long time.

The path of alchemy begins by selecting seven plants, one for each of the Seven Planets, and preparing them spagyrically. These are gradually worked with over time, progressively purifying each layer of the astral body, organ, system, and tissue of the physical body, and each level of our psychological and spiritual self. In order to magnify the effects, they are ingested during the planetary day and time of the corresponding Planet. This progressive purification liberates us from the stagnant patterns preventing us from living in accordance with our true nature and consciously moves us into a spiritual awareness of the visible and invisible worlds. We are realigning our whole being with the highest virtues of each archetypal force, strengthening our inner starry sky. From the Qabalistic perspective, we are building our own internal Tree of Life, a perfect mirror image of the macrocosm within us.

In his book *The Path of Alchemy*, Mark Stavish describes the spiritual goal of plant-based alchemy:

> *1) To utilize the energy bound in the matter of the material world (Assiah) to purify the material body and its etheric link to the astral world (Yetzirah). 2) To open up conscious experiences in the astral world that bring emotional and psychic harmony to our being. 3) To assist in bringing mastery over our emotional and psychic nature as expressed through our psychic body—our chief mechanism of spiritual, astral and psychic connection to the material world and the invisible worlds—and in doing so, prepare us for inner spiritual initiation. This initiation is the awakening of the Inner Alchemist, or, in magical terms, "Knowledge and Conversation with One's Holy Guardian Angel."[10]*

Thus we see the gradual process of working through the body, spirit, and soul, opening us into a greater spiritual understanding of ourselves and the world. In this way, alchemy is not just a system of medicine but a spiritual path.

Many practitioners of alchemy and spagyrics think that the moment of cohobation (that is, the recombining of the Sulfur, Mercury, and Salt of the plant) is the completion of the spagyric process. From my perspective, that is merely the end of the first half of the process. Everything in alchemy must always be resolved to the core axiom "As above, so below," or put another way, "As within, so without." Once one side of something is done externally, it must be flipped upside down, reversed, and done internally. As we distill the plants in the laboratory, we must do our internal distillation work. As the plant passes into the lower world through fermentation, so too must we turn and face our shadow side. And as we separate, purify, and recombine the plants in the lab externally, so too must we allow them to separate, purify, and recombine our own Sulfur, Mercury, and Salt internally. In this way, the spagyric process is not complete until we ingest the medicine and it *becomes a part of who we are*, realigning our inner microcosm with the outer macrocosm. I believe this is the true meaning of cohobation.

The art of spiritual pharmacy is not only the process of preparing holistic herbal medicines in the laboratory, but the cultivation of the highest medicinal virtues within ourselves and direct communion with the forces of energetic architecture. Just as we prepare medicines in the lab by harnessing the archetypes within them, the process is not complete until they prepare *us* into medicine ourselves. It is at this point that we walk across the bridges they build within our microcosm and enter the archetypal landscape of the macrocosm.

Initiatic Medicine and
the Archetypal Landscape

*The Tree of Life, astrology, and the Tarot are not three mystical
systems, but three aspects of one and the same system, and each is
unintelligible without the others.*

—DION FORTUNE[1]

In the course of this work, we have explored a multifaceted approach
toward developing a system of herbalism that balances the science,
medicine, and spirituality of plant medicine. Through perceiving the
signatures and correspondences between plants and the energetic
architecture model, we hold the key that bridges their invisible and
visible worlds.

As we sensitize ourselves to this invisible spiritual territory, we begin
to enter the archetypal landscape. It is in this place that we contact the
spirits of the plants, where we dream and vision into worlds outside our
ordinary reality, where we see the roots of disease that reside beyond the
body and directly experience each facet of energetic architecture. We
are walking in new territories of herbalism here, but we need not traverse them without maps, for these places have been walked by others
before, and luckily for us, some of them charted their way.

As we see energetic architecture within the botanical kingdom, we are left with the big question: *how* will a plant evolve the corresponding facets of our architecture? In what *specific* way will a Venusian plant influence Venus within us? We understand that spagyrics will trigger transformational healing, but how do we understand the *specific nature of that transformation?* Each Planet, Element, and Principle is massive in its scope of symbolism and evolutionary functions, and each remedy corresponding to them will function slightly differently than another. If someone needs a Venusian plant, how do we know when it's more appropriate to use Wild Rose versus Pulsatilla versus Lady's Mantle? While this can often be determined by selecting the plant that matches constitutional and organ system patterns, it's also important to consider the plant's specific psychological and spiritual influences.

These initiatic virtues, or evolutionary functions, are central to alchemical medicine. They are triggered because the plant functions as a bridge to a specific force of the macrocosm, and on that sphere dwell the archetypes. As we connect to these forces in the macrocosm, they influence the corresponding force in our microcosm, based on sympathy.

Archetypes are expressed universally throughout the mythologies, religions, and great pantheons of the world, and they directly correlate to the forces of the Elements, Planets, and Principles, as well as the zodiac. As we have discussed in this book, those forces are directly imprinted within plants, seen within people, and concentrated into spagyric medicines. This gives us a botanical key that opens doorways between ourselves as microcosm and the macrocosm. And when we step through, we enter the invisible landscape of the archetypal realm.

Within this context, the term *archetype* is not necessarily referring to the contents of the collective unconscious spoken of by Jung. It belongs rather to the context of the traditional Western philosophy posited by Plato, Aristotle, Paracelsus, and Jacob Boehme. They understood archetypes as spiritual qualities existing independently of the human unconscious, regarded as real entities, not just aspects of the mind, but forces that influence it.

While the Planets, Elements, and Principles are represented in many herbal and spiritual traditions, they are also the foundation of two unique systems—two maps—used in the Western esoteric traditions for a very long time: the tarot and the Qabalistic Tree of Life. These map the archetypal landscape and the evolutionary pathways our souls traverse throughout life. These areas of study are each massive unto themselves, and unfortunately there isn't enough space to cover them in significant detail here. My intent is to introduce them on a foundational level, show their reflections of energetic architecture, and illustrate how they can be used to understand the initiatic virtues of plants and the transformational cycles of people.

The Tarot

The use of tarot cards was first documented in the mid-1400s throughout Europe, primarily as a card game, though they gradually evolved into a system of divination based on the archetypal principles represented in the cards, said to be encoded with ancient Egyptian knowledge. In the early nineteenth century, the famous occultist Eliphas Lévi correlated the cards to the Qabalistic Tree of Life, revealing a key to esoteric knowledge and linking the cards to religions, pantheons, and mythologies of the world. Tarot cards represent the sequential stages of development within human consciousness, along with the underlying architecture of reality itself.

This is represented on the cards through symbols, which are considered the "language of the birds"[2] in the alchemical tradition. Indeed, many alchemical secrets are hidden within symbols to protect the sacredness of these mysteries, as seen in many gothic cathedrals in France.[††††††] As we have seen throughout our studies of

---

[††††††] See *Fulcanelli: Master Alchemist: The Mystery of the Cathedrals,* translated by Mary Sworder.

signatures and correspondences in people and plants, the language of Nature is encoded in symbols that reveal the deeper meanings embedded within form. From the perspective of esoteric traditions, meditating and reflecting upon these symbols opens doors into the archetypal landscape, lucid dreams, or the imaginal realm. Henri Corbin refers to this as the *mundus imaginalis*.[3]

The primary division of the seventy-eight cards rests in an initial separation of the major arcana (twenty-two cards) and the minor arcana (fifty-six cards). This could be seen as the above (spiritual, major arcana) and below (physical, minor arcana) separation of the cards. Some prefer a threefold level of division, further separating the sixteen royalty cards from the minor arcana, making the latter forty cards instead of fifty-six. These three divisions of the cards generally correlate to Sulfur, Mercury and Salt, relating to the major, royalty, and minor cards, respectively.

The twenty-two cards of the major arcana represent fundamental archetypal forces of life and specific stages, or paths, in the development of consciousness. Each card is a sole embodiment of one of the archetypes associated with the twelve signs of the zodiac, the Seven inner Planets, and the Three Philosophical Principles, giving us twenty-two cards (12 + 7 + 3). Each of these forces represents an integral facet of the self that must be developed in its purest form for us to become whole.

MAJOR ARCANA CARD	ARCHETYPAL FORCE
0- The Fool	Mercury (Principle)
1- The Magus	Mercury (Planet)
2- The Priestess	The Moon
3- The Empress	Venus
4- The Emperor	Aries

MAJOR ARCANA CARD	ARCHETYPAL FORCE
5- The Heirophant	Taurus
6- The Lovers	Gemini
7- The Chariot	Cancer
8- Lust	Leo
9- The Hermit	Virgo
10- The Wheel of Fortune	Jupiter
11- Adjustment	Libra
12- The Hanged Man	Sulfur
13- Death/Rebirth	Scorpio
14- Art/Temperance	Sagittarius
15- The Devil	Capricorn
16- The Tower	Mars
17- The Star	Aquarius
18- The Moon	Pisces
19- The Sun	The Sun
20- The Aeon/Judgment	Salt
21- The Universe	Saturn

Figure 34. The energetic architecture of the major arcana

While the major arcana reflects the pattern of the twelve signs, Seven Planets, and Three Principles, the minor arcana is abstracted from the Four Elements, shown in the four suits, each corresponding to a particular Element: discs/pentacles = Earth, cups = Water, swords = Air, and wands = Fire. Each of these suits contains ten cards, ace through 10, which represent the cosmology of each Element in its formation in the macrocosm and development within the microcosm. The ace represents the Quintessence of each Element, which moves from the 2 down to the 10, where it manifests in the material plane. In Aleister Crowley's Thoth deck, each of these minor arcana cards (with the exception of the aces) has particular astrological correlations represented by a Planet residing in a certain sign, further detailing its specific qualities and characteristics.

The cards of the minor arcana reflect the life experiences we go through to develop each archetypal force represented by the major arcana. They are the specific worlds we live in throughout our daily lives—both internally and externally—that serve to teach us the bigger life lessons that move us forward on our pathway of healing and growth. As such, they reveal the development of our practical lives (discs/pentacles), emotions (cups), mind (swords), and spirit (wands).

CARD	THE SUIT OF DISCS (EARTH)	THE SUIT OF CUPS (WATER)	THE SUIT OF SWORDS (AIR)	THE SUIT OF WANDS (FIRE)
Ace	Root Powers of Earth	Root Powers of Water	Root Powers of Air	Root Powers of Fire
Two	Change Jupiter in Capricorn	Love Venus in Cancer	Peace Moon in Libra	Dominion Mars in Aries
Three	Work Mars in Capricorn	Abundance Mercury in Cancer	Sorrow Saturn in Libra	Virtue Sun in Aries
Four	Power Sun in Capricorn	Luxury Moon in Cancer	Truce Jupiter in Libra	Completion Venus in Aries
Five	Worry Mercury in Taurus	Disappointment Mars in Scorpio	Defeat Venus in Aquarius	Strife Saturn in Leo
Six	Success Moon in Taurus	Pleasure Sun in Scorpio	Science Mercury in Aquarius	Victory Jupiter in Leo

CARD	THE SUIT OF DISCS (EARTH)	THE SUIT OF CUPS (WATER)	THE SUIT OF SWORDS (AIR)	THE SUIT OF WANDS (FIRE)
Seven	Failure Saturn in Taurus	Debauch Venus in Scorpio	Futility Moon in Aquarius	Valor Mars in Leo
Eight	Prudence Sun in Virgo	Indolence Saturn in Pisces	Interference Jupiter in Gemini	Swiftness Mercury in Sagittarius
Nine	Gain Venus in Virgo	Happiness Jupiter in Pisces	Cruelty Mars in Gemini	Strength Sun in Sagittarius
Ten	Wealth Mercury in Virgo	Satiety Mars in Pisces	Ruin Sun in Gemini	Oppression Saturn in Sagittarius

Figure 35. The minor arcana with astrological correspondences

We can organize both arcana based on their zodiacal correspondences as in figure 36.

SIGN	MAJOR ARCANA	MINOR CARD 1	MINOR CARD 2	MINOR CARD 3
Aries	The Emperor	2 of Wands- Dominion. Mars	3 of Wands- Virtue. Sun	4 of Wands- Completion. Venus
Taurus	The Hierophant	5 of Discs- Worry. Mercury	6 of Discs- Success. Moon	7 of Discs- Failure. Saturn
Gemini	The Lovers	8 of Swords- Interference. Jupiter	9 of Swords- Cruelty. Mars	10 of Swords- Ruin. Sun
Cancer	The Chariot	2 of Cups- Love. Venus	3 of Cups- Abundance. Mercury	4 of Cups- Luxury. Moon

SIGN	MAJOR ARCANA	MINOR CARD 1	MINOR CARD 2	MINOR CARD 3
Leo	Lust	5 of Wands-Strife. Saturn	6 of Wands-Victory. Jupiter	7 of Wands-Valour. Mars
Virgo	The Hermit	8 of Discs-Prudence. Sun	9 of Discs-Gain. Venus	10 of Discs-Wealth. Mercury
Libra	Adjustment	2 of Swords-Peace. Moon	3 of Swords-Sorrow. Saturn	4 of Swords-Truce. Jupiter
Scorpio	Death	5 of Cups-Disappointment. Mars	6 of Cups-Pleasure. Sun	7 of Cups-Debauch. Venus
Sagittarius	Art	8 of Wands-Swiftness. Mercury	9 of Wands-Strength. Sun	10 of Wands-Oppression. Saturn
Capricorn	The Devil	2 of Discs-Change. Jupiter	3 of Discs-Works. Mars	4 of Discs-Power. Sun
Aquarius	The Star	5 of Swords-Defeat. Venus	6 of Swords-Science. Mercury	7 of Swords-Futility. Moon
Pisces	The Moon	8 of Cups-Indolence. Saturn	9 of Cups-Happiness. Jupiter	10 of Cups-Satiety. Mars

Figure 36. The twelve signs within the major and minor arcana

The nine cards (2–10) in each minor arcana suit correspond to a Planet and sign, the latter of which is associated with its particular Element, with three cards relating to each sign.§§§§§§ For example, the suit of wands (Fire Element) has three cards relating to each of the three Fire Signs: Aries, Leo, and Sagittarius. This threefold division of the signs is referred to as decadents in astrology.

---

§§§§§§ Note that the aces do not have zodiacal correspondences because they are of a quintessential nature, meaning they exist beyond the sphere of the twelve signs.

PLANET	THE SUN	MOON	MARS	VENUS	JUPITER	SATURN	MERCURY
Major Arcana	The Sun	The Priestess	The Tower	The Empress	Fortune	The Universe	The Magus
Minor Arcana	3 of Wands-Virtue: Aries	2 of Swords-Peace: Libra	2 of Wands-Dominion: Aries	4 of Wands-Completion: Aries	6 of Wands-Victory: Leo	5 of Wands-Strife: Leo	8 of Wands-Swiftness: Sagittarius
	9 of Wands-Strength: Sagittarius	7 of Swords-Futility: Aquarius	7 of Wands-Valour: Leo	5 of Swords-Defeat: Aquarius	8 of Swords-Interference: Gemini	10 of Wands-Oppression: Sagittarius	6 of Swords-Science: Aquarius
	10 of Swords-Ruin: Gemini	4 of Cups-Luxury: Cancer	9 of Swords-Cruelty: Gemini	2 of Cups- Love: Cancer	4 of Swords-Truce: Libra	3 of Swords-Sorrow: Libra	3 of Cups-Abundance: Cancer
	6 of Cups-Pleasure: Scorpio	6 of Discs-Success: Taurus	5 of Cups-Disappointment: Scorpio	7 of Cups-Debauch: Scorpio	9 of Cups-Happiness: Pisces	8 of Cups-Indolence: Pisces	10 of Discs-Wealth: Virgo
	4 of Discs-Power: Capricorn		10 of Cups-Satiety: Pisces	9 of Discs- Gain: Virgo	2 of Discs-Change: Capricorn	7 of Discs-Failure: Taurus	5 of Discs-Worry: Taurus
	8 of Discs-Prudence: Virgo		3 of Discs- Work: Capricorn				

Figure 37. The Seven Planets within the major and minor arcana

Figures 36 and 37 provide excellent reference points for studying the archetypal forces associated with each tarot card. For example, when you are working with the influences of the Sun through both study and experience, such as working with solar herbs, you can work with the symbolism represented on the seven cards with solar correspondences. This also lends a useful approach to studying potential relationships of herbs to the cards when deciphering the energetic architecture of a plant.

Rather than studying each card in isolation, it's beneficial to orient your studies of them into patterns, or constellations. One way we can see these patterns between the major and minor arcanas is through numerical correlations. For example, card 5 of the major arcana, the Emperor, is directly correlated to the 5 of cups (disappointment), 5 of discs (worry), 5 of swords (defeat), and 5 of wands (strife). It is also connected to card 14 of the major arcana, Death, as $1 + 4 = 5$. These reveal *constellations of influence* that correlate the cards in ways that help us understand the specific stages of developing a particular archetypal force. Another way of thinking of this is that the minor arcana cards reveal the physical (discs), emotional (cups), mental (swords), and spiritual (wands) levels of development associated with a particular archetypal force, represented in the major arcana cards.

The sixteen royalty cards are a fractal pattern of the Elements, with four cards (the knight, prince, queen, and princess) associated with each suit (discs, cups, swords, and wands). They are essentially "Elements of the Elements." Thus, there is a Fire of Earth, Air of Earth, Water of Earth, and Earth of Earth, as represented by the knight, prince, princess, and queen of discs. These are the archetypal forces that compose the Elemental beings.

Thus we can see how the pattern of energetic architecture rests at the very foundation of the organization and structure of the tarot cards. When you determine the architecture of a plant, you can start to translate that architecture over to the tarot and see the specific psychological, emotional, and spiritual qualities that *may* correlate to that plant. This underlying architecture is precisely the same pattern as outlined in the ancient glyph known as the Qabalistic Tree of Life.

Qabalah and The Tree of Life

The Qabalah is considered by many the fountainhead of Western mysticism, with its roots in the substratum of Western religion—most notably, Judaism. The Hebrew religion has three books at its core: the Torah (the Old Testament), the Talmud (commentaries on the Torah), and the Kabbalah****** (the mystical interpretation of the Torah). Because of Moses's direct connection with Egypt, this tradition is said to be heavily influenced by Egyptian cosmology, mysticism, and philosophy. Historically, this mystical tradition has been integrated into the Western mystery and esoteric schools, most specifically the diagram known as the Tree of Life *(Otz Chaim)*.

The Qabalah is commonly referred to in esoteric traditions as the "yoga of the West." This is an apt definition, for its sole purpose is the same as the *original* purpose of true yoga, which is union with God. The Tree of Life represents the entire pattern of the macrocosm—or the energetic architecture of life—and directly relates it to every force and form in the visible and invisible worlds. It is a system of correspondence, one that enables us to see the web of relationships within life and how we are intimately connected to everything.

****** The spelling of the word *Qabalah* differs depending on what element of the tradition is being observed. In Judaic mysticism, it is typically spelled with a *K* and referred to as the Kabbalah. In Western esoteric and magical traditions, it is spelled with a *Q* and referred to as the Qabalah. Often Christian interpretations spell it Cabbalah.

Paracelsus defined the use of the Qabalah quite succinctly when he said:

> But the cabala, by a subtle understanding of the Scriptures, seems to trace out the way to God for men, to shew them how they may act with Him, and prophesy for Him; for the cabala is full of divine mysteries.... Its operation consists in knowing the inner constitution of all creatures, of celestial as well as terrestrial bodies what is latent within them; what are their occult virtues; for what they were originally designed, and with what properties they are endowed. These and the like subjects are the bonds wherewith things celestial are bound up with things of the earth.... Hence ensued the excellent commixtures of all bodies, celestial and terrestrial, namely, of the sun and planets, likewise vegetables, minerals and animals.[4]

In this way, the Qabalistic Tree of Life enables us to understand correspondences between the macrocosm and the microcosm. As Paracelsus states, this includes not only people but also "vegetables, minerals, and animals." This speaks to reading signatures inscribed within the natural world to understand their physical, energetic, and spiritual properties. A study of the Qabalah is said to be an integral aspect of the path of alchemy, as it, along with astrology, is considered one of its "sister sciences" that guides our explorations of the inner and the outer worlds, their connection, and the pathways of the soul's evolution. Dion Fortune explains this well in *The Mystical Qabalah:* "The Tree, considered from the initiatory standpoint, is the link between the microcosm, which is man, and the Macrocosm, which is God made manifest in Nature."[5]

Because the Tree of Life is directly based on the foundational patterns laid out in the energetic architecture model, you already have the key that unlocks these esoteric mysteries within the botanical kingdom. You have the Rosetta Stone that allows you to effectively translate the holistic properties of plants to the spiritual teachings laid out by the Tree of Life.

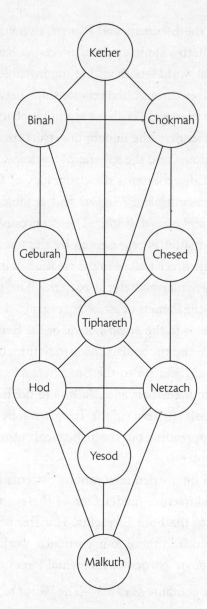

Figure 38. The Qabalistic Tree of Life

The foundation of the Tree of Life is represented by ten spheres (called *sephiroth*), which are connected by twenty-two pathways. Each pathway and *sephira* contains associations to various aspects of Nature, from the Elements and Planets, to mythological deities and pantheons, herbs, stones, colors, angels ... basically anything within the natural world—both visible and invisible—has its placement upon the Tree through the relationships between consciousness, energy, and matter. It is also a map that charts the evolution of human consciousness, the underlying structure of our energetic and physical anatomy, and the spheres of the mind.

The Tree of Life represents the cosmology of Creation, beginning at the topmost *sephira (Kether)* and gradually materializing into the lowest *sephira (Malkuth)*. The progressive manifestation from spirit into matter is represented by the ten *sephiroth* on the Tree, reflecting the precise steps in the creation of life. As such, each sphere holds particular archetypal patterns. The ten *sephiroth* are corresponded to the Planets of astrology, organized in the Ptolemaic order: *Kether* relates to the *prima materia* or the Source of Creation, *Chokmah* to space and the zodiac, *Binah* to Saturn, *Chesed* to Jupiter, *Geburah* to Mars, *Tiphareth* to the Sun, *Netzach* to Venus, *Hod* to Mercury, *Yesod* to the Moon, and *Malkuth* to the Earth. This forms the "lightning flash" pattern on the Tree. It can be thought of as a different way of spreading out the alchemical cosmology of Nature discussed in chapter 4.

The Tree can be divided into various patterns that correlate to the energetic architecture model. One of these is the four worlds, which correlate to the Four Elements. The Tree of Life as a whole can be segmented into these four particular worlds, which correspond the *sephiroth* to particular Elemental forces.

Assiah/Earth, contains *Malkuth*—The World of Action

Yetzirah/Water,[†††††††] contains *Yesod, Hod,* and *Netzach*—The World of Formation

---

[†††††††] This is based on Mark Stavish's work as outlined in *The Path of Alchemy,* which follows the alchemical designations of the order of the Elements from volatile to fixed (Fire-Air-Water-Earth). Most Qabalists switch the Elemental correspondences between *Binah* (Water) and *Yetzirah* (Air).

*Briah/*Air, contains *Tiphareth, Geburah,* and *Chesed*—The World of Archetypes

*Atziluth/*Fire, contains *Binah, Chokmah,* and *Kether*—The World of Spirit

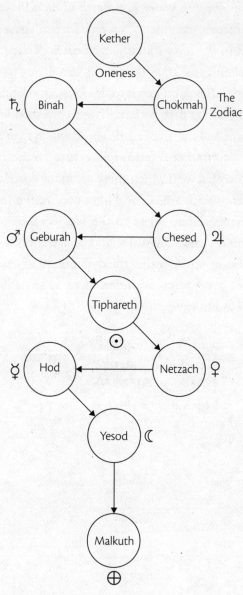

Figure 39. The lightning flash and planetary correspondences

The Elemental pattern has a deeper level of specificity, whereby each individual *sephira* is split into the four worlds. Thus, there is an *Assiah, Yetzirah, Briah,* and *Atziluth* of each sphere on the Tree, for a total of forty possible energetic dynamics (10 spheres × 4 Elements = 40). This is the Fire, Air, Water, and Earth of each Planet, commonly described as different "continents" on each Planet. These forty dynamics correspond to the forty minor arcana cards of the tarot, with the four aces correlating to *Kether,* the four *2*s correlating to *Chokmah,* the four *3*s relating to *Binah,* on down to the four *10*s relating to *Malkuth,* following the lightning flash pattern. These correspondences between the minor arcana and the Tree of Life are shown in figure 40.

Another pattern of energetic architecture on the Tree of Life is the Three Principles, with which there are many correlations. One is the three pillars, which are vertical lines connecting the left, center, and right spheres. These relate to the *ida, pingala,* and *sushumna* channels of energy that flow through the astral body according to the Vedic tradition, representing the dynamic, magnetic, and central channels. They are commonly referred to as the Pillar of Mercy, Severity, and Equilibrium.

	DISCS/ EARTH/ ASSIAH	CUPS/ WATER/ YETZIRAH	SWORDS/ AIR/ BRIAH	WANDS/ FIRE/ ATZILUTH
Kether (Aces)	Root Power of Earth	Root Power of Water	Root Power of Air	Root Power of Fire
Chokmah (Twos)	Change	Love	Peace	Dominion
Binah (Threes)	Works	Abundance	Sorrow	Virtue
Chesed (Fours)	Power	Luxury	Truce	Completion
Geburah (Fives)	Worry	Disappointment	Defeat	Strife
Tiphareth (Sixes)	Success	Pleasure	Science	Victory

	DISCS/ EARTH/ ASSIAH	CUPS/ WATER/ YETZIRAH	SWORDS/ AIR/ BRIAH	WANDS/ FIRE/ ATZILUTH
Netzach (Sevens)	Failure	Debauch	Futility	Valor
Hod (Eights)	Prudence	Indolence	Interference	Swiftness
Yesod (Nines)	Gain	Happiness	Cruelty	Strength
Malkuth (Tens)	Wealth	Satiety	Ruin	Oppression

Figure 40. The minor arcana of the tarot and the Qabalistic sephiroth

The center Pillar of Equilibrium is the most direct pathway to union with the divine and is the root of the mystical path. It connects *Malkuth* (physical body), *Yesod* (emotional body), *Tiphareth* (the heart), and *Kether* (spiritual consciousness). The Pillar of Mercy contains the dynamic energies of *Binah, Geburah,* and *Hod,* or the powers of Saturn, Mars, and Mercury. The Pillar of Severity relates to the magnetic energies of *Chokmah, Chesed,* and *Netzach,* correlating to the powers of the zodiac, Jupiter and Venus. The three pillars form an organizational understanding of the connecting *sephiroth* and how they work together to form particular pathways we tread through life on our evolutionary journey.

Another threefold pattern involves the three triads, which are three spherical trinities on the Tree. The supernal triad contains the spheres *Kether, Chokmah,* and *Binah,* representing the fundamental principles of life: Source and the grand dance of yin and yang. The ethical triad contains the spheres of *Chesed, Geburah,* and *Tiphareth,* which form the evolving individuality or the spiritual soul, where force begins to crystallize into form—the mirror image of the supernal triad. The last is the astral or magical triad, which contains *Netzach, Hod,* and *Yesod,* which are associated with the egoic self that ultimately manifests into the physical body in the final sphere of

Malkuth, the only sphere that doesn't exist within a triad. These patterns of relationship form a central understanding of the Tree, for each sphere can only be understood in its relationship to the others.

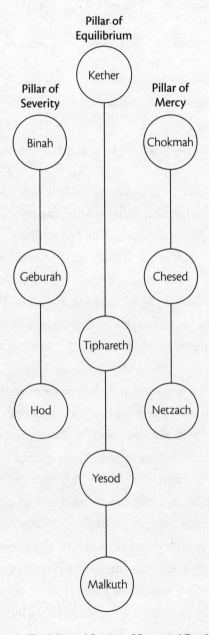

Figure 41. The Pillars of Severity, Mercy, and Equilibrium

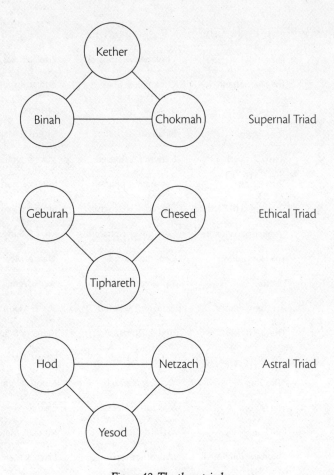

Figure 42. The three triads

The twenty-two pathways that connect the *sephiroth* correlate to the twenty-two cards of the major arcana. The ten *sephiroth* themselves are considered pathways 1–10, and the twenty-two lines that connect the spheres are pathways 11–32.

PATHWAY	TAROT CARD	SEPHIROTH	PLANETS
11	The Fool	Kether & Chokmah	Source & Zodiac
12	The Magus	Kether & Binah	Source & Saturn
13	The Priestess	Kether & Tiphareth	Source & Sun
14	The Empress	Chokmah & Binah	Zodiac & Saturn

PATHWAY	TAROT CARD	SEPHIROTH	PLANETS
15	The Emperor	Chokman & Tiphareth	Zodiac & Sun
16	The Heirophant	Chokmah & Chesed	Zodiac & Jupiter
17	The Lovers	Binah & Tiphareth	Saturn & Sun
18	The Chariot	Binah & Geburah	Saturn & Mars
19	*Lust/Strength	Geburah & Chesed	Mars & Jupiter
20	The Hermit	Chesed & Tiphareth	Jupiter & Sun
21	The Wheel of Fortune	Chesed & Netzach	Jupiter & Venus
22	*Adjustment/Justice	Geburah & Tiphareth	Mars & Sun
23	The Hanged Man	Geburah & Hod	Mars & Mercury
24	Death	Tiphareth & Netzach	Sun & Venus
25	Art/Temperance	Tiphareth & Yesod	Sun & Moon
26	The Devil	Hod & Tiphareth	Mercury & Sun
27	The Tower	Netzach & Hod	Venus & Mercury
28	*The Star	Yesod & Netzach	Moon & Venus
29	The Moon	Malkuth & Netzach	Earth & Venus
30	The Sun	Yesod & Hod	Moon & Mercury
31	The Aeon/Judgment	Malkuth & Hod	Earth & Mercury
32	The Universe	Yesod & Malkuth	Moon & Earth

* These correspondences are based on Aleister Crowley's Thoth tarot, whereby the Star and the Emperor, and Adjustment and Lust were switched in their pathway correspondences.

Figure 43. The pathways of the Tree of Life and major arcana of the tarot

The Tree of Life provides a framework for understanding the archetypal influences that operate through plants, as summarized by Dion Fortune:

> *The association of plants with different Paths rests upon a twofold basis. Firstly, there are plants traditionally associated with the legends of the gods, as is corn with Ceres and the vine with Dionysus; these we find associated with the Sephiroth, with which the functions of these gods are correlated,*

corn with Malkuth and the vine with Tiphareth.... The arbitrary attribution of drugs cannot always be justified by actual experiment, but we may safely say that whole classes of drugs could be regarded as under the presidency of certain Sephiroth because they partake of the nature of certain modes of activity which are classified under these Sephiroth. For instance, all aphrodisiacs could justly be assigned to Netzach (Venus), all abortifacients to Yesod in her Hecate aspect; analgesics to Chesed (Mercy) and irritants and caustics to Geburah (Severity). This opens up a very interesting aspect of the study of materia medica—the psychic and psychological aspect of drug activity. [6]

This brief description of the Tree is meant to reveal how it is based on the fundamental pattern of energetic architecture, as it is a subject far too expansive to cover in depth here. Recommended reading includes *The Mystical Qabalah* by Dion Fortune, *A Garden of Pomegranates* and *The Tree of Life* by Israel Regardie, and *A Practical Guide to Qabalistic Symbolism* by Gareth Knight.

The Archetypal Influence of Plants

The tarot and Qabalah are incredibly comprehensive in the way they exemplify all the possible forces within the Earth and Cosmos and how they manifest within various forms of life, including people and plants. They are maps of the archetypal world, guiding us towards understanding the specific ways alchemically prepared herbal medicines initiate us and provide transformational healing.

As you deepen your connection to herbal medicines through the heart and learn to see their pattern of energetic architecture, you learn to translate the plants onto these esoteric maps. The specific Planet, Element, and Principle within a plant are keys that unlock your understanding of the particular archetypal influences it connects you to, the spagyric bridges built between the architecture of your microcosm with the celestial influences of the macrocosm.

There are a few ways we can translate the energetic architecture of a plant onto these esoteric maps:

- The Planet, Element, or Principle that governs the plant correlates to one of the major arcana cards of the tarot and pathways on the Tree of Life. These correspondences must be incredibly strong, with the plant embodying the essence of that layer of energetic architecture. This is the case with a remedy like St. John's Wort *(Hypericum perforatum)*, which contains the essence of the Sun, corresponding to card 19, the Sun, or pathway 30 on the Tree of Life, the connection between *Yesod* and *Hod*, or our emotional body with our minds—which can only be done through the heart.

- The Planetary and Elemental correspondences can be combined to reveal the particular sphere and world on the Tree it relates to. For example, a plant such as Nettles, which relates to Mars and the Water Element, initiates us into the *Yetzirah* of *Geburah*, or the Water of Mars. As *Geburah* is the fifth sphere on the Tree, and Water relates to the suit of cups, this translates to the tarot as the 5 of cups, Disappointment. This is a fitting card for Nettles, represented by Mars in Scorpio.

- The Element and Principle within the plant combine to form a particular sign of the zodiac, influenced by the Planetary ruler. This can then be related to a particular card in the minor arcana. Taking our Nettles example, we could say Nettles is Salt-Water, as it operates through the fluids of the body, is diuretic, and contains a high amount of minerals and nutritives. This would lead us to the sign of Scorpio (Fixed-Water). Nettles, being ruled by Mars, could then be said to be Mars in Scorpio (interestingly enough, Scorpio is traditionally ruled by Mars). The card for Mars in Scorpio is also the 5 of cups, which relates to our Qabalistic correspondence revealed in the previous step, showing the precision of these patterns.

- Another consideration is the spectrum of antipathy and sympathy, whereby the energetic architecture of a plant may bring us to a card that doesn't necessarily match the architecture of the plant but rather points to a "challenge card" the plant is remedial for. For example, Milky Oats correlates to the Moon, Air, and Salt Principles. The Moon is the ninth *sephira,* and the Air Element is the suit of swords. This brings us to the 9 of swords, Cruelty, represented by Mars in Gemini. Mars in Gemini can certainly create a great degree of overstimulation of the nerves through mental overactivity, which Milky Oats is specific for.

Through these simple "formulas," we can understand the different ways each layer of architecture combines to point toward the plant's archetypal influences by relating it to the patterns on the Tree of Life and the tarot. This can yield very specific and precise information about the psychological, emotional, and spiritual influences of the plant and how those patterns relate to its physical properties. Let's take a look at a few examples:

Calendula *(Calendula officinalis),* with its bright orange flowers, volatile bitter flavor, and warming energetics, is clearly related to the Sun. Its influence upon damp conditions in the body and specificity for the lymphatics correlates it to the Water Element. Because of its powerful vulnerary (wound healing) properties, and its ability to strengthen physical tissues through astringency, we can relate it to the Salt Principle. Putting the Principle together with the Element gives us Fixed-Water, the Sign of Scorpio. The Sun in Scorpio brings us to the 6 of cups, Pleasure. Interestingly enough, we get to the same card via the route of the Tree of Life. The Sun relates to *Tiphareth,* the sixth sphere on the Tree, in *Yetzirah,* or the Water Element. This also brings us to the 6 of cups.

In short, this card relates to a deep level of emotional pleasure that is both healing and rejuvenating. It is "the new life that

germinates from the putrefaction" as "the water is again in movement, whereby the balance is restored."[7] It relates to the joy of
life, fulfillment, satisfaction, and lifting up the spirit, something
Calendula clearly does in its treatment of melancholy and seasonal
affective disorder. We can see how it brings the internal waters back
into movement through its lymphagogue and cleansing actions.
It's interesting to note that the lotus blossoms on the card are also
orange like Calendula.

Blue Vervain *(Verbena hastata)* has the underlying architecture
of Venus-Air-Salt. This is exhibited in the tall, thin, dainty appearance of the plant, the blue-purple flowers, affinity for the female
reproductive and nervous systems, and overall property of being a
nervine relaxant. Some of the main indications for this remedy are
indeed antipathetic to Venus, being for willful people with incredible drive who tend to push themselves too hard, work themselves
into the ground, and have a difficult time relaxing—all signs of
excess Mars. We can think of this plant as a strong Venusian remedy
for excess Mars patterns. Its Salt/fixed correspondences are shown
in its strong bitterness, which anchors the vital force down and in,
as well as its preference to grow in shady, damp environments.

As we combine the Air Element and the Salt/fixed mode, we get
the sign of Aquarius. This sign is typically quite nervous, tense, and
sensitive in their nervous system. Venus in Aquarius is represented
by the 5 of swords, or Defeat. This card relates to a state of fear, either
of what has occurred in the past or of the unknown. It represents the
experiences that beat us down and make us afraid to get back up and
face the world. It is a contracted state and represents an inner conflict within the mind. Interestingly enough, the goal is "recognition of
one's own limits,"[8] and the classic Blue Vervain person has very weak
limits and boundaries, working themselves into the ground out of a
fear of not being enough, failing, or being defeated. It represents the
transformation of our inner fears and shows the Blue Vervain personality when it has moved into extreme excess.

Motherwort *(Leonurus cardiaca)* has the architecture of Venus-Fire-Salt. The combination of Fire and Salt brings us to Leo, the Fixed-Fire sign. This is in accordance with Nicholas Culpeper, who noted Motherwort being an herb of Venus in Leo. These correspondences are revealed through the sharpness of the leaves and base of the flowers (Fire), as well as its actions as a nervine and antispasmodic, with an affinity for the female reproductive system (Venus) as well as the heart (Leo). The Salt qualities enter when we see that Motherwort helps to establish rhythm within the body, anchoring irregularities and fixing them into a coherent pattern, such as the menstrual cycle and heart rate.

Venus corresponds to the seventh *sephira, Netzach,* and the Fire Element relates to the suit of wands, which brings us to the 7 of wands, Valor, which is represented by Mars in Leo. This is an antipathetic quality, whereby Venus opposes to Mars. The card itself represents bravery, courage, and the ability to assert ourselves even when it seems that our best isn't enough, a certain strength of resolve to fight for our destiny and overcome externally placed obstacles in our path. It is a strength in the heart—a quality highly exemplified by *Leonurus cardiaca* or the "lion-hearted." Mars in Leo could manifest physically as heat, stress, and excitation in the cardiovascular system, a pattern that Motherwort is particularly suited to.

But as Motherwort so strongly relates to the archetype of Leo, she could also correspond to the major arcana card associated with this sign: Lust (or Strength), card 11. This card represents the ability of the self to rise above the internal demons and darkness that want to hold us back from achieving our destiny, from radiating our truth and beauty out in the world. It is when we overcome our "beasts of burden" that we open ourselves to receive the divine light of our heart, truth, and ultimately the essence of Life itself. It is interesting that the root of the word "lust" comes from "lustre," meaning to shine outward by reflecting light.

Motherwort relates to this card in that it opens the heart to our essential self, giving us the courage and strength to be who we truly are. But in order to do this, we have to overcome what we are not: our conditioned patterns, habits, and animalistic instincts. As Culpeper states, "There is no better herb to take melancholy vapors from the heart, and to strengthen it."[9] These "melancholy vapors" could be seen as these subconscious drives that are not in alignment with our true nature that volatilize up and influence the mind.

Motherwort, like the lion, helps us defend our essential self, instilling the strength and courage to rise above the parts of self that want to hold us back, keep us down, and prevent us from fulfilling our destiny. And when we do rise above these parts of the self and integrate them (transmute them into gold, as the alchemists would say), we enter a phase of life fueled by creativity, joy, and self-expression, for our heart is full, clear, strong, and open, allowing something greater to move through us and express out into the world. This ultimately leads to our happiness and success in life as a whole, which matches the dynamics represented by Lust/Strength.

These are a few examples of how we can use the energetic architecture of plants to translate them onto these esoteric maps of the archetypal realm. This rubric takes our physiological knowledge of herbs and enables us to discover their psychological and spiritual properties in a way that is *connected to the fundamental pattern of life*. For the alchemist, this establishes a context for deciphering the precise initiatic virtues of the spagyric remedies they prepare. For the herbalist, it provides a translation mechanism that relates the physical attributes of plants to their spiritual properties by seeing the cards, *sephiroth* or paths it corresponds to. Integrating these patterns into a model of herbalism shows how we can utilize plants to support transformational healing that furthers our soul's evolution and enables us to grasp the essential nature of the plants we work with.

PART V

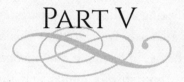

Know Thyself

From this it follows that the human being should receive a knowl-edge from the physician; for god created him in order that he should tell you what you are, by what it is that you are captured and bound, and how you are to be set free. All of this is an arrangement for no other reason than because the human being has been made from external created things, in order that he should study himself and what he has been made of.

—PARACELSUS[1]

We all carry a wound inside of us. It is a part of what makes us human. But for every wound on this Earth there grows a medicine.

For some, the wound is inflicted through acts of horror and vio-lence. For others, it's a harsh word spoken by a relative, the taunts of a mean child on the playground, or the rejection of a lover. Regardless of the nature of our wound, it's something we all carry within us, something that's a part of who we are, something that makes us dis-tinctly human. This wound is not a mere superficial scratch; for each and every one of us, it pierces to our core.

Some carry their wound in a recessed part of the self, unaware of its influence or existence, with no thought toward the need to heal it. When left unattended, this wound festers, putrefies, and spreads into the bloodstream of our lives, touching every facet of our hearts and minds, manifesting as the deepest struggles we face.

But we have a choice. We can allow this wound to permeate throughout our being, influencing our unconscious reactions, the thoughts moving through our minds, and the emotions flowing through our hearts. We can choose to drag our shadows behind us and let them weigh us down, blaming our life circumstances on the traumas we have suffered and what others have done to us. We can let our shadow block the light of our hearts from shining out into the world by stuffing it inside the closets of our interiority. We can allow the trauma of our past infect the present.

If this wound is left unattended, it traps us in our perpetual patterns, the mistakes we repeat, the lessons we never seem to learn. There will forever be a sense of incompletion, not being whole unto ourselves, striving toward something that remains just out of reach. The ancestral patterns that stretch back throughout our lineage are passed down to our future generations. We unconsciously reap the karma we sow, whether in this life or the next. If we don't tend to it, this wound will poison the waters of our lives.

Or we can turn around and open the doorway into our interiority and face what we spend most of our lives trying to avoid. We can be humble before the parts of ourselves we don't want to see and acknowledge them as our teachers. We can reorient how we perceive our traumas in a new light of awareness, shining it into the dark patches and blind spots of our lives. We can clean out the wound, purify it, and heal ourselves. *We can take our trauma and turn it into our transformation.*

For this wound is sacred. It's the key that opens the doorway into our deepest inner territories. We have walked that landscape before, escaping with this wound—and it is only in that place where the specialized medicine grows to heal it. We need only to develop the courage to return and attend to it.

To heal this sacred wound, we must strengthen our hearts to honestly look at our lives. We must go back to where we acquired the wound—our homes, our childhood, our families—and perceive *everything* with new eyes. We must see our lives through the eyes of our parents, see their lives through the eyes of our elders, and see all of our lives through the eyes of the Creator and thus understand everyone in their humanity. The healing of this wound entails separating our perception from our isolated stories and seeing life from a wider perspective—how each struggle is an opportunity for our growth and transformation. *We learn to see that everything has unfolded in the precise pattern needed for us to heal and grow as a soul.*

As we move through this internal landscape, we absolve those who harmed us, retract our judgments and preconceived notions of how things *should* have been, and accept everything for how it is and how it was. We enter the territory of forgiveness. For it is only through the selfless act of forgiving each and every person in our past and present that we can liberate our hearts and minds, and we can free our soul from the past and move forward into the future.

And one of the most important people to forgive is none other but ourself. As we forgive, we do not forget; we simply move on. We learn to honor our past, as it shaped and molded us into who we are today. We make the best from what life has presented to us, and we ultimately learn to be grateful for each and every trauma, struggle, frustration, and suffering we have experienced. For that's the grit that builds us into someone with strength, character, compassion, and something to offer the world. For healers, it is this deep process of healing that gives us the power to serve others. *To know thyself is to heal thyself.*

The practice of evolutionary herbalism rests in the alchemical transformation of this wound into your courage and strength, your faith and belief. Your wound is the gift from life that teaches you to become an embodiment of the medicinal force if you change how you see it. Through this transformation, poison is turned into medicine, fear into courage; doubt becomes faith, and judgment becomes compassion. You take an honest look at your life, reenter the inner landscape where the wound was inflicted, and gather medicine from that place. As you consciously tend to it, you ignite your deepest healing work. From tissue to fat, muscle to bone, this fire purifies you down to the essence of who you are. And it kindles within your heart, where it grows, illuminating and healing the world around you.

The medicine you offer to another will only penetrate as deep as you have healed yourself. The only way you can cultivate the compassion necessary to care for, love, and tend to the sick and wounded is if you have been sick and wounded yourself. The only way you can transform the spirit and soul of another through the power of the plants is if you have first been transformed by them in this way yourself. *We are all wounded healers because we are supposed to be, for to heal the other in this way, we must first heal and know ourselves.*

In this way our soul's evolution and our healing path are one and the same. As we heal we evolve, and as we evolve we are forced to heal. By tending to our own personal healing, we ultimately come to know ourselves. As we heal ourselves of what is false, the truth of who we truly are steadily becomes revealed and we discover the unique medicine we carry. This is what generates the virtues of a healer, the true plant doctor who has been transformed by the touch of the medicine plants. *Through your own healing you become an embodiment of the pure medicinal force of Nature, which reaches through you to heal those that sit before you and ask, "Can you help me?"*

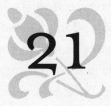

From Trauma to Transformation

We are the people of the Alder. Our roots convert toxic cultural waste into vibrant life force, providing nutrients necessary for your strong growth. Our roots dive deep and spread wide to break up compacted, hard-pan soils of ideology.... We purify and clarify atmospheres of mind with the greenness of our leaves so that you can focus on the great work ahead.

—SCOTT KLOOS[1]

To heal the soul of another, you must heal your own soul first to understand the territory they walk. The only way someone will open their inner landscapes to you is if they trust that you've walked there yourself. They need to know that you have been down this path before, that you know the way, and that you'll stand beside them as they face the wound they have worked so hard to avoid. They need to know that you know where to gather the medicine that will heal them.

Stages of Transformation

The transformation of our trauma doesn't happen overnight; it's a cyclical process. Time is commonly thought of as linear, so that when we heal ourselves of a certain pattern, it's done and over, never to be seen again. But time is not a line; it's a circle, a spiral, and we return to these themes of transformation over and over again throughout our lives. But upon our return, if we navigate the territory well, we carry a greater degree of wisdom than before, and we know how to travel through our trigger points with greater awareness. We learn how to respond to them in the moment, rather than react to them from our past wounding. If the wound reopens, as they so often do throughout life, we know the specific medicines that will heal it.

The human struggle is universal, and our traumas are not unique to us. While we all have our distinct stories of wounding, certain archetypal themes exist behind them that have repeated throughout time. Whether our trauma involves our mothers or fathers, sexual abuse, power issues, violence, or isolation, these thematic elements are represented in the old stories and myths of the world. Indeed, they are facets of the archetypes. Venus, Mars, Saturn, the Sun— each archetypal force has its embodiment of a traumatic theme, or certain ways they can afflict us. And they also carry the medicine to heal us. In alchemical medicine, the healing journey is the transformation of each archetypal force from its traumatic embodiment to its most evolved, virtuous expression.

There are certain stages in the transformational process of healing that lead to greater self-knowledge. Understanding these stages helps us engage in our personal healing process, and it helps us better serve others. As we are speaking of healing our sacred wounds, we can use a physical wound as a metaphor for this process. When treating an infected wound, we do not start by stitching it up or applying something to immediately regenerate the tissues. We take certain steps to ensure that the wound will heal in its entirety, from the inside out.

The process begins with **opening**. We open ourselves to the understanding that we are wounded, acknowledging the wound's existence, and we gently begin to look at it, for these are often the parts of ourselves and elements of our lives we do our best to avoid.

Transformation begins by opening ourselves to face our shadow, remembering what we try to forget, and learning to re-vision our past in a new light of awareness infused with forgiveness. The opening phase is an exploration of life experiences that affected us deeply in "negative" ways, causing pain or suffering, sadness or isolation, fear, shame, or regret. This isn't about reopening old wounds to just feel their pain again or reliving past traumas and getting stuck there; in fact, it's being stuck in the past that allows our wounding to unconsciously permeate our lives. Our goal to is to go back with the conscious intent to heal so we can move *forward*.

The second stage is **cleansing**. Similar to lancing an abscess or cleaning an infected wound, so too do we need to cleanse these traumatic events from our memories—not in the sense of erasing them, but rather *cleansing our perceptions of them*. As the wound is purified and the torrent of emotional charge moves through us, we do not suppress it into our subconscious but allow it to move through us, letting ourselves feel and witness it. This involves a high degree of self-awareness, as we allow ourselves to feel what needs to be felt without the intrusion of the labeling or judging mind. It's this re-visioning of our perceptions of the emotional charge within the wound that ultimately leads to its healing.

The third stage is **healing**. After a wound has been cleansed of infection, we initiate the process of healing it, stitching the tissues back together so they can be whole again. This is best achieved by stepping outside our story and seeing the sequence of events in our lives within the greater context of everyone else's story—and thus everyone else's trauma, too. We step outside of our blame and judgments, fear and regret, shame and anger, all of which perpetuate the wound, as well as that of others. As the wound is cleansed of its emotional charge, we see our experiences with new eyes. We have greater compassion and understanding for the man who abuses his children, especially when we understand how much he suffered when he was a child and his own father unbuckled his belt. We are not making excuses for people; we are developing the ability to realize that *we are all doing the best we can with the tools we are given*. The healing of this trauma is rooted in an incredibly deep process of forgiveness, both for those who played a role in our wounding and for ourselves.

The fourth stage is **rejuvenation**. This phase involves moving forward with our lives. As we cleanse and heal our wounds through reorienting our perception and releasing our negative emotional charges around it, we step into the innate power our traumas hold. The rejuvenation stage sees the teachings behind them, understanding how they have shaped our character in a positive way. Rejuvenation involves taking the poison and turning it into a medicine, reflecting upon how we can learn from our experiences so we can do something good with them. Our fear becomes our trust. Our anger become our confidence. Our blame becomes our compassion.

The final stage is **protection**. This is not simply putting up walls around ourselves because we're afraid of being hurt again. Rather, it's a protection of our newfound clarity and insight into our wounding. *We must defend our forgiveness and protect our compassion.* We must stand strong in our resolve not to allow our wounding to get the best of us and dominate our lives. If we reflect upon our trauma and feel the maelstrom of emotions rise to the surface, that means we still have inner work to do. Protection within this context means that every time the memories resurface—every time we go home and see our father wearing his belt—we consciously maintain our connection to the lessons we've learned and the positive outcomes of our inner work. We ultimately learn to be *grateful* for the challenges we face in our lives, honoring the struggle, for they are the sculptors that shape our being. Difficult as this is, we learn to see the positive in everything on a deep and fundamental level.

This is the work we must do to heal ourselves so we may better heal others. It's not achieved in a singular flash of insight or during a weekend self-help workshop; it's the constant inner work that constitutes the foundation of our spiritual development. While these psychological issues are often worked through via therapy, healing them with plants is superior to those methods because plants treat not only the psychological wound but also the corresponding physical memory, thus ferreting out the wound from its core.

We can only rise up into the heights of the Heavens as far as we journey deep into the roots of our inner underworld. As patterns resurface throughout the course of our lives—each time we face them with strength, forgiveness, and compassion—we grow in our wisdom, understanding, and medicinal potency. As Matthew Wood says, "In dealing with our wound we become the incarnation of the archetype that stands behind that wound, as a positive beacon leading us, plants, animals, humans, creation, to cure."[2] That's the essence of what makes a potent person of medicine.

This process is the foundation of the great work that constitutes inner alchemy, which transforms the base metal of our trauma into the gold of our true, authentic self. In the same way that we gather plants from the forests and prepare them into medicines, so too must we allow plants to prepare us into living medicine. As herbalists, we rely on the healing wisdom of the plants to take our trauma and turn it into our transformation.

The Plant Path

One day at Bastyr University, while I was having lunch with my herbal first-aid teacher, Karyn Schwartz, she looked at me and asked, "Have you ever heard of a plant named Wood Betony?"

This question caught me off guard because it came out of nowhere and was completely irrelevant to the conversation we were having. "No," I replied, "never heard of it."

She looked at me intently and said, "I think you should look into this plant." So I jotted it down in my notebook before heading down to the herb lab for my next class in medicine making.

At the end of the class, feeling guilty for composting the herbs I had pressed from my tinctures (this was before I knew spagyrics), a dear friend and classmate approached me with a basket full of bottles and jars and said, "Hey, I just finished all this medicine, and have more than I know what to do with. You want a bottle of something?"

This was a silly question, because what herbalist would *deny* a bottle of medicine? "Of course," I answered. "Whatever you want to give, I'll take!" She reached into her basket, blindly pulled out a bottle, handed it to me and walked away. "Enjoy!" she called out over her shoulder.

I looked down and turned the bottle to read the label. To this day I can remember the distinct shiver that ran down my body as I saw the words: *Wood Betony*.

What were the odds that the plant Karyn had just mentioned would be the same one my friend randomly handed me a bottle of?

After school I went to work at the local coffee shop where I worked as a barista, and then I returned to my small one-bedroom apartment, exhausted from yet another long day of school and a full-time job. I got into bed and performed my nightly ritual, which was to read a chapter in my favorite herb book at the time (and still to this day), *The Book of Herbal Wisdom* by Matthew Wood. I'd open it to a random page, and whatever plant I landed on that was the herb I'd study.

I grabbed the book from my nightstand, stuck my finger in and opened the page ... right to the beginning of the chapter on none other than Wood Betony. I still get a chill thinking of that moment.

As I read through Matthew's in-depth analysis of this plant— its unique effects upon the digestive and nervous systems, the way it influences the mind and emotions, its spiritual dynamics—tears welled up in my eyes. *Everything* I read spoke to the deepest challenges I was currently facing in my life. Through my focus on making myself a better person, I had come to realizations about myself and how I wanted to grow. But I didn't know how to go about making the changes I knew I needed to make. I needed help.

As I read about the unique medicine of Wood Betony, I realized there was something in this plant that provided the precise healing I needed, as if it carried an essential part of myself that was missing.

Over the ensuing months as I worked with Wood Betony, drinking the tea, taking the tincture, making offerings and wrapping my heart around it in the Bastyr herb garden, those patterns started to shift. My mind started thinking differently. My heart opened in new ways. My body started to change. The things that were holding me back loosened their grip on my soul. Something fundamental inside me transformed as I integrated this plant into my being.

I realized that Wood Betony had come to me. Through my prayer to be in relationship with the plant kingdom, through my dedication to heal myself so I could better heal others, this plant magically wove its way into my world, synchronistically making me aware of its presence. There was something within this plant that mirrored an essential part of myself that I needed to reclaim. Something I had lost along my pathway through life. Something I had forgotten. Some hole inside of me that only Wood Betony could fill. The pattern in this plant matched my own physical, psychological, and spiritual patterns that needed healing. Through my commitment to understanding this plant, its medicine grew inside of me. And I carry Wood Betony in my heart to this day.

It's experiences like these that are the substratum of the plant path—the foundation of cultivating our inner medicine. As you move through the territory of your life, certain plants will make themselves known to you. *They will stand up in the forest and call your name.*

These plants that speak to you, that draw your senses toward them and synchronistically emerge in the pattern of your life, are those that contain the specific medicine for your sacred wound. There is something within them sympathetic to your nature, matching the architecture of your essential self. They are those specific medicines that mirror facets of your being back to you and support the ecological reclamation of your soul, repatterning the architecture of your being into accordance with the pattern of the macrocosm.

This is because plants, too, have their own "trauma." They have faced challenges in their lives they had to overcome and therefore carry a specific medicine for a physical "wound." This is analogous to a psychological wound as well, and if we experience "plants as people," as so many herbalists do, then we understand that they also have suffered and have overcome an analogous wound of the soul. They incarnated the strength of an archetype by having been through the exact problems that the constitutional pattern is susceptible to.

Plant by plant you walk this path, progressively healing the deepest parts of yourself. As you do so, these plants *become* a part of who you are. You carry their medicine within you. They reassemble the integrity of the architecture of your soul realigning your inner nature with outer Nature. Their essence and your essence become one.

At some point, another person will recognize this medicine you carry within. Some part of them yearning to be reconnected with the Earth and their own internal nature will see something in you. They will ask you for help.

Through the magic of this work, as they tell their life stories and open their interiority to you, you will find something of yourself in them. Perhaps they have a similar story; perhaps their trauma is resonant with yours. There will be something distinct about what they are going through that you understand, because you have traversed that inner landscape yourself. Through the opening, cleansing, healing, and rejuvenation of your own sacred wound, they trust that you know the way and will guide them through to the other side. Through what you gathered in transforming your trauma, through coming to know yourself, you carry the specific medicine that they need to heal.

22

Walking the Plant Path
through the Inner Forest

Our ability to journey into the archetypal realm, to vision into the energetic architecture of Nature, depends on our capacity to contact the essence of our own internal nature—for they are merely reflections of one another. We must first come to know ourselves before we can come to know the plants and the archetypal forces that operate through them. To walk the plant path is to heal ourselves so we may better heal others, or rather, to let the plants make us like hollow bamboo, so they can heal through us. Our essence becomes plantlike as they become a part of who we are. An inner forest grows inside of us.

—AUTHOR'S JOURNAL, 2014

Sometimes a plant will stand up in the forest and call your name. You have felt its calling, echoing from the forests at the perimeters of the world and into your heart. Leaving behind the hardened concrete shell of the world, you entered the wild territory of the Earth; through deserts of expansive, starry nights and the carved barks of ancient forests, to the peaks of snowcapped mountains and the depths of fertile valleys. The plant path is one we tread both outside in the landscapes of the

Earth and within the inner forest of our being. When they come together, we are initiated at the hand of Nature.

Traversing these wild places of the world, you see the luminous plant, so perfectly poised between Heaven and Earth. Its language is at first foreign, speaking unknown dialects. Its syntax becomes known when you offer your senses to its intelligence, through yielding your heart to its essence. Understanding of its true nature dawns as you merge with its living language, allowing it to pour into you, to fill you, *to become you*. The plants distill their wisdom into your mind and condense it into your heart, cohobating their teachings upon your soul. You feel their stems and vines growing through your blood, their roots pressing into your bones, their flowers opening in your heart, their seeds dispersing in your mind as they become a part of who you are.

An inner forest begins to grow inside of you.

As we merge our consciousness with plants, we see them containing all of the Heavens and the Earth. As we see their wholeness from the quintessence of our awareness, we see them as a constellation of the fundamental pattern of life itself. As we receive the vision of their architecture, their inner macrocosm, spiritual seeds are sown within us. Every time we sit with the plants, take them into our bodies, pray to them, and develop relationships with them, we water those seeds within us.

And over time they sprout and grow as we tend to our inner forest, shining the light of our awareness upon them. As plants grow within, they take on a new form, operating through a new body, using us to fulfill their medicinal purpose. In one way, we use the plants to heal, and in another, *they are using us*. For they understand that to heal the world, they need a human instrument to work through, a bridge to cross from the Earth and into the world. This is the ecological function of the *herbalist*.

The plants that stand up and call your name hold a special resonance with you, a sympathetic connection to your inner constellation of energetic architecture. They reflect certain facets of your soul as a still pond reflects the stars on a clear winter night, each one a key that opens a doorway into the archetypal landscape. In this place, you reclaim essential parts of yourself, realigning your body, spirit, and soul with the macrocosm of life itself. It is this invisible world, operating through the life of plants, that shapes our ability to transform lives.

The roots of our inner forest grow through this ecological reclamation of our soul. We return to the truth of Nature within, perceiving the outer world within us. Each tree, each plant, every root, leaf, flower, and fruit along this path teaches a different form of wisdom, integrates a different medicinal specialty.

The leaves of our inner forest sprout as we internalize this botanical wisdom. Through them we are healed, transformed, and imbued with new levels of understanding from Nature and how we are intricately interwoven into it. We till the soil of our souls to make space for the wisdom of the plants to grow inside of us. Cleaning our sacred wound, rejuvenating our bodies, purifying our minds and hearts, we let go, forgive, and heal our past. We heal ourselves so we can better heal others. Or, more rightly, we heal ourselves so we can become an instrument for the plants to heal others.

The flowers of our inner forest unfold as we are turned into a living medicine ourselves. From this depth of communion and unity with Nature, a calling emerges—a different calling from what we heard at the concrete perimeter of the world when we began this journey. That calling is to share the healing we have received with the people in the world who need the medicinal touch of the Earth. It is our duty, our purpose, our path to be a bridge between the world and the Earth, between plants and people. *We become the forest. We become an embodiment of the medicinal force.*

The fruits and seeds of our inner forest extend beyond us, sown into the bodies and hearts of the people who come to us asking for help. As the remedies we administer germinate and grow, they replace the sickness and suffering within people, healing their sacred wounds, strengthening their inner nature, rejuvenating their bodies. As Nature reaches into people through our medicinal art, the spiritual sickness of the world is cleansed as people are reconnected to the Earth they are part of.

Our understanding of this medicinal force growing within our inner botanical kingdom is not figured out, it is *revealed*. This revelation occurs to those with the courage to see the world anew, to drop down from the mind and perceive through the eyes of the heart. To walk the plant path means we are first, foremost, and forever students of Nature. For when our understanding is rooted in Nature, it will always be true, and the true physician is always true to Nature, for it is she who cultivates true healers.

As this inner forest grows roots and leaves, flowers and fruits, we develop faith and trust in our medicines. We know they will heal others because they have healed us. We know they will transform the person asking for help because they have transformed us. Faith and trust in our medicines are the sun and water that nourish the inner forest, and they instill faith and trust in those we serve. *For how can they trust us and the plants if we ourselves don't trust in our medicines?*

We learn to care for the plants. We pray to them. We harvest them with reverence, prepare them with respect, and administer them with understanding. Our relationship with the plants becomes the power of our herbal art, for we know where they came from, how they were tended, and the potency of their medicine. Through this, we trust and believe in them, and we yield ourselves to their healing power.

Through our humility we know that it's the plants themselves that do the healing. It's our job to merely be their stewards, their translators, their bridges to walk from the Earth into the world. We become humble servants of the Earth, *for the Earth,* because we are part of the Earth. And in this way as we heal ourselves, our families, our communities, we contribute to the healing of the Earth. And as we collectively heal and transform, we contribute to the evolution of consciousness of the whole, stitching the human heart and mind back into the pattern of Nature and mending the soul of the world.

To walk the plant path through the inner forest—to be an evolutionary herbalist—is to offer ourselves to the medicinal force within the plants to become healers in service to the Light of Nature.

A plant has stood up in the forest and called your name. The time is now to heed its calling.

Now that you've read *Evolutionary Herbalism,* be sure to download the step-by-step integration plan to help you get started on implementing these teachings in your plant path.

Go to

www.evolutionaryherbalism.com/book-bonuses

to get your free PDF integration plan as a gift for reading this book.

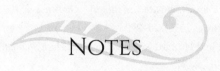

NOTES

Introduction: Ancient Teachings for a New Paradigm of Plant Medicine

1. Terence McKenna, *Food of the Gods* (New York: Bantam Books, 1992).

Part I: The Light of Nature

1. Jolande Jacobi, ed., *Paracelsus, Selected Writings* (Princeton: NJ: Princeton University Press, 1951), 49.

Chapter 1. Natura Sophia

1. Matthew Wood, *Vitalism* (Berkeley: North Atlantic Books, 1992), 10–11.
2. Stephen Harrod Buhner, *Plant Intelligence and the Imaginal Realm* (Rochester, VT: Bear and Company, 2014), 83.
3. Rudolf Steiner, *Theosophy* (Hudson, NY: Anthroposophic Press, 1994), 16.
4. Jeremy Narby, "Intelligence in Nature" (lecture presented at the Bioneers Conference, San Rafael, CA, 2005).
5. *Merriam-Webster,* s.v. "intelligence," accessed July 26, 2018, https://www.merriam-webster.com/dictionary/intelligence.
6. Jan Walleczek, *Self Organized Biological Dynamics and Nonlinear Control* (Cambridge, UK: Cambridge University Press, 2000).

Chapter 2. Gnosis Cardiaca

1. AZQuotes.com, Wind and Fly Ltd., accessed May 24, 2018, http://www.azquotes.com/quote/666043.

2. Doc Childre, Howard Martin, Deborah Rozman, and Rollin McCraty, *Heart Intelligence: Connecting with the Intuitive Guidance of the Heart* (Cardiff, CA: Waterfront Press, 2016), 28–29.

3. Doc Childre and Howard Martin, *The HeartMath Solution* (New York: Harper-Collins, 1999), 28–34.

4. Rollin McCraty, "A Public Statement by Rollin McCraty, PhD, Institute of Heartmath," HeartRelease, accessed May 24, 2018, http://www.heartrelease.com/coherence-3.html.

5. Childre and Martin, *HeartMath Solution,* 27.

Chapter 3: Synderesis Botanica

1. Rudolf Steiner, *Theosophy* (Hudson, NY: Anthroposophic Press, 1994), 25.

2. Stephen Harrod Buhner, *The Secret Teachings of Plants* (Rochester, VT: Bear and Company, 2004).

3. Pam Montgomery, *Plant Spirit Healing* (Rochester, VT: Bear and Company, 2008).

4. Stefano Mancuso and Alessandra Viola, *Brilliant Green* (Washington, DC: Island Press, 2015), 34–36.

5. Richard Karban, *Plant Sensing and Communication* (Chicago: University of Chicago Press, 2015), 9–29.

6. Charles Darwin, *The Power of Movement in Plants* (London: John Murray, 1880), 573.

7. Stephen Harrod Buhner, *Plant Intelligence and the Imaginal Realm* (Rochester, VT: Bear and Company, 2011), 117–24.

8. Henry David Thoreau, "Thoreau's Journal (Part IV)," *The Atlantic,* accessed May 24, 2018, https://www.theatlantic.com/magazine/archive/1905/04/thoreaus-journal-part-iv/542109/.

9. Buhner, *Secret Teachings,* 189.

Part II: Energetic Architecture

1. Brainyquotes.com, Brainy Media Inc., accessed June 2, 2018, https://www.brainyquote.com/quotes/paracelsus_176282.

Chapter 4. The Cosmology of Nature

1. Dion Fortune, *The Mystical Qabalah* (Glastonbury: Fraternity Sanctum Regnum, 2008), 173.

2. Gen. 1:1–2.

3. Andrew Weeks, ed. and trans., *Paracelsus (Theophrastus Bombastus von Hohenheim, 1493–1541): Essential Theoretical Writings* (Leiden: Koninkiijke Brill, 2008), 448.

4. Gen. 1:4–5.

5. Matthew Wood, *Vitalism* (Berkley: North Atlantic Books, 1992), 18.

6. Brainyquotes.com, Brainy Media Inc., accessed June 2, 2018, https://www.brainyquote.com/quotes/luther_burbank_277483.

7. Franz Hartmann, ed., *Life and the Doctrines of Philippus Theophrastus Bombast of Hohenheim Known as Paracelsus* (Whitefish, MT: Kessinger Publishing, 1992), 72–73.

8. Hartmann, 72–73.

9. Julia Graves, *The Language of Plants: A Guide to the Doctrine of Signatures* (Great Barrington, MA: Lindisfarne Books, 2012).

10. Fortune, *Mystical Qabalah,* 13.

11. William H. Gass, *Habitations of the Word* (New York: Simon and Schuster, 1985), 207–9.

12. Jacob Boehme, *The Signature of All Things* (Whitefish, MT: Kessinger Publishing, 2010), 11–12.

13. Matthew Wood, "The Doctrine of Signatures," accessed July 27, 2018, http://www.naturasophia.com/Signatures.html.

14. Matthew Wood, personal communication with author.

15. Matthew Wood, *The Book of Herbal Wisdom* (Berkeley: North Atlantic Books, 1997), 34.

Chapter 5. The Five Elements

1. Tenzin Wangyal Rinpoche, *Healing with Form, Energy and Light* (New York: Snow Lion Publications, 2002), 1–2.

2. David Frawley and Vasant Lad, *The Yoga of Herbs* (Twin Lakes, WI: Lotus Press, 1986), 9–10.

3. Matthew Wood, *The Practice of Traditional Western Herbalism* (Berkley: North Atlantic Books, 2004), 31–32.

4. Frawley and Lad, *Yoga of Herbs*, 10.

Chapter 6. The Three Principles

1. Mantak Chia, *Fusion of the Five Elements* (Rochester, VT: Destiny Books, 1989), 1.

2. "Ayurvedic Doshas—Vata, Pitta, Kapha," Pitta Ayurveda, accessed June 12, 2018, https://www.pittaayurveda.com/ayurveda-doshas-vata-pitta-kapha/.

3. Todd Caldecott, *Inside Ayurveda* (New Westminster, BC, Canada: Phytoalchemy Press, 2014), 54.

4. Vasant Lad, *Ayurveda: The Science of Healing* (Twin Lakes, WI: Lotus Press, 2004), 109–11.

5. Judith Hill, *The Astrological Body Types* (Eureka, CA: Borderland Sciences Research Foundation, 1997), 28.

6. Ted Kaptchuk, *The Web That Has No Weaver* (New York: Contemporary Books, 2000), 58.

7. Kaptchuk, 43.

8. Chia, *Fusion*, 3.

9. Matthew Wood, *Vitalism* (Berkeley, CA: North Atlantic Books, 1992), 70.

10. Matthew Wood, *The Practice of Traditional Western Herbalism* (Berkeley, CA: North Atlantic Books, 2004), 121–33.

Chapter 7: The Seven Planets

1. Three Initiates, *The Kybalion* (New York: TarcherPerigee, 2018), 14.

2. David Osborn, "Nicholas Culpeper, English Herbalist and Astrologer," GreekMedicine.net, accessed July 28, 2018, http://www.greekmedicine.net/whos_who/Nicholas_Culpeper.html.

Part III: Universal Herbalism

1. Michael Tierra, *Planetary Herbology* (Twin Lakes, WI: Lotus Press, 1992), 31.

2. Tierra, 31.

3. Matthew Wood, *The Practice of Traditional Western Herbalism* (Berkeley, CA: North Atlantic Books, 2004).

Chapter 8: The Principles of Vitalism

1. Paul Bergner, *Materia Medica Intensive* (Boulder, CO: North American Institute of Medical Herbalism, 2006), compact disc, disc 1, track 5.

2. Franz Hartmann, ed., *Life and the Doctrines of Philippus Theophrastus Bombast of Hohenheim Known as Paracelsus* (Whitefish, MT: Kessinger Publishing, 1992), 223.

3. Paul Bergner, *Advanced Herbal Actions and Formulation* (Boulder, CO: North American Institute of Medical Herbalism, 2006), compact disc, disc 1, track 3.

4. "Yuan Qi," TCM Wiki, accessed May 28, 2018, https://tcmwiki.com/wiki /yuan-qi.

5. David Frawley, *Soma in Yoga and Ayurveda* (Twin Lakes, WI: Lotus Press, 2012), 96.

6. Vasant Lad, *Ayurveda: The Science of Self-Healing* (Twin Lakes, WI: Lotus Press, 1984), 110.

7. Hartmann, *Life and the Doctrines,* 221.

8. Vasant Lad and David Frawley, *The Yoga of Herbs* (Twin Lakes, WI: Lotus Press, 1986), 72.

Chapter 9: The Holistic Person

1. Franz Hartmann, ed., *Life and the Doctrines of Philippus Theophrastus Bombast of Hohenheim Known as Paracelsus* (Whitefish, MT: Kessinger Publishing, 1992), 211.

2. Matthew Wood, *The Practice of Traditional Western Herbalism* (Berkley: North Atlantic Books, 2004), 100.

3. Vasant Lad, *Ayurveda: The Science of Self-Healing* (Twin Lakes, WI: Lotus Press, 1984), 45.

4. Vaidya Madhu Bajra Bajracharya, Alan Tillotson, and Todd Caldecott, eds., *Ayurveda in Nepal,* vol. 1, *Ayurvedic Principles, Diagnosis and Treatment* (Shelbyville, KY: Wasteland Press, 2009), 46, 60–61, 70–71.

5. Judith Hill, *Medical Astrology* (Portland: Stellium Press, 2004), 10–13.

Chapter 10: The Elemental Human

1. Jolande Jacobi, ed., *Paracelsus: Selected Writings,* trans. Norbert Guterman (Princeton: Princeton University Press, 1951), 63.

2. Vaidya Madhu Bajra Bajracharya, Alan Tillotson, and Todd Caldecott, eds., *Ayurveda in Nepal,* vol. 1, *Ayurvedic Principles, Diagnosis and Treatment* (Shelbyville, KY: Wasteland Press, 2009), 70–71.

3. Bajracharya, Tillotson, and Caldecott, 46.

4. Bajracharya, Tillotson, and Caldecott, 60–61.

Chapter 11: The Triune Human

1. Michael Tierra, *Planetary Herbology* (Twin Lakes, WI: Lotus Press, 1992), 39.
2. Vaidya Madhu Bajra Bajracharya, Alan Tillotson, and Todd Caldecott, eds., *Ayurveda in Nepal,* vol. 1, *Ayurvedic Principles, Diagnosis and Treatment* (Shelbyville, KY: Wasteland Press, 2009), 39.
3. Bajracharya, Tillotson, and Caldecott, 59.

Chapter 12: The Celestial Human

1. Samuel Sagan, *Planetary Forces, Alchemy and Healing* (Sydney, Australia: Clairvision School Foundation, 1996), 1.
2. Judith Hill, conversation with the author, June 2018.
3. Tyler Penor, conversation with the author, May 2018.

Chapter 13: The Holistic Plant

1. Matthew Wood, conversation with the author, May 2018.
2. David Frawley and Vasant Lad, *The Yoga of Herbs* (Twin Lakes, WI: Lotus Press, 1986), 24.
3. Michael Tierra, *Planetary Herbology* (Twin Lakes, WI: Lotus Press, 1988), 33.
4. Frawley and Lad, *Yoga of Herbs,* 31.
5. Vasant Lad, *Ayurveda: The Science of Self-Healing* (Twin Lakes, WI: Lotus Press, 1984), 44–47.
6. Paul Bergner, *Advanced Herbal Actions and Formulation* (Boulder, CO: North America Institute of Medical Herbalism, 2006), compact disc, disc 1, tracks 4–5; Bergner, *Materia Medica Intensive* (Boulder, CO: North American Institute of Medical Herbalism, 2006), compact disc, disc 1, tracks 8–10.
7. Matthew Wood, conversation with the author, May 2018.
8. Matthew Wood, *The Practice of Traditional Western Herbalism* (Berkeley: North Atlantic Books, 2003).
9. Frawley and Lad, *Yoga of Herbs,* 25–26.
10. Matthew Wood and Judith Hill, conversation with the author, May 2018.
11. Lindsay M. Biga et al., eds., *Anatomy and Physiology* (Corvallis, OR: Oregon State University, 2018), http://library.open.oregonstate.edu/aandp.
12. Bergner, *Advanced Herbal Actions,* disc 2, tracks 1–6; Bergner, *Materia Medica Intensive,* disc 2, track 1.
13. Frawley and Lad, *Yoga of Herbs,* 27–28.

14. Frawley and Lad, 27–28.

15. Frawley and Lad, 28.

Chapter 14: The Elemental Plant

1. Dion Fortune, *The Mystical Qabalah* (Glastonbury: Fraternity Sanctum Regnum, 2008), 186.

2. Matthew Wood, *The Earthwise Herbal* (Berkeley, CA: North Atlantic Books, 2008), 1:508.

3. Başar Altınterim, "Cayenne, Capsaicin and Substance-P," *Research & Reviews: Journal of Herbal Science* (2013):11–14, https://www.researchgate.net /publication/268515427_Cayenne_Capsaicin_and_Substance-P.

Chapter 15: The Triune Plant

1. Jacob Boehme, *Aurora,* Jacob Boehme Online, accessed August 9, 2018, http://jacobboehmeonline.com/yahoo_site_admin/assets/docs/AURORAjbo .77133023.pdf.

Chapter 16: The Celestial Plant

1. Franz Hartmann, ed., *Life and the Doctrines of Philippus Theophrastus Bombast of Hohenheim Known as Paracelsus* (Whitefish, MT: Kessinger Publishing, 1992), 75.

2. Matthew Wood, conversation with the author, May 2018.

3. Judith Hill, conversation with the author, May 2018.

4. Matthew Wood, conversation with the author, May 2018.

5. Matthew Wood, conversation with author, May 2018.

6. Judith Hill, conversation with author, May 2018.

Chapter 17: The Energetic Architecture of People and Plants

1. Franz Hartmann, ed., *Life and the Doctrines of Philippus Theophrastus Bombast of Hohenheim Known as Paracelsus* (Whitefish, MT: Kessinger Publishing, 1992), 76–77.

2. Andrew Weeks, ed. and trans., *Paracelsus (Theophrastus Bombastus von Hohenheim, 1493–1541): Essential Theoretical Writings* (Leiden: Koninkiijke Brill, 2008), 131.

Part IV: Transformational Medicine

1. Jolande Jacobi, ed., *Paracelsus: Selected Writings,* trans. Norbert Guterman (Princeton: Princeton University Press, 1951), 49.

Chapter 18: Therapeutic Strategies: Tending to the Inner Cosmos

1. Franz Hartmann, ed., *Life and the Doctrines of Philippus Theophrastus Bombast of Hohenheim Known as Paracelsus* (Whitefish, MT: Kessinger Publishing, 1992), 210.
2. Hartmann, 211.
3. John M. Swan, *Prescription Writing and Formulary* (Philadelphia and London: W. B. Saunders Company, 1910), 12.

Chapter 19: Spagyrics: The Art of Spiritual Pharmacy

1. Johann Wolfgang von Goethe, as quoted in Stephen Harrod Buhner, *The Secret Teachings of Plants* (Rochester, VT: Bear and Company, 2004), 37.
2. Robert Bartlett, lecture, *Prima* Workshop, International Alchemy Guild, Seattle, WA, May 2013.
3. Andrew Weeks, ed. and trans., *Paracelsus (Theophrastus Bombastus von Hohenheim, 1493–1541): Essential Theoretical Writings* (Leiden: Koninkiijke Brill, 2008), 195.
4. Eleni Christoforatou, conversation with the author, May 2017.
5. Matthew Wood, conversation with the author, May 2018.
6. Matthew Wood, conversation with the author, May 2018.
7. Dennis William Hauck, *The Emerald Tablet* (New York: Penguin Books, 1999), 251–52.
8. Hauck, 175.
9. Charles Waters, *Minerals for the Genetic Code* (Austin, TX: Acres USA, 2006).
10. Mark Stavish, *The Path of Alchemy* (Woodbury, MN: Llewellyn Publications, 2006), 44–45.

Chapter 20: Initiatic Medicine and the Archetypal Landscape

1. Dion Fortune, *The Mystical Qabalah* (Glastonbury: Fraternity Sanctum Regnum, 2008), 49.

2. Mark Stavish, *The Path of Alchemy* (Woodbury, MN: Llewellyn Publications, 2006), 170.

3. Henri Corbin, "*Mundus Imaginalis,* or the Imaginary and the Imaginal," Hermetic Library, accessed October 21, 2018, https://hermetic.com/moorish /mundus-imaginalis.

4. Arthur Edward Waite, ed., *The Hermetic and Alchemical Writings of Paracelsus* (London: James Elliot and Co., 1894), 51–52.

5. Fortune, *Mystical Qabalah,* 51.

6. Fortune, 67.

7. Akron and Hajo Banzhaf, *The Crowley Tarot,* trans. Christine Grimm (Stamford, CT: U.S. Games Systems, 1995), 147.

8. Akron and Banzhaf, 164.

9. Nicholas Culpeper, *Culpeper's Complete Herbal* (London: W. Foulsham and Co., n.d.), 239.

Part V: Know Thyself

1. Andrew Weeks, ed. and trans., *Paracelsus (Theophrastus Bombastus von Hohenheim, 1493–1541): Essential Theoretical Writings* (Leiden: Koninkiijke Brill, 2008), 193.

Chapter 21: From Trauma to Transformation

1. Scott Kloos, "We Welcome You to This Life," School of Forest Medicine, February 15, 2018, accessed August 9, 2018, https://forestmedicine.net/blog/2018/2/15/we-welcome-you-to-this-life.

2. Matthew Wood, conversation with the author, May 2018.

INDEX

A

acceptance, Saturn qualities, 254–255

acquired constitution (*vikruti*), Ayurveda, 182–183

actions
Air Element and, 305–307
applying Five Keys to remedy selection, 392, 394
categories of, 272–273
energetics and, 273
Fire Element and, 310–311
important types, 274
Jupiter-related, 351–352
Mars-related, 342
Mercury-related, 363–364
Moon-related, 336–337
overview of, 272
as physiological process, 272
Saturn-related, 355–356
Sun-related, 331–332
synergy with energetics, 287–289
therapeutic strategies related to *kapha dosha*, 322–323
Venus-related, 347–348
Water Element and, 299–300

adaptogens
actions of Fire plants, 312
Mars plant qualities, 342
Sun plant qualities, 331
tonics compared with, 284

addiction, Jupiter-related qualities, 250

adrenals
associated with Fire Element, 214, 216
systems ruled by Mars, 239–240

affinities
actions and, 272
applying Five Keys to, 392, 394
by body's organizational systems, 270
determining, 271
doctrine of signatures, 269
Moon-related, 337

to plants with *vata* characteristics, 320–321
taste and, 269–270

agni (digestive fire)
in Ayurvedic system, 185
center of solar force in body, 231
contrasted with *ama*, 236
metabolic flame of body, 215

Air Element
assessing excesses/deficiencies, 220
in Ayurveda, 117
in Chinese medicine, 121
constitutional qualities, 209
correspondence to nervous system, 190
deriving remedies, 398–399
doctrine of emanations and, 88–90
dosha modes expression, 189–190
evolutionary teachings of, 213
as Metal Element (Chinese medicine), 118
as Movement of Creation, 110
Mullein example, 308–309
organ systems governed by, 209–211
overview of, 112, 209
in people and plants, 122–123
plant qualities, 304–307
psychological and emotional qualities, 212
table of elemental correspondences, 114–115
tissue states and, 211–212
vata and, 224–225, 320
volatility of, 116
zodiac signs under, 121

Aires, organ systems and, 192

aisthesis, 54–55

ajna chakra, planetary associations, 149

Albertus, Frater, 404

alchemy
body quality. *see* Salt (body)

caput mortuum ("death's head"), 413–414
as "consciously assisted evolution," 402
cosmology of Three Principles, 126–127
elements, 116–117
Jung as student of, 122
kapha qualities and, 226
"language of birds," 447
pitta qualities and, 228
preparation of botanical medicines. *see* spagyrics
principles. *see* Three Philosophical Principles
soul quality. *see* Sulfur (soul)
spirit quality. *see* Mercury (spirit)
traumatic themes, 476
vata qualities and, 225

alcohol
manifests Mercury principle in plants, 129–130
purification of Mercury (rectification) and, 427–429

alkali minerals, Salt principle and, 131

allopathic medicine
comparing with holistic approach, 395, 403
herbalism based on symptoms, 164–165
overrides innate intelligence of vital force, 164

Aloe *(Aloe vera)*, 105

alteratives
Burdock *(Arctium lappa)* as, 297
Earth Element and, 295
Jupiter plant qualities, 352
Lymphagogues, 299–300
Mars plant qualities, 342

ama (mucus accumulation), in Ayurveda, 236

anatomy, key area of study for herbalists, 184

ancestral patterns, Saturn plant qualities, 359

ancient teachings, 1–3

ABOUT THE AUTHOR

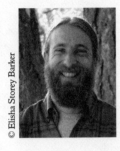

SAJAH POPHAM's, mission is to create a new paradigm of plant medicine based on the synergy of herbal traditions from across the world with modern science and spirituality. His approach is to work with plants to not just heal the body, but to attend to our psychological, emotional, and spiritual health—using plants to facilitate the soul's evolution. Popham is the founder of the School of Evolutionary Herbalism, where he trains herbalists in the practice of transformational healing through the integration of clinical herbalism, medical astrology, and spagyric alchemy. He is also the founder of Organic Unity Spagyrics, a practitioner-grade spagyric herbal product line specializing in traditional alchemical extracts used by herbalists, doctors, and naturopaths around the world. He lives with his wife, Whitney, on their homestead in the forests and mountains of the Pacific Northwest. To follow Sajah and Whitney's work, visit www.evolutionaryherbalism.com and their podcast, *The Plant Path*.

Transform the lives of the people you serve through the practice of Evolutionary Herbalism.

The School of Evolutionary Herbalism offers in-depth, comprehensive online education in the art and practice of clinical herbalism, medical astrology, Ayurveda, and spagyric alchemy, giving you the skills and strategies to bring the deepest levels of healing possible to yourself and your family, community, and clinical practice.

From monthly subscriptions and audio courses to comprehensive membership programs, our courses are designed to give beginners and advanced practitioners alike a solid foundation in the practice of holistic transformational herbalism.

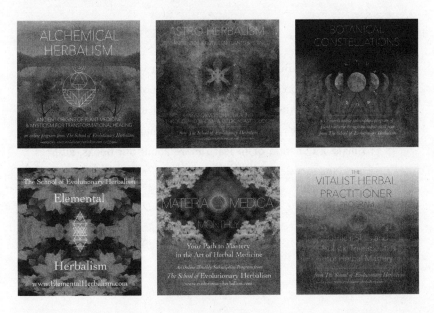

For a free in-depth training series on the practice of herbal alchemy, go to www.evolutionaryherbalism.com/herbal-alchemy-training-sessions. Visit our blog at www.evolutionaryherbalism.com/blog for tons of free videos, and subscribe to our podcast, *The Plant Path,* on iTunes or Stitcher. To connect with us and the Evolutionary Herbalism community, follow us on Facebook and Instagram.

About North Atlantic Books

North Atlantic Books (NAB) is a 501(c)(3) nonprofit publisher committed to a bold exploration of the relationships between mind, body, spirit, culture, and nature. Founded in 1974, NAB aims to nurture a holistic view of the arts, sciences, humanities, and healing. To make a donation or to learn more about our books, authors, events, and newsletter, please visit www.northatlanticbooks.com.